Psychodynamic Concepts in General Psychiatry

Psychodynamic Concepts in General Psychiatry

Edited by

Harvey J. Schwartz, M.D.

with
Efrain Bleiberg, M.D.,
and
Sidney H. Weissman, M.D.

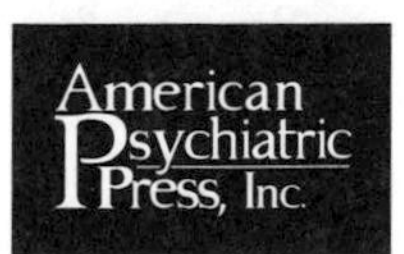

Washington, DC
London, England

Note: The authors have worked to ensure that all information in this book concerning drug dosages, schedules, and routes of administration is accurate as of the time of publication and consistent with standards set by the U.S. Food and Drug Administration and the general medical community. As medical research and practice advance, however, therapeutic standards may change. For this reason and because human and mechanical errors sometimes occur, we recommend that readers follow the advice of a physician who is directly involved in their care or the care of a member of their family.

Books published by the American Psychiatric Press, Inc., represent the views and opinions of the individual authors and do not necessarily represent the policies and opinions of the Press or the American Psychiatric Association.

Manufactured in the United States of America on acid-free paper
98 97 96 95 4 3 2 1
First Edition

American Psychiatric Press, Inc.
1400 K Street, N.W., Washington, DC 20005

Library of Congress Cataloging-in-Publication Data
Psychodynamic concepts in general psychiatry / edited by Harvey J. Schwartz, Efrain Bleiberg, Sidney H. Weissman.
p. cm.
Includes bibliographical references and index.
ISBN 0-88048-536-1
1. Psychiatry. 2. Psychodynamic psychotherapy. 3. Mental illness—Etiology. 4. Psychodynamic psychotherapy—Case studies. I. Schwartz, Harvey J. II. Bleiberg, Efrain, 1952- . III. Weissman, Sidney H.
[DNLM: 1. Mental Disorders—therapy. WM 400 P9735 1995]
RC454.4.P792 1995
616.89—dc20
DNLM/DLC 94-34974
for Library of Congress CIP

British Library Cataloguing in Publication Data
A CIP record is available from the British Library.

To Our Patients

Contents

Section III: Clinical Syndromes

Harvey J. Schwartz, M.D., Section Editor

Contributors

Elizabeth L. Auchincloss, M.D. Clinical Assistant Professor of Psychiatry, Cornell University Medical College, Ithaca, New York; Faculty, Columbia University Psychoanalytic Center for Training and Research, New York, New York

Richard S. Blacher, M.D. Professor of Psychiatry, Tufts University School of Medicine, Boston, Massachusetts; Member, Boston Psychoanalytic Society, Boston, Massachusetts

Efrain Bleiberg, M.D. Dean, Karl Menninger School of Psychiatry and Mental Health Sciences, Topeka, Kansas; Instructor, Topeka Institute for Psychoanalysis, Topeka, Kansas

Fredric N. Busch, M.D. Instructor in Psychiatry, Cornell University Medical College, Ithaca, New York; Candidate, Columbia University Psychoanalytic Center for Training and Research, New York, New York

Martin Ceaser, M.D. Clinical Professor of Psychiatry, Georgetown University Medical Center, Washington, DC; Teaching Analyst, Baltimore-Washington Institute for Psychoanalysis, Laurel, Maryland

Arnold M. Cooper, M.D. Stephen P. Tobin and Arnold M. Cooper Professor in Consultation-Liaison Psychiatry, Cornell University Medical College, Ithaca, New York; Training and Supervising Analyst, Columbia University Center for Psychoanalytic Training and Research, New York, New York

Aaron H. Esman, M.D. Professor of Clinical Psychiatry, Cornell University Medical College, Ithaca, New York; Faculty, New York Psychoanalytic Institute, New York, New York

Abraham Freedman, M.D. Honorary Clinical Professor of Psychiatry and Human Behavior, Jefferson Medical College, Thomas Jefferson University, Philadelphia, Pennsylvania; Faculty, Institute of the Philadelphia Association for Psychoanalysis, Philadelphia, Pennsylvania

Eugene L. Goldberg, M.D. Associate Clinical Professor of Psychiatry, Albert Einstein College of Medicine, New York; Training and Supervising Analyst, Columbia University Center for Psychoanalytic Training and Research, New York, New York

Howard B. Levine, M.D. Faculty, Boston Psychoanalytic Institute and Massachusetts Institute for Psychoanalysis, Boston, Massachusetts

Jacob D. Lindy, M.D. Training and Supervising Analyst, Cincinnati Psychoanalytic Institute, Cincinnati, Ohio

Elena G. Lister, M.D. Clinical Instructor in Psychiatry, Cornell University Medical College, Ithaca, New York; Lecturer in Psychiatry and Collaborating Psychoanalyst, Columbia University Center for Psychoanalytic Training and Research, New York, New York

Ken Marcus, M.D. Lecturer in Psychiatry, Yale University School of Medicine, New Haven, Connecticut; Deputy Commissioner for Clinical Services, Connecticut Department of Mental Health, New Haven, Connecticut

Gerald A. Melchiode, M.D. Clinical Professor of Psychiatry, Southwestern Medical Center, Dallas, Texas; Training and Supervising Analyst, Dallas Psychoanalytic Institute, Dallas, Texas

Robert Michels, M.D. The Stephen and Suzanne Weiss Dean, Barklie McKee Henry Professor of Psychiatry, Cornell University Medical College, Ithaca, New York; Training and Supervising Analyst, Columbia University Center for Psychoanalytic Training and Research, New York, New York

Ira L. Mintz, M.D. Associate Clinical Professor of Psychiatry, New Jersey College of Medicine, Newark, New Jersey; Supervising Child Psychoanalyst, Columbia University Center for Psychoanalytic Training and Research, New York, New York

Fred Moss, M.D. Resident, Department of Psychiatry, University of Connecticut, Storrs, Connecticut

Richard L. Munich, M.D. Professor of Clinical Psychiatry, Cornell University Medical College, Ithaca, New York; Training and Supervising Analyst, Columbia University Center for Psychoanalytic Training and Research, New York, New York

Philip R. Muskin, M.D. Associate Professor of Clinical Psychiatry, College of Physicians and Surgeons, Columbia University, New York, New York; Collaborating Faculty, Columbia University Center for Psychoanalytic Training and Research, New York, New York

Wayne A. Myers, M.D. Clinical Professor of Psychiatry, Cornell University Medical College, Ithaca, New York; Training and Supervising Analyst, Columbia University Center for Psychoanalytic Training and Research, New York, New York

Malkah T. Notman, M.D. Clinical Professor of Psychiatry, Harvard Medical School, Cambridge, Massachusetts; Training and Supervising Analyst, Boston Psychoanalytic Society and Institute, Boston, Massachusetts

Arlene Kramer Richards, Ed.D. Faculty, Smith College School for Social Work, Northampton, Massachusetts; Training and Supervising Analyst, New York Freudian Society, New York, New York

Arnold D. Richards, M.D. Assistant Clinical Professor of Psychiatry, New York University School of Medicine; Training and Supervising Analyst, New York Psychoanalytic Institute, New York, New York

Harvey J. Schwartz, M.D. Clinical Professor of Psychiatry and Human Behavior, Jefferson Medical College, Thomas Jefferson University, Philadelphia, Pennsylvania; Member, Institute of the Philadelphia Association for Psychoanalysis, Philadelphia, Pennsylvania

Theodore Shapiro, M.D. Professor of Psychiatry, Cornell University Medical College, Ithaca, New York; Training and Supervising Analyst, New York Psychoanalytic Institute, New York, New York

Howard Silbert, M.D. Adjunct Assistant Professor of Clinical Psychiatry, New York University School of Medicine, New York, New York; Senior Candidate, Psychoanalytic Institute at New York University Medical Center, New York, New York

Melvin Singer, M.D. Associate Clinical Professor of Psychiatry, University of Pennsylvania School of Medicine, Philadelphia, Pennsylvania; Faculty, Institute of the Philadelphia Association for Psychoanalysis, Philadelphia, Pennsylvania

William H. Sledge, M.D. Professor of Psychiatry, Yale University School of Medicine, New Haven, Connecticut; Graduate, Western New England Institute for Psychoanalysis, New Haven, Connecticut

Louis Spitz, M.D. Training and Supervising Analyst, Cincinnati Psychoanalytic Institute, Cincinnati, Ohio

Alan Tasman, M.D. Professor of Psychiatry, University of Louisville School of Medicine, Louisville, Kentucky; Graduate, Western New England Institute for Psychoanalysis, New Haven, Connecticut

Robert S. Wallerstein, M.D. Emeritus Professor of Psychiatry, University of California, San Francisco; Training and Supervising Analyst, San Francisco Psychoanalytic Institute, San Francisco, California

Sidney H. Weissman, M.D. Professor of Psychiatry, Stritch School of Medicine at Loyola University of Chicago; Graduate, Institute for Psychoanalysis of Chicago, Chicago, Illinois

David S. Werman, M.D. Professor Emeritus of Psychiatry, Duke University Medical Center, Durham, North Carolina; Training and Supervising Analyst, University of North Carolina–Duke Psychoanalytic Education Program, Durham, North Carolina

Thomas Wolman, M.D. Clinical Assistant Professor of Psychiatry and Human Behavior, Jefferson Medical College, Thomas Jefferson University, Philadelphia, Pennsylvania; Faculty by Invitation, Philadelphia Psychoanalytic Institute, Philadelphia, Pennsylvania

Edward A. Wolpert, M.D., Ph.D. Professor of Psychiatry, Rush University, Chicago, Illinois; Member, Chicago Psychoanalytic Society, Chicago, Illinois

Leon Wurmser, M.D. Clinical Professor of Psychiatry, University of West Virginia, Morgantown, West Virginia; Training and Supervising Analyst, New York Freudian Society, New York, New York

Acknowledgments

I would like to express my appreciation to my coeditors, Drs. Efrain Bleiberg and Sidney H. Weissman, and to the many contributors to this book who generously gave of their wisdom and clinical experience to make this text a reality. The concept for this book emerged out of discussions held by the Subcommittee of Psychoanalytic Directors of Residency Training of the American Psychoanalytic Association. We were seeking to make an active and concrete contribution to psychiatric education and to emphasize the richness and clinical utility of a psychodynamic approach to patients. The members of this subcommittee offered attentive and constructive input throughout the shaping and creation of this project. I would like to thank my co-chair, Dr. Nada Stotland, along with Drs. Stephen Bauer, Clyde Flanagan, David Goldberg, Lee Harris, David Joseph, Ronald Krasner, Jim Lomax, Grace Mushrush, and Allan Tasman. Special thanks go as well to Dr. Arnold Cooper, the chairman of the American Psychoanalytic Association's Committee on University and Medical Education, for his strong support both for the work of the subcommittee and for the compilation of this text.

I would also like to acknowledge the assistance I received from a number of senior residents in my program at Thomas Jefferson University who shared with me their perspectives on the text as it was being written: Drs. Daniel Block, Sean Coldren, Douglas Cosgrove, Nancy Dunbar, Edward Goebel, Doris Mirowski, Timothy Smith, Cynthia Theiss, Judith Watt, and John Zebrun.

Finally, I would like to thank Dr. Carol Nadelson of the American Psychiatric Press, Inc., who supported this effort from its very beginning.

Harvey J. Schwartz, M.D.

Foreword

Recent history has moved psychiatry toward a medical model whose adoption has led to an enormous misunderstanding, neglect, and trivialization of psychodynamics and psychoanalysis. This change, over 30 years, from a psychodynamically dominated psychiatry to one in which pharmacology, a multiplicity of conscious and manipulative psychotherapies, and a lack of understanding of human mental processes prevail is startling if one tries to capture the past and the present within a single frame and attempts to make any comparisons between psychiatry's perception and treatment of patients then and now.

The reality is that we have an opportunity to seize the moment and to lay claim to the best of both worlds. The integration of biology and psychological mental functioning offered by the biopsychosocial paradigm, developed over recent years through the meticulous interviewing techniques and awareness of symbolism of George Engel and carried along by the interest and involvement of many significant thinkers in psychiatry, represents the most vital and perhaps even the most exciting way to address the needs of emotionally disturbed and mentally ill patients.

This book represents an opportunity for mental health professionals from diverse fields to recognize the value that psychodynamic principles bring to the understanding of human mental functioning. The four sections contain a richly representative sampling of information and technique that provides a methodological way of thinking about patients, regardless of how much of the psychodynamic theoretical principles are actually used in the care of the various groups of patients described. Looking not only at the basic concepts but also at the use of applied psychoanalysis in clinical settings and clinical syndromes, one can begin to appreciate the value of understanding the underlying motivations and psychological precursors to adult behavior. If nothing else, psychoanalysis has given us a deep understanding of a basic truth—that "the child is the father of the man," that all people's personalities represent a synthesis over a lifetime of habits, beliefs, perceptions, and fantasies developed in childhood and carried on into adult behavior. That fact not only enables the therapist to understand some of the antecedents to specific clinical syndromes but also provides him or her with an intelligence that cannot, in my opinion, be received through any other methodology.

In essence, this book enables all therapists to develop a psychodynamic perspective. Because the reader is not commanded to follow rules of analytic therapy or to employ stereotypical approaches, maximal flexibility can be exercised in the treatment of people who are ill and disturbed, using all of the techniques at our disposal, from medication to social rehabilitation to various types and levels of psychotherapy, but enriched with a basic understanding of and a search for information and facts that tell us what precipitated the recurrence of depression or the episode of psychosis, what was behind the escalation into mania or the exacerbation of the panic disorder—and, digging still deeper, what are the underpinnings of dissociative disorders, of borderline conditions, of posttraumatic stress, and of the other clinical entities addressed in Section III of this book by some of the most prominent and well-published analysts in the country.

Understanding patients' stimuli to illness as well as their negative and pathological responses to those stimuli enables the therapist to reach beyond simple, conscious formulas that, in many instances, lead to unsuccessful treatment and unfortunate recurrences. Some of the basic psychodynamic principles—not only those about patients but also those about treatment (e.g., attachment, types of anxiety, transference and countertransference, the therapeutic setting as a holding environment)—are taken for granted in most training programs and, at this point in our history, are even seen as givens. This book will assist the reader in expanding those fundamental principles into a broad-based understanding of the application of psychodynamic principles to the practice of general psychiatry.

As I view trainees throughout the United States and see programs in which a resident can spend 4 years and never be touched by the psychodynamic paradigm (which, in fact, means never being exposed to a biopsychosocial approach or to an effort to look at patients by making a biopsychosocial formulation), I cannot help but feel that this situation represents a tragic consequence of the biological reductionism and trivialization of psychoanalysis that have been growing over the past two decades. We are in a position to use psychodynamics rather than dispose of them. Throwing the baby out with the bathwater and creating a false either–or dichotomization penalizes trainees and therapists and renders the practice of psychiatry repetitive and dull. This book takes lofty rhetorical statements about biopsychosocial issues and concretizes them in a way that has the potential to be both productive and practical.

The editors and authors, under the leadership of Harvey J. Schwartz, M.D., have prepared a book that is practical and instructive without resorting to oversimplification and that is comprehensive enough to provide a true flavor of the excitement of "applied psychoanalysis."

Paul Jay Fink, M.D.

Introduction

This text is intended as an invitation—an invitation to get to know how a number of psychoanalytic psychiatrists perceive their patients and their work, as well as how they think within the psychotherapeutic process itself. It is an opportunity to hear them speak frankly about their experiences in the intimate chamber of the therapeutic relationship and their observations about what in that process proves useful for their patients. The work of these practitioners demonstrates that considerable clinical benefit may be gained from the application of a psychodynamic understanding in all settings and for all patients who come to us seeking relief.

The many psychoanalytic psychiatrists who have shared their clinical knowledge in these pages do not speak with one voice. Although all of these authors have a traditional analytic background, they each bring a unique self to their theoretical understanding of emotional pain, to their clinical practice, and to their chapters. The editors have allowed the authors to be themselves. Rather than composing a homogenized norm, this book represents the full range of dynamic styles that actually exist in the professional community. This reflects our acknowledgment that each participant in the therapeutic dyad of necessity brings all of who he or she individually is to the encounter.

It is for this reason that we have decided not to focus on the descriptive phenomenology of patients. Others have addressed that area with admirable thoroughness. We have set ourselves a different task—one that emphasizes the understanding that patients do not experience themselves as diagnostic labels, but instead come to us with subjective experiences of pain. We therefore begin where our patients begin. We follow their internal sense of themselves and seek to expand it. With remarkable regularity, this type of active listening leads patients to recognize a deep and complex set of feelings toward their therapist—and from him or her to their pathogenic, unconscious past.

Although the authors' approaches to patients vary somewhat, they all have in common this appreciation of the fundamental importance of the role of transference and of the impact on later life of the key developmental stages and fantasies of childhood. One might say that this book traces how these two themes manifest themselves in the many clinical settings in which we work and in the multiple symptoms and character pictures that patients bring to us. We are suggesting that these both quite simple yet inordinately subtle appreciations need to remain paramount in our psychiatric listening as we approach all of our patients with a healing intent.

This book is organized to parallel the clinician's psychiatric education. The Basic Concepts section begins with an overview of the psychodynamic model. This chapter demonstrates how the dynamic perspective differs from commonsense psychology in that it recognizes both the bedrock quality of subjective mental phenomena and the fact that all mental events are related to antecedent mental events. This perspective shows that the mind is made up of unrecognized, conflicting wishes and fears that lead to the character traits and symptoms that trouble our patients. The next chapter applies this psychodynamic model to patients in the form of the dynamic formulation. Such a written formulation can organize one's thinking about the patient's intrapsychic struggles as well as foreshadow the nature of the relationship that will be created with the doctor. The vehicle that allows for the emergence of the patient's affect-filled unconscious life is the peculiar participant-observer stance of the clinician. This studied use of the self as a clinical instrument, as described in the chapter by that title, is unique to analytic therapy. It entails an empathically spontaneous yet self-conscious attitude that has the capacity to reveal resistances in either of the parties.

The therapist's encounter with the patient is preceded and framed by the meaning of where and how they meet. The inpatient unit, the emergency room, the medical ward, the community clinic, the health maintenance organization, and the outpatient clinic all contribute both real and imagined contexts to the clinical encounter, as is illustrated in the section on Clinical Settings. The dynamic psychiatrist strives to appreciate the various meanings of such settings to both participants and thereby works to create a therapeutic metaphoric space in any of the physical environments.

The patients we meet in our offices come to us in many kinds of distress. We try to understand both the state and the trait dimensions of their presentations. In so doing, we hope to help them acknowledge those unrecognized aspects of themselves whose strivings so commonly contribute to their difficulties. The contributors to the Clinical Syndromes section review the current dynamic understanding of a wide range of difficulties with which patients present. Each chapter in this section includes a historical review of dynamic perspectives on the topic disorder as well as a discussion of differential dynamic diagnosis. Illustrated in this section is the basic truth that it is the patient's underlying ego structure—not his or her specific descriptive syndrome—that most informs treatment selection and prognosis. Each clinical chapter also presents patient vignettes that are designed to demonstrate the vibrancy, nuances, and therapeutic power of the psychodynamic relationship.

As detailed in the concluding section of the book, the overall orientation of this work is that brain and mind provide complementary perspectives on the human condition. Just as childhood environmental traumas—and, undoubtedly, transference-related affects—impact neurochemical functioning, so, too, does the unconscious meaning patients attach to a medication have a great deal to do with compliance and outcome. Meaning and biology are thus inextricably linked. The clinical applications of this integrated model are discussed in the chapter on the psychology of prescribing and taking medication.

Many therapeutic treatments are characterized by interruptions. Indeed, these events are built into training programs and are more common in all facets of clinical work than is usually recognized. Such arbitrary terminations evoke powerful reactions in patient and clinician alike that can serve to affectively coalesce many of the insights gained throughout the time of the relationship. The meaning, impact, and usefulness of such separations is reviewed in the chapter on interruptions in treatment.

The challenges and accomplishments of research in psychodynamic therapy are discussed in the next chapter. Especially noteworthy are the cost-offset studies that document the savings in medical treatment for those patients in psychiatric care. It appears that when—in a treatment setting—patients' transference desires are allowed to be object directed, the body itself is spared the ravages of their aggressive impulses.

In the final chapter of this volume, a recommended curriculum in psychodynamic psychiatry is offered to stimulate the thinking of psychiatric educators. Such a curriculum is needed to adequately equip the next generation of psychiatrists who will be asked to understand both the new findings in neurochemistry and the timeless insights of unconscious functioning.

This book invites the reader to consider the valuable contributions—and the continuing relevance—of psychodynamic concepts to general psychiatry.

Harvey J. Schwartz, M.D.

Section I

Basic Concepts

Efrain Bleiberg, M.D.,
Section Editor

Chapter 1

Basic Principles of Psychodynamic Psychiatry

Robert Michels, M.D.

History

In 1883 a Viennese physician, Joseph Breuer, told a younger colleague, Sigmund Freud, about a fascinating patient—an intelligent young German woman, Bertha Pappenheim, who in later years was to become one of the founders of psychiatric social work. Breuer's clinical observations on this patient, who suffered from the symptoms of what was then called hysteria, led to a new theory about the nature of the disorder and some suggestions for a possible new treatment. Breuer himself stopped working in this area, perhaps in part because of his discomfort over the intense personal feelings stimulated by his relationships with his patient and his inability to understand those feelings. Freud explored Breuer's method further with other patients, continued to develop the theory, and in time even came to understand the meaning of Breuer's discomfort. The theory and the treatment based upon it were the beginning of psychoanalysis and psychodynamic psychiatry.

Bertha Pappenheim, like other patients diagnosed with hysteria, had multiple symptoms related to several organ systems, altered states of consciousness, and disturbances of thought, affect, and communication. Nineteenth-century psychiatry had understood these symptoms as reflecting abnormalities of the nervous system—that is, as signs of an underlying neuropathology that had not yet been identified. First Breuer and then Freud began to employ a practice that grew out of the tradition of 19th-century medicine far more than that of 19th-century psychiatry: they spent many hours talking with their patients—or, to be more precise, listening to them. As they listened, they noted a relationship between their patients' symptoms and what was on their patients' minds, and—particularly exciting—they discovered that talking about these issues actually influenced the symptoms. Freud and Breuer reconceptualized the symptoms as communications—symbolic expressions of thoughts and memories of which the patient might not be aware, rather than signs of a disordered nervous system. In brief, the meaning of the symptoms and the cause and treatment of the patient's disorder were to be discovered through a dialogue between the patient and the therapist rather than by a dissection of the patient's brain and nervous system. Psychodynamic psychiatry was to be a science of mental life: in Freud's famous formulation, his patients suffered not from brain disease but from "reminiscences."

Psychoanalytic theory grew out of clinical observation, but it also brought its own models and concepts to the clinical data. Freud's background as a neurologist and neurobiologist shaped much of his early thinking; he initially attempted to formulate his theory as a neuropsychology, a project that quickly ran into difficulties because of the then primitive understanding of the nervous system. Freud was also interested in evolutionary biology, cultural anthropology, and history, and one can trace each of these themes, as well as the ideas of late 19th-century positivist science, throughout his work. All of this is to say that psychoanalytic theory has been richly informed by the dominant ideas that influenced its creators and the intellectual climate in which it developed. In recent years, developmental psychology has largely replaced neurobiology and evolutionary biology as the source of conceptual models, and linguistics, information theory, group dynamics, and clinical psychopathology have contributed to these models as well.

Basic Principles

Mentalism

Psychodynamics is about the psyche—the mind. It is about thoughts, feelings, experiences, wishes, fears, fantasies, and memories. It is not about the brain or the body, except insofar as these are seen as the substrate of mental activity or as being represented in mental imagery. It is also not about behavior viewed "objectively," as by a behaviorist, seen as the activity of an organism without regard to the realm of subjective experience. Contemporary psychiatry often pushes neurobiological reductionism to the extreme, regarding mentalist concepts as referring to epiphenomena, with the "real" action occurring at the level of the nervous system. Psychodynamics regards mental phenomena as its subject matter, and therefore it is of greatest value in understanding the world of inner experience. It is not our major tool in approaching brain dysfunction, seizure phenomena, or psychological defects caused by the biological diatheses that underlie the major psychoses. It *is* a major tool in understanding wishes, fears, fantasies, and the relationships among them—how these phenomena arise from earliest experiences, are transformed in the course of development, predispose to both adaptive and maladaptive behavior, and change in response to meaningful human relations. If we want to understand mental life and mental symptoms, we must employ mentalist models.

Psychic Determinism

Commonsense psychology is, like psychodynamics, mentalist—that is, it explains people and their behavior in terms of thoughts, wishes, fears, fantasies, and the interplay among these elements. However, commonsense psychology, unlike scientific thinking, is not strictly determinist; although it explains many things, it accepts that other things might not be explainable—they just happen! For example, most people eat because they feel hungry and stop eating because they feel satisfied; their behavior reflects a mental experience. However, some people stop eating while still hungry and others keep eating although sated. These behaviors can be labeled pathological—anorexic or bulimic—and attributed to a neurobiological abnormality or an unspecified "disease," but there is no commonsense psychological explanation for them. Even more familiar are so-called Freudian slips (psychoanalysts call them "parapraxes"). Most often we say what we are thinking, but sometimes we "just make a mistake," as when a woman got "mixed up" while comparing her sister-in-law with her husband and said, "Judy is just a masculine version of George." Other mental phenomena that seem to commonsense psychology to be without psychic determinism include dreams and most forms of neurotic symptomatology, such as obsessions or phobias.

Psychodynamic theory is different from commonsense psychology in that it asserts a strict and all-embracing psychic determinism—all mental events can be understood as the result of antecedent mental events, not as epiphenomena of brain events (except perhaps for the behavioral aspects of a seizure) and certainly not as without cause. An individual who doesn't eat may have the unconscious fantasy that food is poison; one who overeats may see food as evidence of love. The woman described above who made the parapraxis may have secretly believed her sister-in-law to be overly aggressive and her husband overly passive. In short, dreams and symptoms are symbolic representations of disguised thoughts. Psychodynamic theory argues that determinism is pervasive, and in doing so accepts that self-awareness, or consciousness—a characteristic of mental life that commonsense psychology views as constant—is in fact only intermittent. The anorexic or bulimic individual, the dissatisfied sister-in-law, the dreamer, and the person with a neurosis all share a lack of awareness of the mental forces that govern their experience, and through it, their behavior. From a psychodynamic perspective, these individuals' behavior is totally determined, although the determinants are unconscious. The psychoanalytic method allows us access to unconscious mental life and thereby permits us to fill in the gaps of the incomplete psychic determinism of commonsense psychology.

Mental Dynamics

The psychodynamic approach is not only "psycho"—that is, mentalist—but also "dynamic"—about forces, about motives, and inevitably, because multiple forces have multiple goals, about conflict. Psychodynamic thinking views mental life as the product of conflicting mental forces, wishes, fears, and emotions, each of which "presses" and all of which together direct thoughts and behavior. One of the ongoing theoretical dialogues in psychoanalysis relates to how such forces are best conceptualized. Freud thought of these mental dynamics as biologically rooted drives that unfold in a largely predetermined maturational sequence. Others have emphasized socially and culturally determined attitudes and desires. The classification of mental forces, their origins in biology or social experience, their development over the life span, their plasticity, and their basic content—sexuality, aggression, mastery, curiosity, self-fulfillment, and others—have been ongoing major themes of psychodynamic and psychoanalytic discourse. The dispute in psychoanalytic theory largely relates to the basic nature of these forces. There is much more agreement as one moves from theoretical concepts to clinical phenomena and observes the organizing role of wishes and fears in patients' mental lives.

The Unconscious

Recognition of unconscious mental processes long antedates psychoanalysis. People frequently remember things they had previously forgotten and that must have been "stored" somewhere in the mind during the interval. Furthermore, they can be shown to know something they weren't aware of knowing, by hypnosis or by less exotic means such as behavioral responses to subliminal stimuli. However, unconscious mental processes assume a unique importance in psychodynamic thinking because not just casual memories but major dynamic forces—the wishes and fears that shape our lives and, particularly, our neurotic symptoms and character traits—are believed to be unconscious. That mental processes could occur without our awareness was known to Aristotle; that many of the determinants of our major life choices are unknown to us, but nonetheless—and even because of this—exert powerful influence on us was one of Freud's great discoveries. Psychoanalysts further differentiate unconscious mental activity into "preconscious" (i.e., out of awareness but easily accessible if attention is directed) and "unconscious" in the narrow sense (i.e., inaccessible to the individual under normal circumstances). The clinical psychoanalytic method, with its free association and dream analysis, is designed to facilitate the exploration of unconscious mental activity, making it preconscious and thus accessible to consciousness.

Repression and Defense

Why are mental themes unconscious? The most obvious answer—and the one largely accepted by commonsense psychology—is that they are likely to be forgotten if they are unimportant. However, this cannot explain why major dynamic forces that shape our lives are unconscious. Freud recognized that dynamic unconscious forces are unconscious for the very reason that they *are* important and would cause distress if they were to become conscious. The psychological mechanism that actively keeps powerful and potentially disturbing wishes or fears unconscious is called *repression.* First Freud himself, and then his daughter Anna and other psychoanalysts, came to recognize that repression was only one of the mental mechanisms available to avoid conscious distress engendered by the emergence of disturbing unconscious mental themes, and the term *defense* was introduced to encompass all such mechanisms, with repression as the prototype. In contemporary psychoanalytic thinking, defense is a function that may be served by almost any mental activity that is used to avoid conscious awareness of a disturbing unconscious theme. Whereas early models of psychodynamic therapy focused on helping people become more aware of forbidden unconscious wishes and fears, contemporary views emphasize helping people understand their defensive strategies and diminish the power that these strategies exert in their mental lives.

The Present and the Past

Psychodynamics is about the dynamic mental forces that shape behavior, forces that are very much alive in the present. It has no interest in the past except insofar as that past is preserved in these present dynamic forces. In their earliest inquiries into the unconscious forces that determined psychopathological symptoms, Breuer and Freud had no special interest in childhood. However, within a few years, Freud discovered—and countless psychoanalysts since him have confirmed—that the persistent wishes and fears of childhood are the major themes of unconscious mental life. Thus, the study of psychodynamics, which is the study of unconscious mental forces, became of necessity the study of childhood psychology. The influence of unconscious forces on behavior is the influence of persisting themes of the mental life of the child on adult life. One of the important issues in contemporary psychoanalytic theory is the relationship between the scientific study of the psychology of children and those themes of adult mental life that can be traced back to childhood. The inner subjective record of the past is not the same as the past that would have been observed by a contemporary onlooker. The record is constructed, shaped, and reshaped by the recorder as well as by the circumstances in which it is eventually recounted. Thus, although the study of developmental psychology has relevance for psychodynamics, it is by no means synonymous with the clinical exploration of persisting infantile themes in unconscious mental life.

The concept of transference refers to a particularly important instance of the role of the past in shaping the present. Emotionally charged personal relationships, such as the relationship between a patient and a doctor, are always shaped by the capacity for and the style of relatedness that the patient acquired in childhood. Thus, all important relationships are to some extent repetitions of primary relationships, and a patient's relationship with his or her doctor reflects that patient's relationship with earlier caregivers, particularly parents. An appreciation of this process of transference is vital to our understanding of how therapy works, why it helps patients, and why they often struggle against it.

Infantile Sexuality

Adults generally think of infants and small children as having bland and innocent thoughts—if, indeed, they have any thoughts at all. However, the truth appears to be quite different, based on the observations of experienced infant caregivers and developmental psychologists and, most importantly, on the persisting unconscious fantasies of adults. Children's mental life is driven by elemental passions and primitive terrors, unchecked by the understanding of reality available to adults. Their experience of the external world is organized in terms of the role it plays in the gratification and frustration of basic needs. Freud emphasized the sensual pleasures of bodily experience, which he labeled by the name of the bodily pleasure central to adult experience, sexuality. Other psychoanalysts have emphasized aggressive as well as sexual drives, and the psychological meaning of attachment to and separation from primary caregivers. These themes—sexual, aggressive, clinging, and autonomy-seeking wishes and fantasies persisting from the mental life of childhood as unconscious dynamic forces in adults—are the building blocks of psychodynamic models of psychic conflict.

Mental Structures

Psychodynamic models of mental life focus on dynamic forces. However, certain patterns of mental activity are stable over long periods of time, and the concept of structure has seemed more appropriate than that of force to describe such stable patterns. Motivational systems such as sexuality and aggression, believed by many to stem from the neurobiological organization of the nervous system, are structures. Patterns of defense resulting from innate styles and developmental experiences are structures. Freud's so-called structural model organized mental activity into three overarching structures. One was the id, which referred to the organismic and biologically rooted drives and their psychological representations. Second was the ego, which referred to the adaptive and external reality-oriented aspects of the mind, including perception, cognition, memory, motor control, and adaptive behavior. Finally, there was the superego, a specialized portion of the ego that tended to function as a coherent, organized system, and that was often in conflict with the rest of the ego as well as with the id. The superego encompasses values and standards, notions of good and bad, right and wrong, approval and disapproval, and the inner source of guilt, shame, and pride. The commonsense psychology notion of "conscience" refers to that small aspect of superego functioning that is conscious. Psychodynamic developmental theory views the primary origin of the superego as the child's internal psychological representation of the parent—approving and disapproving, loving and criticizing, rewarding and punishing. Some psychoanalytic writers separate the positive ideals from the critical injunctions of the superego and call the former the "ego ideal."

Adaptive Function of Behavior

Commonsense psychology views most behavior as adaptive, but sees some behavior differently—as a mistake, wrong, stupid, or pathologic. In many ways, this view is a corollary to seeing some behavior as not fully determined. Psychopathology, from a commonsense perspective, is not adaptive; it is wrong, and the goal of treatment is to correct it.

Psychodynamic psychology differs. All behavior, including pathological behavior, is seen as adaptive. Instead of being a mistake, pathological behavior involves the effective pursuit of goals concealed both from the patient and from the rest of the world. Such behavior constitutes an adaptive component of an unconscious strategy. The central goal of treatment is not to expunge the behavior, but rather to identify the secret goal and bring it into the open. When the goals of pathological behavior become known to the patient, the patient is freer to integrate them with the rest of his or her life, and their maladaptive impact is diminished.

Modern clinical psychiatry classifies the phenomenology of psychopathology according to the familiar diagnostic categories. Psychodynamic psychiatry, by contrast, sees behavioral phenomenology as the product of underlying mental forces. Whereas a clinical psychiatric diagnosis is a summary description of pathological phenomena, a psychodynamic formulation is a statement of the major mental themes, wishes, fears, conflicts, and compromises leading to that behavior and the history of their development. Diagnosis focuses on the boundaries and discontinuities between health and pathology; in contrast, psychodynamic formulations focus on the continuities and similarities.

Conflict and Compromise; Symptom and Character

Psychodynamic psychology views behavior as the product of conflicting and often unconscious mental forces. Psychological conflicts produce internal signals of potential dysphoria, anxiety, and depression—signals that will lead to conscious distress and the disruption of functioning if other psychological strategies are not called into play. Most often these signal affects do elicit coping strategies, such as the so-called defense or mental mechanisms—strategies for constructing compromises among the conflicting dynamic themes, wishes, and fears. Typically, such compromises manage to keep the potentially most disturbing themes unconscious while partially and symbolically gratifying the wishes and accommodating to the fears. These compromise structures may sacrifice adaptation to reality in order to satisfy unconscious needs, in which case they can lead to pathology. If the compromise structures are integrated into the individual's experience of self, they are called character traits. If they remain psychologically sequestered and alien from the sense of self, they are called symptoms. Paradoxically, an early task in the psychodynamic psychotherapy of symptoms is to demonstrate to the patient that his or her symptoms are meaningful products of inner psychological themes (i.e., they are linked to character), whereas an early task in the psychotherapy of pathological character traits is to establish some potential dystonicity from the patient's sense of self (i.e., to support the patient's image of a possible self without the undesirable trait).

Alternate Theoretical Schools of Psychodynamics

Most of the theoretical concepts outlined thus far would be shared by the several contemporary schools of psychodynamics, with the major differences residing in the relative emphases given to different themes and the choices selected where possible alternative ideas have been outlined. The dominant psychodynamic school in the United States has been called ego psychology. It emphasizes Freud's structural theory of id, ego, and superego and the central role of conflict among mental themes representing these structures and the compromise formations that result. A second major school, object relations theory, grows out of the work of Melanie Klein and her followers; this school is prominent in England and dominant in Latin America, with Otto Kernberg a major North American spokesman. The object relations group thinks of the mental representations of self, others, and relationships as more fundamental than the organismic drives of the "id" of ego psychology. Object relations theorists have been particularly interested in more serious psychopathology, including severe character disorders and psychoses; in aggressive motivations; and in developmental psychodynamic models that trace mental themes back to the preoedipal themes of the first few years of life. A third school of psychodynamics, which developed around the work of the late Heinz Kohut and his followers, is called self psychology. It places the maturation and development of an organized sense of self at the center of psychodynamic thinking. Relations with others are essential to support that development, and failures in those relationships can lead to developmental defects and arrests. Psychological conflicts are primarily understood as the product of such developmental defects. Sexual, aggressive, and other motivational systems are integrated into the functioning of the self, and emerge as discrete motivational themes only secondary to disturbances of the self. This group has been particularly interested in narcissistic character pathology and the affects and symptoms commonly associated with narcissism, as well as the adaptive capacities and creativity that stem from these dynamics.

Conclusion

The psychodynamic model provides a way of studying and understanding behavior that leads to a strategy for treating some patients and some problems. It is not the only model in psychiatry, nor is it always the best. However, psychodynamics is the preeminent conceptual system that links behavior in general, and pathology in particular, to mental life—thoughts, feelings, wishes, and fears. As such, it is the dominant model guiding the talking therapies—those based on a systematic theory of how people's inner life is related to their behavior and how talking to someone might lead to change.

Chapter 2

The Psychodynamic Formulation

Elena G. Lister, M.D.,
Elizabeth L. Auchincloss, M.D.,
and Arnold M. Cooper, M.D.

Although the psychodynamic formulation is an important part of patient evaluation and treatment, it is often only implicit and not clearly stated. As Perry and colleagues (1987, p. 543) noted, "a psychodynamic formulation is seldom offered [by supervisees] and is almost never incorporated into the written record" of a patient. This omission stems in part from a lack of understanding of just what a psychodynamic formulation is and in part from lack of experience in making formulations of patients' psychodynamics. As a result, the beginning therapist may be fearful about succinctly articulating, especially in written form, what he or she understands about a patient, and a formal written psychodynamic formulation may seem like a daunting and tedious task. It may also seem unclear just how useful a psychodynamic formulation can be for many kinds of treatment.

It is a common misconception of the psychodynamic formulation to see it as demanding a total, comprehensive, and advanced theoretical understanding of one's patient. In fact, however, every therapist makes informal and unwritten psychodynamic formulations all the time to account for how a patient's behavior relates to the patient's mental life. As human beings, we are probably unable to interact with each other without making continuous informal dynamic formulations that attempt to account for behavior. For example, if a spouse comes home from work and, in an uncharacteristic way, yells about a minor mishap, we almost intuitively understand that this foul mood has more to do with a rough day at the office than with the mishap at home. Without full awareness of our thinking, we understand the behavior as an instance of the use of the defense mechanism of displacement. As clinicians, however, we must be as explicit as possible about the similar assumptions and formulations that we use to guide our interactions with patients. Writing a psychodynamic formulation will help us to be more alert to what we are already thinking about the patient, and it will help us to become aware of those aspects of the patient that still puzzle us and for which we want to find answers.

The origins of the concept of the psychodynamic formulation are not clearly identifiable but probably lie in Freud's landmark conceptualizations of psychopathology. Prior to Freud and the birth of the psychodynamic school of psychiatry, the major psychiatric tradition was descriptive, classifying diseases according to observed behavior. Freud offered ways to understand many of these surface behaviors as arising from hidden or unconscious conflicting wishes and fears. He clustered symptoms—and later, personality traits—on the basis of similar unconscious motives and identifiable defensive patterns, thereby defining the major neuroses. With DSM-III-R and DSM-IV (American Psychiatric Association 1987, 1994), psychiatry has sought to recapture some of the benefits of the descriptive approach. The two approaches—*psychodynamic,* based on inner mental life, and *descriptive,* based on external behavior—complement each other, offering different kinds of clustering that mutually enhance our grasp of a patient's difficulties. For example:

> A young woman with depressed mood and vegetative symptoms diagnosed with a major depression attempts suicide by overdose on her prescribed antidepressant when her psychiatrist is about to go on vacation. Certainly, suicidal behavior is part of the depressive syndrome. However, understanding that this particular gesture expresses this patient's rage at being abandoned and the secondary fear and guilt induced by that rage is crucial in guiding our interventions, both for the patient's immediate safety and for helping her to understand her response, so that in the future, she may be able to tolerate or express that rage in less self-destructive ways.

The psychodynamic formulation can be distinguished from other kinds of assessments that we as clinicians make. The psychodynamic formulation is a brief narrative. It is an attempt to understand the patient's current behavior in terms of his or her conscious and unconscious mental life. It is neither a mental status examination nor a case summary; these summarize and detail the observed data. It is likewise neither a diagnosis nor a differential diagnosis; these help us to label and sort the observed behavior. In the psychodynamic formulation, we must try to understand how a patient's mental construction of his or her world—including representations of him- or herself and of the people in that world—helps to shape the behaviors that make the patient unique—provide his or her character—and that contribute to the symptoms that bring the patient to seek help. This formulation constitutes a preliminary attempt to explain the data of observation by linking those data to the patient's underlying psychological world. Using our knowledge of the patient's past and present mental life, and guided by psychological theories, we generate hypotheses to account for and explain observed behavior. These hypotheses constitute the psychodynamic formulation; all clinicians make them all the time, formally or informally.

Although therapists from different schools of thought may offer somewhat differing paradigms to account for behavior, most therapists share certain basic assumptions (see Chapter 1 of this volume) and have expectations about current and future behavior based on past behavior. The psychodynamic formulation is not a long treatise, nor does the psychodynamic formulation stand as the final word on a patient. Rather, our experience with the patient in the office and the psychodynamic blueprint that we construct constantly interact with and influence each other. For example, consider the following:

> Your patient, a young executive, describes difficulty maintaining a job, a depressed mood, and low self-esteem. At first, he seems eager to please you, and your initial hypotheses center on the patient's inhibition in self-assertion. Over time, however, you find yourself becoming irritated with him. Thus alerted, you begin to notice his more subtle denigration of you and his air of self-importance and aloofness. You therefore reconsider the source of the patient's work difficulties, and hypothesize that some portion of those difficulties is created by his arrogance, of which he appears to be unaware. You are then able to generate new ideas as to the origins of his problems at work and their functions for him.

Thus, the psychodynamic formulation represents a plastic model of the patient's inner life, modified in direct relation to the clinician's experience with the patient and to the clinician's increasing sophistication in understanding the patient's psychodynamics.

What do we listen for during our work with patients in order to identify the central themes and conflicts of the patient's life? In addition to the history and descriptions we elicit, patients will naturally convey to us a great deal of information about their mental makeup in their modes of verbal and nonverbal behaviors, in the stories they choose to tell (as well as those they do not tell), in their choice of words, and in their subtle and overt bodily actions and facial expressions. As clinicians, we also have a valuable tool in our self-observations and our intuition. As we listen and learn to trust our inner reactions to patients, we make available to ourselves a greater understanding of who our patients are and how their difficulties have arisen.

The Psychodynamic Formulation

The psychodynamic formulation has four parts: 1) summary of the case, 2) discussion of nondynamic factors, 3) psychodynamic explanation of central conflicts, object relations, and defenses, and 4) prediction of how the patient's dynamics will affect the therapy.

Part 1: Summarizing Statement

This part of the psychodynamic formulation addresses what it is that we will try to explain and understand about the patient. In this section, we construct a very brief outline of the patient's history and major difficulties, paying particular attention to major relationships, affective tone, and the patient's sense of self.

Part 2: Description of Nondynamic Factors

In this second part, we discuss nonpsychological factors that impinge on the psychiatric disorder and its treatment. These include genetic vulnerabilities, physical trauma, and organic factors that affect the brain, such as drugs, physical illness, and mental retardation. These nondynamic elements are important, both because they may provide an adequate explanation for certain phenomena without further search and because such major historical events may be the foci for many of the patient's unconscious conflicts and defenses. For example, when evaluating a depressed woman with an alcoholic father, we must consider the patient's genetic predisposition as well as the potential emotional and social deprivations that may have occurred in early childhood.

We must also try to understand the meaning to the patient of these nondynamic factors, often in a developmental perspective. Past traumata may have a particular subjective meaning in relation to the developmental stage at which they occurred. For example:

> A female patient, incapacitatingly anxious about beginning graduate school, mentions to you in an offhand way that because of a severe injury at puberty, she had to wear a massive back brace throughout her early teens. Although you may treat her anxiety with anxiolytic medication, it would seem important to attempt to account for why this young woman's anxiety is overwhelming her now. In a brief conversation, it becomes apparent that the patient feels that entering graduate school represents the real end of her handicapped and necessarily sheltered childhood. She is fearful of being independent, worried about sexual encounters, angry over how much she missed as an adolescent, and frightened that if she misbehaves she will again injure her back and be locked in a brace.

On the basis of this bit of dynamic formulation, it may seem quite likely that this patient will respond to brief psychotherapy and thereby avoid long-term medication, with its potential side effects and its connotations of physical illness, which are specially significant to her.

Part 3: Psychodynamic Exploration of Central Conflicts, Object Relations, and Defenses

All human beings have similar basic wishes and fears. These include the wish for attachment to others; the longing for dependency; the fear of separation from loved ones; fears of loss or harm to oneself or others; strivings for autonomy, mastery, and self-esteem; wishes for sexual and aggressive gratification; and moral concerns. Many of these wishes are incompatible with each other or with reality, and each person creates his or her own compromises to resolve the conflicts between unacceptable wishes, conscience, and the demands of reality. Such compromises, usually created outside awareness, represent the best possible adaptive effort to resolve the conflict by gratifying, even unconsciously, some portion of consciously unacceptable wishes without grossly violating moral and reality standards. When the compromise solution is reasonably adaptive, the individual enjoys a rich and active life with intimate relationships, a wide range of available affects and pleasure, and a cohesive sense of self. Patients present with psychiatric illness when their intrapsychic solutions have inhibited these capacities.

The psychodynamic formulation is an attempt to understand the major conflicts of a particular patient, the compromises arrived at, the defensive structures used to maintain the compromises, and the ways in which these structures serve or subvert healthier adaptations, as reflected in the quality of relationships, achievements, and satisfaction. These intrapsychic solutions involve defenses that have usually been established earlier in life, in childhood or adolescence, and that have become enduring as the individual brings his or her past expectations to new situations, leading to a continual reliving of the past in the present. For example, the irritable spouse mentioned earlier invoked the defense of displacement, expressing aggression outwardly to his partner when it was actually intended for the boss, whose retaliation and loss of love are excessively feared and resented. The spouse is reacting psychologically as though the boss is the all-powerful, punitive parent of childhood, at whom one dare not be angry. This minor example illustrates that in psychodynamically understanding any piece of psychological behavior, we note the wishes (to yell at, humiliate, or murder the boss), the fears (guilt for being a bad child, loss of love and security), the defensive compromise (displacement toward the partner), the distortions of the internal representations of self and object ("I am still a child and the boss is my all-powerful parent who may discard me"), and the state of the self ("I lack the sturdiness to support my self-esteem with realistic actions and so must resort to maladaptive defenses").

In formulating a model of the patient's psychodynamics, the therapist may give different stress to the ego-psychological description (wish, prohibition, defense), the object-relational model (internal structures of interactions of self and other), the self-psychological model (the structure and deficits of the self), or the interpersonal model (the ways relationships are conducted), depending on which models or areas of focus best describe the patient's psychological state. The ego-psychological description of the patient's forbidden desires and internal self-punishment for those desires may guide the therapist's understanding of the patient. Or it may be most useful to emphasize the nature of the internal images of self and others, especially parents, and how these distorted images create disturbances in the patient's experience of him- or herself and others. This object-relations focus can be especially helpful in explaining the fragmented inner worlds of borderline and psychotic patients. Alternately, we may choose to highlight the development of vulnerabilities in the sense of self as a key to understanding the patient's psychiatric difficulties. Narcissistic problems in patients with all types of illness can be understood from this self-psychological perspective. The therapist may wish to emphasize the interpersonal point of view—examining how patients mold their actual interactions in the world to bring about outcomes that are both desired and feared. Not all perspectives are equally relevant for all patients. As clinicians thinking psychodynamically, we use an admixture of emphases, depending on what is most relevant to each patient's difficulties. A psychodynamic formulation is intended to be helpful to the therapist in his or her day-to-day encounters with patients. It is not necessary to be overly inclusive to satisfy this goal.

Part 4: Prediction of How the Patient's Dynamics Will Affect the Therapy

In this final portion of the psychodynamic formulation, we attempt to anticipate how the patient will behave in treatment. On the basis of the hypotheses put forward in Part 3, the therapist makes predictions about transference, positive and negative; about resistances, including acting out; and about his or her own countertransference. These predictions rest on the assumption that for all individuals, our major modes of responding to new situations will recapitulate those adaptations, both useful and harmful, that we have used in the past. We therefore assume that the patient will respond to us in therapy with the same array of conflicts, distorted inner representations, and attempts at compromise solution that we have learned about in the patient's history and observed in the patient's interactions with us, and that we have described in Part 3 of our psychodynamic formulation. Within the patient's relationship to the therapist—the transference—the patient will relive his or her past experiences and prior attempts at conflict resolution. For example, with psychodynamic understanding, the therapist of the young executive with difficulties on the job due to his subtle arrogance is equipped to predict power struggles within the therapeutic relationship and potential disruptions in therapy, just as occurred in work situations. As another example, a patient who is unconsciously ashamed and frightened of her dependency needs, and who in reaction responds to authority with automatic defiance, can rather reliably be predicted to be noncompliant with medication. Depending on our immediate and long-range goals, we may attempt to help the patient to understand and change her inner defensive structure so that she can make a more enlightened decision about taking medication, or we may use our knowledge of the patient to help her feel that medication is her idea, not the therapist's, thereby bypassing an area of potential conflict.

A reasonable knowledge of our own conflicts and defenses will enable us to predict our own responses to a patient's behavior. Furthermore, these countertransference responses are an important source of data concerning the patient. Noting our rising irritability during a session, or becoming aware of starting to dread the appointment with a particular patient, or recognizing the special pleasure with which we anticipate certain patients' appointments are opportunities to understand some of the dynamic interaction of doctor and patient. Are we irritated by the patient's defensive use of narcissistic devaluation, or do we dread seeing a patient who has made us feel therapeutically impotent, reproducing his conviction that his parents lacked the power to protect him, or are we excited about seeing a patient who acts in a seductive manner? In each of these instances, a knowledge of the patient's major psychodynamics and the ability to recognize our own responses enables us to understand and respond therapeutically to the patient's complex and sometimes destructive therapeutic behaviors.

Finally, we emphasize once again that the dynamic formulation is intended to be useful—and thus should be as brief as it can be, and no more inclusive than it need be. Any formulation is tentative and readily subject to change as we learn more about the patient.

Case Example

History

When Ms. A entered treatment in 1989, she was 24 years old, unemployed, and living alone. Ms. A was the youngest of three daughters from an upper-class German-Jewish family. Her father was a surgeon and her mother a fundraiser for charitable causes. Ms. A had many reasons for seeking treatment, but foremost on her mind was an eating problem described as bingeing followed by vomiting two times a month for 2 years. This was a deep secret, never told to anyone before.

Ms. A also complained of confusion about career goals, fearing that any career choice would "swallow her up." She had worked briefly as a hospital aide since graduating from college but had hated the job because she felt "consumed with worry" and "eaten up inside" about whether she was caring properly for patients. Although Ms. A had written several screenplays, she feared trying to sell any of these lest her ideas be stolen.

Ms. A also suffered from social isolation, which was largely self-imposed. Although superficially popular and well liked, she avoided anything but casual contact with friends. Despite being lonely, she did not want a roommate, fearing that she would be watched all the time, especially when eating. Ms. A was unable to eat in front of others, feeling that they monitored her intake and were contemptuous of her lack of control. At other times, she feared that friends would steal her tricks for successful dieting. If a friend expressed ideas different from her own, she would often break off the relationship to avoid feeling forced to "swallow their opinions." Ms. A found solace and strength in competitive sports, at which she excelled. She spent most evenings and weekends in her parents' home and was financially supported by her father.

Ms. A had had few and only brief romantic attachments with "boys" and dreaded trying to talk to them. In conversation she exerted herself to be "bland and agreeable." Despite her lack of involvement with men, Ms. A was preoccupied with a fantasy in which she was married to a wealthy, athletic, well-educated professional whose background would be as much as possible like her own. She had had few sexual experiences.

Ms. A described the precipitating event for seeking help as the experience she had had breaking her back in a lacrosse game "with some boys" the week before her graduation from college. Ms. A was forced by her injury to move back home. She became upset when she experienced how her parents neglected her. Instead of caring for her, her mother asked her to babysit for her niece. Ms. A developed bulimia during this time.

Ms. A described her mother as an insecure, controlling woman determined for her daughters to succeed socially, but totally unable to function as a mother of three. Ms. A described her home as dirty and messy, full of unwashed children with unplanned lives, who were served meals at odd times. The prevailing mood of the house was one of tension and depression. Ms. A's mother complained constantly that her children made life impossible with their incessant demands. She punished them by locking the refrigerator and the linen closet. She also set a timer during meals and threatened to serve uneaten food for breakfast. Her mother would become enraged if the children ate food without telling her; she often went through the garbage to find out what they had been eating.

Ms. A described her handsome, athletic physician father as laconic, with a tendency to withdraw from problems. She loved her father intensely and saw him as strong and self-sufficient. Ms. A enjoyed going to sporting events with him. She was the "good girl" in her family, seeking always to mediate between her enraged mother and her rebellious, runaway sisters. Ms. A had spent her childhood striving for moral excellence, good grades, and perfection in competitive sports.

Psychodynamic Formulation

Part 1: Summarizing statement. Ms. A is a 24-year-old single, unemployed woman who presented with chief complaints of bulimia, confusion about career goals, and social isolation with paranoid thinking. Although eager to marry a handsome, wealthy, athletic man with a background as similar to her own as possible, she had had only distant, nonsexual relationships with men. The precipitating event for her seeking treatment was a back injury that required Ms. A to depend on her dysfunctional mother, for whom food was a battleground, and her withdrawn father. Prior to this injury, Ms. A had been relatively successful in achieving an ideal of self-sufficiency, good behavior, strength, and success in school and athletics.

Part 2: Nondynamic factors. Ms. A's paternal family had a history of alcoholism. There was affective disorder on her mother's side of the family: her maternal uncle had committed suicide. One of her sisters had a problem with drug abuse. This family history of affective illness and substance abuse may be related genetically to Ms. A's bulimia. It may also contribute to her history of deprivation and neglect.

Part 3: Psychodynamic exploration of central conflicts, object relations, and defenses. At the moment when she came for treatment, Ms. A had given up all serious pursuit of romantic or professional ambitions and was immersed in conflicts over basic dependency needs, separation, and autonomous functioning. When her back injury led her to be thrown into a state of dependence on her dysfunctional mother, it awakened frustrated, hungry rage from a lifetime of deprivation. Ms. A's lifelong strategy had been to renounce need and anger in favor of self-control, goodness, and self-sufficiency, and in the past, she had felt good only when feeling strong. Her broken back threatened this strategy when, thrown back on her mother's care, basic dependency longings were aroused and again frustrated. Ms. A clearly resented being placed in a caregiver role as babysitter and, later, as hospital worker. It was during this time that she became bulimic. She experienced outbursts of greedy hunger, which led to despair at feeling out of control, weak, and full of hated food. Ms. A quickly learned that she could regain control by vomiting and ridding herself of the unwanted food, which clearly represented a bad maternal object tainted with the poison of her angry frustration. Ms. A's unemployment allowed partial gratification of her dependency needs in terms of financial support. Her difficulty in separating from her parents represented both a continued effort to gratify frustrated longings and a need to cling to an object tie (with her parents) that was jeopardized by her destructive rage.

Ms. A's paranoid ideation resulted from the projection of her greedy, devouring hunger onto other people and situations that she feared would "swallow her up" and reject her after stealing her best ideas and leaving her depleted. The image of others who spy on her and watch what she eats was probably related both to aspects of her actual mother and to a projected critical superego.

On entering treatment, Ms. A's oedipal strivings seemed to be on hold. No doubt she experienced her broken back as the punishment for her attempted separation, for having already achieved more than the other women in her family, and for having had a fun, sexy time with her peers. Her back injury probably symbolized a warning of the dangers she could expect if she continued to pursue achievement and sexuality. Currently, Ms. A views men vaguely and from a safe distance; she seeks someone as close as possible to her own ideal self and to her ideal picture of her father, a choice that serves to repair a damaged, weak, and vulnerable self.

Part 4: Prediction of how the patient's dynamics will affect the therapy. In the treatment setting, it is likely that Ms. A will reproduce her friendly but distant attitude toward others in her relationship with the therapist. The therapist will feel friendly toward Ms. A but frustrated at how hard it is to know more about her inner life. Secret-keeping will likely be an issue, as Ms. A can be expected to hide some of her less "bland" thoughts from the therapist, whom she will expect to watch her with a critical eye. The patient's anger over frustrated dependency needs and failures on the part of the therapist to make her perfect will probably result not in the overt expression of anger but rather in increased withdrawal and superficiality. Frustrated dependency needs and separations will likely lead to increased bulimia. Any improvements in Ms. A's life will lead to fears of the therapist's hungry envy and fears of further bodily harm.

Discussion of Case Example

In this example of psychodynamic formulation, the therapist was able to find a connection between apparently unrelated presenting complaints by listening closely to Ms. A's use of language in describing her troubles. The use of metaphors related to eating was pronounced. By noting them, the therapist was able to arrive at a formulation connecting Ms. A's bulimia, her fears of intimacy, and her fear of taking a job to conflicts about her underlying hunger and the projection of that hunger.

Whether the experience of hunger resulted from frustrated dependency needs, from the activation of a feeling of starvation as part of a genetic, biological disorder in the form of bulimia, or from both of these dynamics would be difficult to say. Nevertheless, psychodynamically it was possible to link many of Ms. A's concerns to symbolic transformations of the idea of hunger and to fears about this hunger.

As discussed above, a psychodynamic formulation must account for the fact that important ideas, feelings, fantasies, and symptoms represent compromise formations between many conflicting motives. For example, Ms. A's bulimia represented a partial gratification both of her overwhelming hunger and need and of her need to control that hunger by purging and vomiting. The guilt and despair she felt over this behavior stemmed from her own inner disapproval of her wishes to eat and her dependency needs. The social isolation that accompanied her bulimia served to protect others from her neediness, which she feared would destroy them, provoke their retaliation, or, at the least, lead to their disapproval and rejection.

In a similar vein, the image of the roommate who spies and steals secrets was created as a compromise between a wish (id) component (i.e., the patient's own hungry desire to eat and steal) and a moral or conscience (superego) component (i.e., the hovering eye that criticizes). A complete formulation of the image of the spying roommate would include the "ego" component, which, in this case, would be the defense mechanism of projection that serves to help Ms. A avoid the painful awareness of her own greedy wishes to steal from and to devour others, as well as the awareness of her own inner disapproval of these same wishes.

Formulations such as these of Ms. A's bulimia and suspiciousness—of symptoms and fantasies in terms of compromises between conflicting motives—demonstrate how the psychodynamic formulation makes use of ego psychology. However, in addition to descriptions of conflicting motives, the psychodynamic formulation presented here also contains many references to self-images and to images of others; such images are the main focus of the object relations model. An example, of course, is the image of the spying roommate discussed above. In preparing the formulation, the therapist listened carefully to Ms. A's descriptions of her parents, her siblings, her friends, and others of importance, as well as to her descriptions of herself. Important similarities should be noted. For example, in Ms. A's description of the roommate she fears or the boyfriend she longs for, it is possible to detect similarities to her descriptions of her mother and her father, respectively. In the same way, in Ms. A's description of her "ideal self" as having perfect self-control and self-sufficiency, the therapist could detect elements of the patient's descriptions of her "ideal" father. From the point of view of a self psychologist, Ms. A's image of ideal self-sufficiency would be seen as an attempt to compensate for a damaged and vulnerable sense of self resulting from the failures of her dysfunctional parents to provide sufficient "empathic mirroring" necessary for the creation of a strong sense of self. From this point of view, the patient's search for an "ideal" husband could also be seen as an attempt to make up for her profound sense of insecurity and weakness.

Discussion

Although theoretical influences are not always explicitly spelled out, it is clear that the psychodynamic formulation will depend on some working knowledge of various theories of mental functioning. The dominant theories we have alluded to include those of ego psychology, object relations theory, self psychology, and interpersonal dynamics. As mentioned above, in any psychodynamic formulation, the influences of clinical theory are likely to be many. Which theories appear most useful in any given case formulation will depend on the orientation of the therapist and the prominent concerns of the patient involved. The psychodynamic formulation will result from an interaction between clinical data and available theoretical models. Increased clinical experience will enable the therapist to "hear" the data in more complex ways and to make more complex formulations, leading to formulations of greater depth and sophistication. Similarly, increased knowledge of clinical theory will increase the range of possible formulations that can be made.

The relevant literature clearly suggests that it is beneficial to patient care to construct a formal psychodynamic formulation (Friedman and Lister 1987; MacKinnon and Yudofsky 1991; Perry et al. 1987). More accurate psychodynamic understanding leads to better clinical practice. By clarifying central issues and conflicts, the formulation provides a blueprint or guide to the patient's inner world that allows the clinician to distinguish, from the great mass of clinical information, those elements of the history and current functioning that are likely to be essential from those that are secondary. With such a blueprint, the clinician is better equipped to choose the best treatment modality for a given patient and, within that treatment, to choose the proper timing and form of interventions. The blueprint not only helps the clinician to feel that he or she understands the patient, but also provides the warning signals for when he or she misunderstands the patient and a change of plan is needed. When our treatment predictions are wrong, we must go back to the drawing board and seek a different way to understand the patient. Empathy and enhanced understanding stabilize the therapist and the therapy, "discouraging a change in tack with each slight shift in the wind" (Perry et al. 1987, p. 543).

Contrary to common misconceptions, the psychodynamic formulation is not solely for patients in long-term expressive psychotherapy. The success of any kind of therapy involves supporting, modifying, or managing some aspect of the patient's personality. For example, to maximize compliance with psychopharmacological interventions in a paranoid patient, it is useful to be able to formulate the unconscious motives of that patient's fears and conflicts about ingesting a foreign substance. In the case of Ms. A, the formulation will be helpful in understanding her responses to any type of treatment, whether it be psychotherapy that seeks to explore her inner fantasies and fears or cognitive behavioral therapy and medication for controlling her bulimia. Even if nondynamic factors have played a major role in causing psychiatric symptoms, the therapist attending to the patient's psychodynamics will be better equipped to choose and implement specific treatment interventions. For example, a "pseudohumanitarian approach"—a verbal kindly handholding—that does not consider the character style of the patient may be experienced by paranoid patients as intrusive, by histrionic patients as seductive, by obsessive patients as demeaning, by depressed patients as undeserved and guilt inducing, and by phobic patients as sanctioning further avoidance, even if the underlying disorder is being treated with medication (Perry et al. 1987). Understanding the range of possible responses to nonspecific interventions can be important in the conduct of every therapy, regardless of its primary orientation.

It is also important to emphasize that the construction of the psychodynamic formulation is not just a training exercise for beginning therapists. All therapists, from the novice to the most seasoned, can benefit from having a psychodynamic blueprint, preferably in written form. By writing a formulation, therapists ask questions about the patient that may not have occurred to them before. No matter how experienced a therapist is, "the written psychodynamic formulation helps [the therapist] . . . to recognize its incompleteness, to inquire about pieces of the puzzle that are missing, [and] to appreciate that not every piece fits neatly into place" (Perry et al. 1987, p. 544). The formulation also serves as a reminder that a patient's behaviors in treatment are manifestations of his or her underlying psychodynamics, and that those behaviors represent the best possible compromise the patient feels he or she can make under current circumstances. Such a reminder helps the therapist remain tolerant of the patient's psychopathology.

Finally, the written psychodynamic formulation is an important potential research tool. It can provide a uniform and clear way for clinicians and researchers to speak to each other about patients, to compare patients, and to study treatment outcomes.

Conclusion

The psychodynamic formulation represents an effort to account for the patient's difficulties and to predict how he or she will behave in treatment based on an understanding of the patient's history and intrapsychic life, including his or her unconscious conflicts and compromises. Therapists construct a formulation by applying their knowledge of psychopathology and their theories of psychodynamics to what they hear, see, and feel with the patient. The interaction of theory with the therapist's direct experience with the patient is an essential component of the psychodynamic formulation. Because the formulation predicts behaviors and interactions in the treatment, it also alerts therapists to omissions and errors in their understanding of the patient, and thus provides cues for changing the formulation when new and unforeseen data arise. A psychodynamic formulation, by providing at least a preliminary understanding of the patient, enables the therapist to stabilize the treatment and to maintain clearer therapeutic aims. A formulation can be helpful in the conduct of a broad array of psychiatric therapies.

References

American Psychiatric Association: Diagnostic and Statistical Manual of Mental Disorders, 3rd Edition, Revised. Washington, DC, American Psychiatric Association, 1987

American Psychiatric Association: Diagnostic and Statistical Manual of Mental Disorders, 4th Edition. Washington, DC, American Psychiatric Association, 1994

Friedman RS, Lister P: The current state of psychodynamic formulation. Psychiatry 50:126–141, 1987

MacKinnon R, Yudofsky SC: Principles of the Psychiatric Evaluation. Philadelphia, PA, JB Lippincott, 1991

Perry SW, Cooper A, Michels R: The psychodynamic formulation: its purpose, structure and clinical applications. Am J Psychiatry 144:543–550, 1987

Chapter 3

The Self as a Clinical Instrument

Malkah T. Notman, M.D.

The "self" is an ambiguous concept with many meanings and uses. One of these uses is to contrast the "self" with the "object world." Kohut (1977) said that the self amounts to one-half of the contents of the human mind; the outside world is the other half. Technically, the self is an abstraction; it is considered a structure within the mind. However, in this chapter the term is used in the more informal sense of a person using his or her own personal powers, skills, and self-awareness in the therapeutic process, with an emphasis on the individual rather than on the techniques of therapy or a specific body of knowledge.

Scharff (1992) describes the therapist's self as consisting of "what I have to offer. I am both myself and the person the patients need me to be" (p. 133). She states that in her interaction with her patients, they "recreate the early experience that has shaped their psychic structures." The therapist's self is the therapeutic instrument. How that instrument is used depends both on the patient and on the therapist's understanding of the patient. Scharff also describes the self-understanding that can come from learning the patient's fantasy about her, and also from the discrepancy between her own concept of herself and the patient's perception of her. The transference consists of the patient's repetition in the therapeutic relationship of early object relationships; it also includes attempts to get the therapist to respond in ways that come from these earlier, internalized relationships.

Jacobs (1991) talks about the therapist's skills and "instrument" as including the therapist's perceptions of the patient's nonverbal behavior, such as body language. This instrument, in turn, "makes contact via associative pathways with visual aspects of memory and stimulates the recall of memories that are linked with the patient's nonverbal communications"; thus, this linkage of the therapist's visual and auditory perceptions of the patient with the therapist's memories of his or her own experience influences the total skills the therapist brings to bear in the treatment. The skill of the therapist also includes a way to draw on the therapist's unconscious reactions. In a similar way, the nonverbal messages communicated by the therapist play a significant role in the total communication that affects the therapy.

With the expansion of biological psychiatry and the shift in orientation from the "mind" to the "brain," there has been concern as to whether we are in danger of losing those aspects of psychiatry we think of as constituting the "mind." One attribute of the mind is the subtle and important interplay between the patient and the psychiatrist—the psychiatrist's reactions to the patient, as well as the patient's to the psychiatrist. In many residency training programs, there has been a sharp decrease in psychotherapy training, with more time being spent on other aspects of the curriculum. Some of these other approaches are quicker, less labor intensive, and perhaps more immediate in achieving symptomatic improvement. As a by-product of these changes and of an orientation to "managing" the patient, there is a tendency to minimize or to leave out altogether a focus on the more complex interactions between the psychiatrist and the patient, even though an understanding of such interactions is actually very useful in all patient-doctor relationships, whether in a formal psychotherapy session, a pharmacotherapy meeting, a therapy group, or any other setting in which patients are seen. Knowledge about oneself and about the underlying dynamic processes in both patient and psychiatrist can be an enormously effective resource. This capacity to look at oneself and to "tune in" to one's own reactions as a sensitive indicator of what is taking place between oneself and another person is important in all aspects of psychiatry. Such an active attunement represents one way that the "self" can be thought of as a clinical instrument.

The following examples illustrate the importance of the therapist's attunement to feelings.

> Dr. B was evaluating a new patient for psychotherapy. The patient, a man about her own age, in his mid-30s, had been referred to her by a well-known psychiatrist, one of Dr. B's former supervisors. Her supervisor did not know the patient directly but had given Dr. B's name to a colleague as someone who was a good therapist and who could see the patient for a low fee, since she was just starting out. Dr. B was flattered by the referral and approached the patient with anticipation as well as some anxiety as to whether she would live up to this recommendation.
>
> The patient began the interview by asking Dr. B about herself—her background, training, and present position. Even though she was uncomfortable at his taking over the interview, Dr. B at first answered these questions since they seemed legitimate and the patient had taken her by surprise. The patient then asked about Dr. B's family—whether she was married and had children. Dr. B became more uncomfortable and decided not to answer these questions, since it seemed they were more personal and she did not think answering them would constitute appropriate

technique. She also became aware of becoming even more anxious, but was not clear about why. Later in the interview, when Dr. B took a family history, the patient commented that she was sitting with one leg crossed under her. He said this reminded him of his mother, who would sit that way in her nightgown. Sometimes he would glimpse her genitals.

Later, as Dr. B thought about the interview, she realized how acutely anxious this information had made her. She asked herself what it meant, and she felt the aggressive, sexualized threat of the patient's behavior. Focusing on her own reaction made it clear to Dr. B what the patient was bringing into the interview. Dr. B's sense of violation and the pressure that she felt from the patient offered an important clue to his intrusiveness and to the aggression that he felt immediately in the transference. She also was aware of the erotic component and could sense this patient's potential problem with boundaries. Because she recognized that this dynamic would be prominent and would be repeated in the therapy, Dr. B had to decide whether she thought she could deal with it effectively.

If Dr. B. had been less attuned to her own responses and less inclined to take these seriously, she could simply have responded to her general discomfort by avoiding the patient, or by taking him into therapy without full awareness of the problems that might be encountered, and would thus be unprepared. Dr. B might have become anxious and defensive and allowed herself to be drawn into an interaction from which it would be difficult to extricate herself. Maybe she would have wanted to prove to the patient that she was not like his mother. Another therapist in this situation might have been motivated to override or deny his or her discomfort and start the therapy without recognizing its potential difficulties. Dr. B's attention to her own reactions as a meaningful piece of information, telling her something about the patient as well as herself, can be viewed as analogous to how one might monitor the movement of a needle on a dial. Such a posture requires the capacity to observe and understand oneself and the ability to take a position of awareness of one's own reactions, sensitivities, and also psychological blind spots, without needing to be defensive about them.

Sonnenberg (1991) points out that the psychoanalytically trained therapist's most unique skill is the ability to think analytically about oneself and others. Thinking about the self also involves thinking about the nature of one's own resistance—that is, one's own defenses that serve to keep uncomfortable or painful material out of awareness. This means that therapists need to recognize the barriers they construct, which can take the form of reluctance to remember, or "stay with," the patient or the patient's story.

Another young psychiatrist, Dr. C, was seeing an elderly woman patient. Over the course of the treatment, Dr. C became aware that she was shortening her interviews with this patient without realizing it. She had cut one of the interviews by 5 minutes and another by 10 minutes. Once, she had confused an appointment time and missed seeing the patient altogether. Sometimes she found her mind wandering while the patient was talking. Dr. C was not aware of having any particular feelings about this patient and was puzzled as to why she was behaving in this uncharacteristic way. She was usually careful and meticulous, concerned with being accurate and punctual, and maintained an even demeanor toward patients.

Dr. C was in therapy herself, and as she described these incidents to her therapist, she began to recognize how impatient and irritated she felt with this patient, who was a woman about her mother's age. As Dr. C talked further about it, she recognized that in her complaining, depressed, and agitated way, the patient evoked Dr. C's relationship with her own mother, a depressed, withholding woman who had refused to come to visit Dr. C because of her phobias. Dr. C had not consciously felt angry at her mother before. To herself she had explained her mother's behavior as caused by illness, and therefore had expected herself to be tolerant and understanding. By becoming aware that the feelings this patient stimulated in her were similar to those evoked by her mother, Dr. C could then recognize her resentment at the patient, which she had expressed by abbreviating the patient's time, and also come to acknowledge her underlying feelings about her mother.

Both of these examples are of interactions in which the therapist becomes aware of an uncomfortable feeling and then uses this awareness in a way that is eventually enlightening. In the first case, this awareness was useful in clarifying what the patient was doing, and in the second, in bringing to light the therapist's previously unrecognized feelings. Such a response calls upon self-observation and self-knowledge as well as the skills that derive from these processes. The therapist must also be willing to not run away from what she sees (it can be very tempting to reject an unwelcome insight). The therapist's responses can then be treated as a source of information about what is happening: what the patient is doing and what the therapist is doing. Although the therapist relies mostly on conscious knowledge, unconscious processes are at work as well, and can sometimes be recognized by their effects. The resentment Dr. C felt toward her mother was unconscious until the patient mobilized it, and as a result of this interaction, Dr. C came to understand her own feelings more deeply.

Another aspect of the therapeutic use of the self involves the capacity to relate to patients in an empathic way. The role of empathy in psychotherapy has been a focus of interest in recent years (Buie 1981; Margulies 1989; Winnicott 1965). Empathy can be thought of as the capacity to feel with patients—to put oneself in their situation—without losing one's own sense of who one is and where the boundaries lie. An empathic relationship can be a major tool in psychotherapy—a way for patient and therapist to connect through the therapist's achieving an emotional grasp of the patient's experience. It provides the validation of the patient's experience that comes from both people acknowledging it. Because empathy is a means of understanding another person's feelings through resonance with one's own feelings, it depends on the capacity to use one's personal experience to appreciate someone else's feelings and perceptions. This does not mean simply being sympathetic, or offering support, or making a patient feel good; rather, an empathic relationship involves achieving understanding through one's own connection with the other person's experience.

Obviously, there are also limits to these empathic connections. Sometimes what seems like an empathic understanding is not, but instead represents more of a projection—that is, one projects one's own reaction onto the other person and perceives it as if it were coming from him or her. Empathy is based to some extent on one's perception of the other person's response, which is then interpreted emotionally through one's own experience (Buie 1981). Perceptions may be inaccurate or misinterpreted. Someone who is very preoccupied with a crisis or with themselves is unlikely to have an easy time being empathic. Someone who is angry at another person, or feeling defensive toward or threatened by them, will also have difficulty. An orientation toward a patient that focuses on understanding the patient's perceptions and modes of experiencing leads to a different way of listening to and hearing the patient's story, and to a different way of organizing what one hears (Schwaber 1986). Such an orientation involves looking for links and connections that give some emotional coherence to the story and that fit with the patient rather than primarily looking for information to fill certain categories on a diagnostic checklist. By contrast, a descriptive approach to a patient places the therapist or evaluator in a position of listening for relevant symptoms or pathology in a particular diagnostic category, rather than of attempting to see how those pieces fit together for that person as an emotional and historical whole. The patient's selection of a material to talk about and the sequence in which he or she presents that material also offer clues to the meanings of events and responses. The way the therapist conceptualizes the emotional or historical coherence of the patient's story also depends on having some theoretical framework into which to fit the data.

Sometimes a beginning therapist, upon hearing a story from a patient that represents an obvious distortion, will be tempted to correct the story, to introduce reality, or even to get into an argument with the patient. For example, a therapist, upon hearing a patient's description of a classroom encounter that was perceived to be attacking, might be tempted to say, "Your teacher could not really have been intending to humiliate you." An empathic response to this patient's story might be to try to understand the patient's experience of feeling humiliated and to focus on that experience, rather than attempting to correct what is judged to be a misrepresentation of reality.

The life experiences of the therapist have a profound influence on the therapist's capacity for empathy with a particular patient. Two people who are very different may not be able to trust each other. Similarities or differences created by race, gender, class, and cultural background have been thought to have a decisive effect on the capacity of one person to understand and be empathic with another. Of course, no two people's experiences are exactly the same. Differences of style, values, and ways of thinking and explaining the world certainly influence the way one person thinks about another and what sense that person can make out of someone else's feelings. Individual differences also play an important role. Even physical differences affect one's body image and determine one's view of the world. A small person can feel vulnerable and out of place among larger ones. A large person can feel awkward and ungainly, particularly if those around him or her are small. It is certainly harder to appreciate the sensitivities created by growing up as part of a minority group if one comes from a privileged and dominant social group. The culture in which one grows up shapes the kinds of perceptions and emotional responses that one has. However, there are important commonalities among people in both life experiences and emotions. It is not so difficult to recognize fear, pride, shame, or agitation, and the attempt to put oneself in someone else's shoes and to understand them is valuable in itself.

The pregnant therapist provides a unique situation of the intrusion of the therapist's self as a reality into the therapy. This situation has received increasing attention as more women have entered psychiatry. Unlike an illness, which can be intrusive but is more often silent, a pregnancy cannot be hidden. The patient is confronted with the reality of the sexual life of the therapist and with the potential for displacement by the baby. For many patients, this situation evokes sibling rivalry and feelings of abandonment. The therapist has the complex task of sustaining her therapeutic investment and role, dealing with her own feelings and stresses, and negotiating commitments with colleagues, particularly if she is a resident or has a job involving covering for others and being on call. It can also be a productive period for the treatment. Many therapists can feel guilty about what seems to be disloyalty to the patient and opting out of responsibilities. Therapists' own conflicts about siblings, parenting, and work can become intense at times. In the face of patients' reactions and sometimes of hostility from staff as well, it is possible to lose sight of the fact that pregnancy is a normal life stage and confrontation of this reality might result in potential gains for the patient.

The therapist's capacity for empathy comes into particular prominence in explorative, uncovering, and expressive psychotherapy. It is helpful to have the freedom to let one's own associations roam, stimulated by the patient's associations, and even to follow thoughts that might create some anxiety, suspending a certain amount of judgment and criticism. Any major problems the therapist has can interfere with this process by causing defensive reactions that make it difficult to sustain empathic involvement.

A therapist's personality and ordinary defensive style also affect the possibility of making an empathic connection with a patient. A therapist can appear threatening to a patient because he or she reminds the patient of a frightening person from the past, or stirs up stereotypes; a patient can evoke similar reactions in a therapist. An example of this phenomenon was the patient who reminded the therapist of her depressed mother, and thus stirred up the therapist's unrecognized anger at her mother, which was then displaced onto the patient, whose hours she shortened. A therapist struggling with a personal problem may have difficulty hearing about a related issue from a patient; for example, a therapist who blocks out thoughts about his or her own homosexual feelings is likely to find it disturbing to hear about the love affairs of a gay patient. Such a therapist would probably be even more disturbed by a homosexual erotic transference. An ambitious, achieving, anxious therapist might dismiss, ignore, or devalue the concerns of a nonintellectual, less ambitious patient, or might be made anxious by a student with whom he or she identifies who threatens to drop out of school. A woman who is concerned with her body image and with keeping thin may find it difficult to remain uninvolved in a fat girl's struggles with her mother around dieting. A therapist's need to maintain control and tendency to become involved in struggles with patients around this issue is another vulnerability that can undermine therapy.

Sometimes the wish to be effective and helpful and thus powerful can merge with wishes and fantasies of being able to perform near-miraculous deeds and rescue or transform a patient. Rescue fantasies can lead a therapist to undertake heroic treatments that become overwhelming or get out of control. Working with difficult patients is challenging and can be frustrating. It can feel defeating. It may seem that by offering more and more or intervening in extraordinary ways, it might be possible to accomplish extraordinary things. Some therapists are persuaded to go beyond appropriate boundaries and do extra things—accepting gifts, giving gifts, extending hours, or meeting the patient in places other than the usual office. If a patient does not respond, the therapist can feel guilty for not doing enough and believe it is necessary to do yet "more." Sometimes these feelings are intensified because they draw on unresolved wishes from the therapist's past—that is, the countertransference can evoke a relationship with a parent one tried to cure, or please, or appease. Therapists need to derive some sense of effectiveness from working with patients, and frustrations can be difficult to tolerate, particularly since the complexity of psychotherapeutic work means that progress is not likely to be even. Knowing one's own feelings and sensitive areas becomes especially important with a difficult and taxing patient. The therapist's own personal psychotherapy is an invaluable resource for achieving such self-knowledge.

Another dimension of the use of the self has to do with the importance of the therapeutic relationship itself in furthering the therapeutic work. This relationship forms the context in which the work takes place, but it is also a "real" relationship with its own vicissitudes. It has been recognized that therapy is a "two-person relationship" in which the therapist is an equal participant, not merely a screen on which the patient projects transferential responses. The therapeutic relationship can rightly be thought of as providing a "holding environment"—a supportive framework, a space where the patient can feel safe, can be assured that he or she will not be subjected to impulsive, irrational behavior, and can feel confident that no retaliations will meet his or her communications. This does not mean that the therapeutic relationship offers primarily warmth and affection or support. Limits are set, boundaries protected, and the recognition and expression of aggression and other "negative" affects are part of the work. Patients sometimes become angry at these boundaries and limits; however, they need to have confidence that the therapist can tolerate their expressions of anger and stress. Although communication in words is a central part of most therapy, the relationship itself is also an important component.

A common therapeutic mistake is to regard the therapeutic relationship as if its function were to provide the "good parent" that the patient lacked in childhood. This perspective is based on the idea that the therapeutic relationship is primarily restorative—that is, that its purpose is to make up for past deficits and to supply the ingredients that were missing from the patient's early experience. According to this view, if a patient had inadequate mothering, the therapist provides a new "good mother." If the patient's early life was chaotic, unpredictable, and disorganized, he or she can "re-do" that early life in the therapy. Although predictability is, in itself, an important aspect of the therapy, and the therapist should indeed aim to provide a consistent and predictable experience, this is not enough by itself. The therapeutic relationship can only provide a field in which the internalized residues of past experience and their developmental effects on the patient's character and defenses can be seen and understood. These dynamics are repeated in the transference and can, therefore, be made accessible to consciousness and reworking. Work is still required to accomplish inner changes. The model of the therapist as someone who seeks only to remain "objective" and to offer interpretations and formulations of the patient's problems is a model of an active therapist and a passive patient. In reality, the therapeutic relationship is interactive; the therapist's job is to focus on the relationship and the transference, but also to be aware of his or her own feelings and role in the interactions.

Many therapists describe their changed relationship to patients after they have gone through a major new experience, such as having a baby. Becoming a parent can shift the therapist's perspective profoundly. Before having a child, the therapist may be very identified with child patients and may tend to see the parents as pathogenic. Parents might appear unfeeling, punitive, or repressive. After becoming a parent, however, the therapist can identify more readily with a parent who is confused, angered, or frustrated by a child who is difficult—or merely stressed, such as a toddler who is pushing the limits. The therapist's understanding of the dynamics of the parent-child relationship is deepened and his or her capacity to empathize with the parent and the parent's dilemmas is usually enhanced. One therapist who had undergone a period of infertility said that this experience had provided her with a bridge to being an adult, by which she meant that it compelled her to deal with the limitations, frustrations, and uncontrollability of much of life—aspects that she, as a successful young woman, had not previously encountered.

It is obvious that therapists need to know about their own blind spots and vulnerabilities—what kind of patients make for boredom, depression, or anxiety; what kind of therapy hours are exhausting and frustrating, or exciting and gratifying; and what kinds of scenarios are related to one's own wishes, conflicts, and history. Therapists need to feel effective and, to some extent, to be liked and to be seen as kind and generous. It is difficult to reconcile a patient's recurrent anger and perception of the therapist as a withholding, frustrating, or inadequate parent with one's own wishes and intentions to be good, helpful, and gratifying. The capacity to assess what is appropriate and to tolerate anxiety, restlessness, and feelings about one's limitations can be achieved only with self-knowledge. To be truly helpful is not compatible with always being liked.

Maintaining objectivity does not mean being uninvolved. It is also important to develop the capacity to see the impact of one's presence and intervention—both positively and negatively. It is not really possible to be just an observer; such a stance ignores the countertransference as well as the transference. Having feelings toward the patient—being interested, sometimes drawn in, sometimes angry, and sometimes attracted (or repelled)—is inevitable. All therapists find that they react to patients. What is important, however, is not to act on these feelings. If they become intrusive, then a consultation is indicated.

The unresponsive therapist of a decade or more ago who had a way of deflecting every question, showed no expression, and maintained a wooden, uncommunicative demeanor was a caricature of therapeutic objectivity. This neutral posture was originally recommended with the goal of not being intrusive, of allowing the patient to focus on his or her issues, and of trying to be "objective." The therapist actually may not be unresponsive or remote or literally not responding. The patient can feel frustrated that the therapist is not giving more. There is an inevitable amount of frustration. Nevertheless, it is not necessary to answer a patient's questions, gratify wishes, or step over boundaries to communicate warmth and the wish to understand or to create an atmosphere of tolerance and interest. The term *countertransference* was originally used in the narrow sense of the therapist's unconscious feelings toward the patient, with the implication that these were neurotic feelings and indications of conflict. The term is now used more broadly to mean all of the therapist's feelings toward the patient.

The supervisory relationship parallels the therapeutic relationship in some ways. The supervisor attempts to understand the patient and the dynamics of the patient's problem as well as to assess the supervisee's therapeutic interventions, technical and otherwise. The supervisor's role also involves forming a relationship with the supervisee-therapist and being available to respond to the subtle dynamics of the relationship between the patient and the therapist that are often repeated with the supervisor. How much the supervisor should intervene in what may be personal issues for the therapist has been a matter of debate. However, when the therapist's own blind spots or dilemmas interfere with or distort aspects of his or her relationship with the patient, it is important for the supervisor to be able to address these issues. The supervisor can help the therapist sort out various responses both to the patient and to the supervisor.

The "self" is thus a valuable and complicated "instrument." It demands involvement and at the same time distance, attention, and awareness—but not intrusiveness. Developing and training this instrument is a challenging and rewarding task.

For Further Study

Jacobs TJ: The Use of the Self. Madison, CT, International Universities Press, 1991

Margulies A: The Empathic Imagination. New York, WW Norton, 1989

Modell AH: Psychoanalysis in a New Context. New York, International Universities Press, 1984

Scharff JS: Projective and Introjective Identification and the Use of the Therapist's Self. Northvale, NJ, Jason Aronson, 1992

Sonnenberg S: The analyst's self analysis and its impact on clinical work: a comment on the sources and importance of personal insights. J Am Psychoanal Assoc 39:687–704, 1991

References

Buie D: Empathy: its nature and limitations. J Am Psychoanal Assoc 29:281–307, 1981

Jacobs TJ: The Use of the Self. Madison, CT, International Universities Press, 1991

Kohut H: The Restoration of the Self. New York, International Universities Press, 1977

Margulies A: The Empathic Imagination. New York, WW Norton, 1989

Scharff JS: Projective and Introjective Identification and the Use of the Therapist's Self. Northvale, NJ, Jason Aronson, 1992

Schwaber E: Reconstruction and perceptual experience: further thoughts on psychoanalytic listening. J Am Psychoanal Assoc 34:911–932, 1986

Sonnenberg S: The analyst's self analysis and its impact on clinical work: a comment on the sources and importance of personal insights. J Am Psychoanal Assoc 39:687–704, 1991

Winnicott DW: The Maturational Processes and the Facilitating Environment. New York, International Universities Press, 1965

Section II

Clinical Settings

Sidney H. Weissman, M.D.,
Section Editor

Chapter 4

The Inpatient Unit

Edward A. Wolpert, M.D., Ph.D.

The Changing Demands of Society

Treatment of patients in psychiatric inpatient facilities has not demonstrated a progressive evolution toward improved care. Throughout history the goals of psychiatric inpatient care have been balanced between the demands of society and the needs of the individual. In the Middle Ages, such facilities were lifelong repositories for those deemed "possessed," and active individual treatment was not possible (Henry 1941). With the enlightenment of the late 18th and early 19th century, this changed. Many mental hospitals in the United States in the 1820s–1840s had high staff-to-patient ratios, with staff at all levels devoted to "moral treatment." An effort was made to understand each patient in the context of his or her own social and life history. Staff members and patients participated as far as possible on an equal basis in the day-to-day activities of the hospital. However, under the impact of social changes in the 1870s–1890s—industrialization, urbanization, and immigration—American psychiatric hospitals degenerated into the huge, poorly staffed institutions of that era, whose purpose seemed to be to protect society from those damaged by the sociocultural changes occurring in the wake of the industrialization of a previously agrarian society (Bockoven 1963). Individual treatment for hospitalized patients was now provided only to a privileged few.

With the developing sophistication of psychological and social theory in the late 19th and early 20th centuries, individualized treatment of the psychiatric patient again became a possibility. Clinicians began to apply a positive set of expectations to inpatient treatment; however, the goals of treatment diverged to coincide with the unstated values of the therapist. Two experiments following World War II demonstrate how great this divergence could become. At Belmont Hospital in England, Maxwell Jones created the Industrial Neurosis Unit, whose purpose was to return English war casualties to productive work through intensive individual, group, and social treatment (Jones 1953). At the University of Chicago, on the other hand, Bruno Bettelheim created in the Sonia Shankman Orthogenic School a milieu whose purpose was to treat severely neurotic or psychotic dysfunctional children so that as adults, they could determine their own goals and lifestyles (Bettelheim 1950).

The consequences for patients, staff, and society of these two disparate goals of treatment were profound. In the Industrial Neurosis Unit, treatment was directed primarily toward the benefit of society, whereas at the Orthogenic School, treatment was directed primarily toward the benefit of the individual. In each case, the secondary goal of the one became the primary goal of the other. At the time that these units were established, few people believed that the good of society could be antithetical to the good of the individual. In today's economic climate, however, it is clear that such treatment goals may indeed be opposed, sometimes totally.

These units diverged in other ways as well. The Industrial Neurosis Unit was highly staffed with a variety of professionals: nurses, psychiatrists, rehabilitation officers, vocational counselors, and social workers. All staff efforts were concentrated on effecting attitudinal changes in the patient so that he or she could obtain and hold a productive job. At the Orthogenic School, the bulk of the work was carried out by schoolteachers and counselors (generally, untrained college students) under the close supervision of Bettelheim, a master clinician of charismatic impact. He focused on helping the staff understand not only the reactions of the children, but their own reactions to the children as well. This emphasis promoted the ego growth of the patient instead of forcing an attitudinal change.

With the advent of effective psychopharmacological treatment of the major psychoses (i.e., effective in controlling symptoms in many, but not in all, patients) and with the spiraling costs of inpatient medical care, attempts to limit lengths of stay in hospitals have increased markedly. Now many patients have insurance programs that mandate external checks on the physician, sometimes to an unacceptable degree. At times the physician is directly faced with a conflict between the individual needs of the patient and the demands of society as enunciated by the third-party payer, private or governmental. A further complication is the court-mandated admission, in which a physician must treat—against their will—patients who lack the objectivity to recognize their need for treatment. We have reached a stage in the development of psychiatric care in which society, as exemplified by insurance companies, governmental agencies, and business concerns, demands quick solutions to problems that have beleaguered physicians for more than 4,000 years (see Wolpert 1993). Naive planners seem to believe that the third great psychiatric revolution—psychopharmacology—has found the answer to mental illness, although it is clear that in many cases, the effects of medications may be worse than those of the disease being treated. (For a striking example of a relatively mild seasonal affective disorder converted by a tricyclic drug into a devastating rapid-cycling process, see Berman and Wolpert 1987.)

The Role of Psychodynamic Understanding in Treatment Planning

Despite third-party wishes to the contrary, it is still true that the inpatient unit is necessary for the treatment of those patients who are a risk to themselves and/or to others outside its confines. Planning appropriate treatment for each patient requires an accurate, unbiased assessment that relies not only on manifest symptoms but also on an understanding of the underlying psychodynamics.

Unconscious fantasies are determinants of behavior; their explanation can remove resistances to treatment. Understanding transference attitudes facilitates the discovery of these unconscious fantasies. It is critical to understand staff reactions to the patient. A dynamic understanding is necessary to make appropriate long-range treatment plans as well as to understand specific resistances. Each patient must be considered as a unique individual and treatment designed for him or her rather than for a given diagnostic or social entity.

An understanding the patient's unconscious psychological dynamics not only plays a critical role in formulating a treatment plan but also provides guidance at crisis points in the ongoing treatment. To illustrate this thesis, I present two case studies of patients with a primary diagnosis of depression (Wolpert 1980).

Case 1

In this case study, the understanding of unconscious psychological forces was critical in the formulation of the entire inpatient treatment plan.

> Mr. D was admitted for a depression unresponsive to tricyclics, monoamine oxidase inhibitors, and psychostimulants. As the depression continued without symptomatic relief, the patient's distress escalated, and his fear that he would jump to his death led Mr. D's outpatient psychotherapist to recommend hospitalization.
>
> Mr. D had been born to a family of great wealth in Austria, and at the time of the *Anschluss* had been a commander in the Austrian Home Guard. When the Nazi troops invaded, he had wanted to "go to the front" to "lead my men." His superiors convinced him that there was no army to lead, and he fled to America. During World War II, Mr. D became an officer in the Office of Strategic Services, often parachuting behind enemy lines and winning many medals for heroism. After the war, he settled down, married, and began to raise a family. Although successful in business, Mr. D always felt that he had failed in some way; however, he was unable to explain just how he had done this.
>
> On admission, Mr. D kept to himself, paced up and down, and obsessively talked of failing, but could not specify in what way he had failed. Interpretations that explained his "failure" as war related, business related, or family related were all brushed off by the patient as not making sense. However, it was noted that Mr. D seemed fearful of a tall, muscular nurse who appeared "Germanic." His treatment

team, frankly desperate because all available medications had been tried without success, formulated the "Germanic" nurse as a transference object representing his "good" Austrian mother on the one hand and a "bad" German mother on the other. Mr. D's "failure" that had resulted in his depression was hypothesized to be the result of unconscious shame in the face of the "good" mother at not having fought the Nazi "bad" mother in 1938. In Mr. D's mind, even his subsequent heroism could not make amends for his earlier failure "of nerve." Consequently, the team decided to treat Mr. D *as if* he had gone to fight the Nazis, failed, been captured, and sent to a concentration camp, on the assumption that under those conditions, these major unconscious issues could be brought dramatically to the fore and become accessible to resolution.

The treatment decided upon was to place Mr. D in a work therapy situation, in which he would be given the task of straightening up the dayroom to an exact order (other patients had other tasks, such as making coffee for the group, arranging the snacks, and so forth). After Mr. D had performed the appointed task, the nurse he seemed to fear would deliberately move one of the ash trays on the table, and he would be asked to reposition it in its place. In this way, an attenuated unpredictable, malignant concentration camp milieu could be suggested. This scenario was enacted daily for 2 weeks without any explanation of the nurse's behavior being asked for or given.

During this "work therapy" treatment, Mr. D reported to his therapist daily a series of dreams. In the first dream, he was vaguely aware of being in a darkened, enclosed place with dank and stale air, and of feeling terror stricken. The next night Mr. D dreamed the same dream, except that now he realized that others were with him. The dreaming continued, each night's dream elaborating on that of the previous night, gradually revealing him to be riding in a crowded railway car in a uniform with others, who turned out to be soldiers, all of them fearful of their destination. The next-to-the-last night in the series, the uniform was revealed to be that of the *Heimwehr.*

In the final dream in the series, the railway car came to a stop, the door opened, and Mr. D realized he was in a concentration camp. The next day his depression was gone, as was his fear of the "German" nurse. He was overjoyed and could finally accept the interpretation that he had harbored shame at not fighting the Germans in 1938. This interpretation, first offered intellectually by his outpatient therapist, had seemed so farfetched that Mr. D had not accepted it, especially since, in reality, his Army superiors had supported his "running away." When, on the other hand, the "Germanic" nurse behaved as if he were in a concentration camp, he was transported back to those dreadful days of 1938. The dream series revealed to Mr. D that he had really gone to the front to fight the Germans but had been captured and punished, and therefore, by implication, he no longer needed to feel shame. He could finally make peace with the historical reality; he now realized that the gesture he would have made if he had gone to the front would have been suicidal (one against thousands) and meaningless. Mr. D was discharged with no sign of depression, and a 10-year follow-up indicated no recurrence and no need for further treatment of any kind.

In this case, the hospital was redesigned by the treatment team for the individual patient to make a psychodynamic point about a past traumatic event that could be partially reexperienced in an attenuated form. In most cases, such a plan to enable a patient to reexperience a serious trauma would not be possible or feasible. The very structure of the hospital, however, allows not only for such a plan to be implemented when indicated, but also for a clearer understanding of unconscious forces than is ever possible in outpatient forms of treatment. The transference becomes clearer in a powerful way. In the directly observable relationship of the patient with staff members and co-patients, feelings from the past about major caregivers and styles of perception from earlier years may be revealed or surmised with a degree of power and immediacy unequaled in other settings. Indeed, the power of such reexperiencing is so great that it must be controlled to prevent the reemergence of affects that are too intense to be therapeutically useful—and that might even be quite dangerous.

Case 2

In the next case study, the reverse occurred: The hospital allowed the patient to come to terms with a depressive illness physiological in origin that he had felt was psychogenic.

> Mr. E, a middle-aged professional man, had been unhappy in his marriage, as had his wife. After several attempts at conflict resolution with professional assistance had failed, Mr. E and his wife obtained a divorce. Inexplicably, during the autumn 3 years after his divorce was finalized, Mr. E became depressed and entered four-times-weekly analysis. Three years into his analysis, he was referred for a consultation by his analyst, who had noted Mr. E's increasingly severe autumn–winter depressions followed by equally severe hypomanic rebounds each spring. No psychotic symptoms were noted at either extreme, and no external precipitants or internal dynamic shifts preceded the change in affective status.
>
> In August, at the time of the consultation, Mr. E was seen to have a mild, asymptomatic obsessive-compulsive character without significant current pathology and with no obvious dynamic reason to explain his progressively severe affective cyclicity. That the regular cyclicity seemed attached to the seasons rather than to any psychological event argued against a psychogenic etiology despite Mr. E's divorce and its attendant problems. A diagnosis of seasonal affective disorder was made and prophylactic use of lithium or lights recommended. The patient refused this treatment, continuing his analytic work. He could not accept the postulated physiological origin to his depression, being more comfortable with a psychogenic causation. That winter, Mr. E's depression deepened. In January, he attempted suicide by jumping into a river in –5°F weather. He was hospitalized and started on an antidepressant (imipramine 50 mg qid). When his depression remitted, the treatment team espoused the view that he had demonstrated a clear-cut history of seasonal affective disorder and would need lithium to protect him from a hypomanic rebound. Light therapy would be instituted in the autumn to prevent recurrences.

Mr. E spent the final weeks of his 3-month hospitalization receiving cognitive instruction about lithium prophylaxis, light therapy, and prodromal signs of impending affective shifts.

Mr. E agreed to the treatment plan and terminated his analysis 3 months after his discharge from the hospital. He began using lights the next autumn and also began taking 2-week vacations during late January–early February instead of in the summer. There have been no recurrences of affective instability, and Mr. E states at yearly follow-up that he feels as well as he ever did and functions better in his profession and with friends and family than before.

Of import in the present context, the first of these two cases of depressive illness demonstrates the critical need for a psychological approach, and the second an equally critical need for a physiological approach. Although the manifest symptomatology in the two patients was identical, Mr. D responded to a manipulation of the environment to allow a (much attenuated) reexperiencing of a past trauma and Mr. E to the institution of physiological treatment that apparently corrected an unknown internal imbalance. In the first case, the depression appeared to be precipitated by a real-life event with attendant shame; in the second, no significant internal or external precipitant could be found.

Despite these patients' differences, both responded to inpatient treatment, the one involving a recreation of the (corrected) past by the treatment team, and the other supportive and educative work by the team. Effective treatment requires effectively assessing the individual patient rather than arbitrarily placing him or her in a group that has similar symptoms. Patients with identical symptoms may be found to require quite different therapies.

Case 3

More often, unconscious forces may be observed that affect one particular aspect of the treatment. A very frequent occurrence in hospitalized patients is the phenomenon of "splitting." In its simplest form, the patient selects one or more staff members to represent the "good parent" and one or more staff members to be the "bad parent." In the extreme form of splitting, at least one staff member from each shift is assigned the "good" role, and at least one staff member from each shift is assigned the "bad" role. Through judicious use of interpretation, patients can be shown that they impose their own schematic view of the world on the staff, and that these mistaken displacements represent attitudes toward significant past parental images rather than accurate observations in the present.

Ms. F, a 30-year-old secretary, was admitted in transfer from a hospital whose administration had recommended transfer because of this patient's "splitting." Ms. F had originally been admitted for a medication overdose that had left her in a comatose condition for 3 days. Once out of danger, her eroticized behavior had maximally threatened the staff and made further treatment at that hospital impractical. When the consultant was first seen at the original hospital during the day shift, he was told by a female nurse that Ms. F refused to talk to staff members. A second consultation was held during the night shift and a male mental health worker on that shift reported that the patient was always verbal. The consultant considered that there must be significance in this discrepancy, but the source of the discrepancy was not apparent.

The initial history revealed Ms. F to be the oldest daughter of four children born to a poor farm worker who had married the daughter of a wealthy landowner. He had physically abused his wife and children, and Ms. F had escaped from the horror of her home by marrying a student she had met in college after her mother and father divorced. The breakup of her own unhappy marriage had precipitated a depressive illness, leading to a series of inconclusive hospitalizations with four successive psychiatrists and the unsuccessful use of all available groups of antidepressants.

Upon transfer, the team, viewing Ms. F's splitting propensity as her most significant resistance, adopted a plan to point it out to the patient whenever it occurred and to attempt to trace its origin. It became clear, through interpretation of the splitting process, that whereas Ms. F was seductive with men, she withheld her feelings from them; conversely, she was quite expressive of her feelings to women, whom she nevertheless depreciated. When this dynamic was brought to her attention, Ms. F responded by revealing—for the first time in more than 3 years of treatment attempts—a history of sexual abuse by her father from ages 12 through 20, which she had found exciting and highly gratifying; she also revealed that she regretted her loss of his attentions when he remarried.

In this case, the splitting could be seen to symbolically refer to the role Ms. F had historically played in the family with the parental dyad, and the explication of its derivative in the hospital prompted her revelation of further history, ultimately leading to a deeper, previously unknown, layer of her pathology. This interpretation of the splitting behavior by no means could in and of itself lead to a resolution of the depression, but it could and did lead to revelation of issues that had to be dealt with before resolution could be possible.

Case 4

The transferences of the patient as well as the countertransference feelings of the staff must be understood to facilitate the patient's recovery. Both block access to important feelings and prevent conflict resolution.

Ms. G, a 78-year-old widow with a history of recurrent depressive illness since age 18, had been successfully managed outside the hospital with supportive psychotherapy and prophylactic antidepressants from ages 56 to 75. Prior to age 56, she had had 17 hospitalizations for suicidal attempts, all of which had seemed serious, but from age 56 to 75 she had been depression free. Between age 75 and 78, Ms. G developed an intractable migrainous headache that was unsuccessfully treated by four neurologists and six internists and that was accompanied by a return of her disabling depression as she felt increasingly isolated with the death of friends and family members. During these 3 years, Ms. G was hospitalized eight times because of suicidal attempts or mild histrionics involving dangerous behavior, and spent no more than 90 consecutive days outside the hospital. The staff began to feel helpless.

When Ms. G was recovering from a depression, she would agree to a move from her own home to a retirement community, where she would have activity and stimulation; however, once the depression resolved, she would renege on her agreement, only to again become depressed. During the last hospitalization, the interpretation was made that Ms. G equated the retirement community with death—that is, with retirement from life; once this was recognized by the staff members, whose own countertransference had interfered with their coming to understand the source of the patient's exasperating behavior, they could address Ms. G's fear by demonstrating that such a community was full of activities and did not mean death. Then and only then was Ms. G able to agree to this interpretation and to carry out her move to the retirement community. Throughout this last phase, Ms. G's transference attitude gradually shifted from a negative to a more positive one, reflecting the change in the staff's attitude, which allowed the discharge plan to be actualized.

In this case, an understanding both of the patient's fears and of the staff's reaction to her fears was necessary to allow the patient to make a successful transition to assisted living.

Case 5

My final case example points both to the direct danger of managed care intruding on a treatment and to the possibility of using even such an event to make a psychodynamically important point to a patient, thereby facilitating recovery.

H was 14 years old when her inpatient therapist asked for a consultation. Although the patient was well insured, the managed care firm managing her case wanted electroconvulsive therapy (ECT) to be used because H had been resistant to adequate treatment agents of four groups of antidepressants (two known to be effective for obsessive-compulsive behavior); had failed to receive benefit from outpatient combined psychotherapy and pharmacotherapy, both at home and at a residential treatment center; and had had two previous hospitalizations (12 weeks for the first, 1 week for the second) without permanent improvement.

As might be expected, H's history was complex. Behavioral abnormalities—tics and rituals—dating from age 2 and 3, respectively, were present. Relations with peers had been disturbed from age 5, and anorexic symptoms had been present from age 10, immediately following her parents' divorce. H's relationship with both her mother and her father was disturbed; she could live with neither. The present admission was precipitated by the patient's loss of control at a residential treatment center.

Examination revealed H as a depressed, frightened girl, caught by ritualistic behavior. She was terrified of ECT. She knew her therapist opposed the procedure and that to avoid a direct consultation with the managed care company's psychiatrist, her therapist had asked two senior psychiatrists, one an expert psychopharmacologist and the other a psychoanalyst, to evaluate her. During the consultation, this writer told the patient clearly that although ECT could be lifesaving to anorexic patients with serious medical complications (abnormal electrocardiograms and abnormal electrolytes, as she had demonstrated on her past admission but not the current admission), since there were two psychopharmacological groups that had not yet been tried (trazodone and quartenary cyclic agents), this should be done before considering ECT. The patient was told that she must also work on her problems, no matter how hard this seemed. With this in mind, the patient arranged for a meeting (lasting 2 hours) of the two consultants; her therapist; the social worker, primary nurse, teacher, and activities therapist from the unit; and her divorced parents. What was most striking was that the patient's father, who lived 1,000 miles away, came for this consultation, although he usually did not participate in his daughter's treatment.

During the consultation, H led the group for most of the time, asking questions about ECT, its dangers, and its possible success. She involved her parents actively in the discussion and clarified everyone's opinions in her mind. Following the consultation, trazodone 50 mg tid was started; on the fourth day, H asked to stop her liquid diet and began to voraciously eat the regular ward diet. In 2 months, she gained 16 pounds and was discharged back to her residential treatment facility, where she continued to do well.

Although we cannot know the ultimate outcome of H's case, it is clear that the intrusion of the managed care company forced two consultations and ultimately led the patient to ally herself more closely with the therapist to prevent the ECT procedure. In the process, she temporarily was the center of a large group process that brought her parents together in their efforts to help her. Significantly, the first of the three wishes she told this author was "to have my parents together again." Once again, the inpatient unit was able to provide—in attenuated form—the dynamic the patient longed to attain.

Conclusion

Psychopharmacotherapeutic agents and psychotherapeutic approaches must be appropriate for the given patient; neither should be applied blindly to all patients fitting some externally postulated "group." It must be remembered that the statement "80% of depressive patients respond to X medication" is a group phenomenon. When faced with a new patient, we do not know whether that patient is in the 80% group that will respond or the 20% group that will not. Hence, the individual's chance of responding is only 50%, not the 80% true for the group. As always, each patient is unique and the treatment appropriate for one patient may fail for another. The psychiatrist must be alert to the patient's psychological (both conscious and unconscious), physiological, and social historic context. In addition, the demands of society may either limit or expand what options are available.

For Further Study

Gralnick A (ed): The Psychiatric Hospital as a Therapeutic Instrument. New York, Brunner/Mazel, 1969

Maxman JS, Tucker G, LeBow M: Rational Hospital Psychiatry. New York, Brunner/Mazel, 1974

Sederer LI: Inpatient Psychiatry: Diagnosis and Treatment. Baltimore, MD, Williams & Wilkins, 1983

Stanton AH, Schwartz MA: The Mental Hospital. New York, Basic Books, 1954

Strauss A: Psychiatric Ideologies and Institutions. Glencoe, IL, Free Press, 1964

Thompson JD, Golding G: The Hospital: A Social and Architectural History. New Haven, CT, Yale University Press, 1975

Ullmann LP: Institution and Outcome. New York, Pergamon, 1967

Zinberg N (ed): Psychiatry and Medical Practice in a General Hospital. New York, International Universities Press, 1964

References

Berman E, Wolpert EA: Single case study: intractable manic depressive psychosis with rapid cycling in an 18-year-old woman successfully treated with electroconvulsive therapy. J Nerv Ment Dis 175:236–239, 1987

Bettelheim B: Love Is Not Enough. Glencoe, IL, Free Press, 1950

Bockoven JS: Moral Treatment in American Psychiatry. New York, Springer, 1963

Henry GW: Mental hospitals, in A History of Medical Psychology. Edited by Zilboorg G, Henry GW. New York, WW Norton, 1941, pp 558–559

Jones M: The Therapeutic Community. New York, Basic Books, 1953

Wolpert EA: On the nature of manic depressive illness, in The Course of Life, Vol 3. Edited by Pollock G, Greenspan SI. Washington, DC, National Institute of Mental Health, 1980, pp 443–452

Wolpert EA: From metapsychology to pathopsychophysiology towards an etiological understanding of major affective disorders, in The Course of Life, Vol 6. Edited by Greenspan SI, Pollock G. Madison, CT, International Universities Press, 1993, pp 451–478

Chapter 5

The Emergency Room

Howard Silbert, M.D.

Whenever an individual feels the need to seek out psychiatric help, the clinician should appreciate the request as evidence that a crisis exists within or around the patient (Tarachow 1963). The trouble may be internal (e.g., mental anguish over a failed relationship) or in the individual's environment (e.g., threat of job loss if he or she does not agree to undergo evaluation). Nowhere is such evidence clearer than in the emergency room.

In recent years, hospital emergency rooms have increasingly come to serve as the initial evaluation and treatment setting of choice for patients experiencing disturbances in thought, feelings, and/or action for which therapeutic intervention may be necessary.

In this chapter I review the emergency psychiatrist's goals and responsibilities in assessing and understanding the patient's acute symptomatology and underlying conflicts. The unique features of the emergency room setting and their impact on the patient and the clinician are explored. Also discussed is the opportunity afforded by the emergency or crisis for the clinician to intervene in the core conflictual areas of the patient, and for the patient to mobilize new mental mechanisms to better manage such conflicts. Finally, it is my hope that this chapter will provide a greater appreciation for the function and importance of emergency room evaluation and intervention in the overall treatment of the patient.

Evaluating the Patient in Crisis

The main goal of an emergency psychiatric evaluation is the timely assessment of the patient in crisis—his or her strengths and weaknesses, motivation for help and/or change, and immediate needs—as well as the identification of the precipitants of the crisis. This assessment will lead the physician to a formulation of the case, a provisional or differential diagnosis, and an initial treatment plan.

Crisis intervention in the emergency room or referral to a more appropriate treatment setting can then be carried out.

A classic psychiatric interview composed of a history, a mental status examination, and—when appropriate—a physical examination with supporting diagnostic tests forms the foundation of the emergency room evaluation. Although the clinician should always be prepared to individualize his or her approach to meet the patient's needs, this is especially important in the emergency room setting—for example, in structuring the interview with an expansive, volatile, bipolar manic patient or departing from conventional standards regarding confidentiality in assessing suicide risk in an uncooperative borderline adolescent. A hallmark of good psychiatric practice is flexibility. In the emergency room, posture should be tempered with pragmatism. The emergency psychiatrist is obliged to make an initial determination of the patient's problems and to address any truly emergent issues in a timely fashion. Any parameter introduced to further this goal whose rationale is described in the medical record is consonant with good clinical practice.

What constitutes a psychiatric emergency is highly subjective. An elderly man with schizophrenia whose pet cat has died may have greater difficulty adjusting to his loss than a healthier obsessional patient facing the breakup of his marriage. The psychiatrist must consider each patient's unique constitutional strengths and weaknesses, as well as the typical psychological mechanisms of response to internal and external stresses and the environmental factors that come together at a particular time in the patient's life, to adequately assess the individual's degree of distress and/or dysfunction. Although this kind of total biopsychosocial formulation is optimal, the emergent status of the patient, concern for the emergency room population at large, and other constraints of the emergency room setting (discussed below) often make this goal an ideal rather than a reality. At a minimum, the following issues should be addressed in every emergency psychiatric evaluation: 1) safety, 2) differential diagnosis, 3) reality testing, 4) potential for violence, and 5) ability to provide self-care.

Safety

The physical well-being of the individual patient, the other patients in the area, the treating physician, and the entire staff are of the highest priority in the emergency room. An adequate evaluation cannot be done unless an atmosphere of safety prevails. The architectural design and decor, staffing patterns, and other features of the treatment setting should convey this concern to the patient (see below). The emotional safety of the patient is equally important.

The psychiatrist, through his or her verbal and nonverbal communications with the patient, must convey an attitude of respect and concern for the patient's life and problems. Winnicott's concept of a holding environment (Modell 1976; Winnicott 1965) is particularly relevant in the emergency room setting. The physician cannot make assumptions about the patient's ability to understand or tolerate the evaluation process. Rather, he or she must be prepared to explain, in jargon-free language at the patient's level of understanding, who he or she is and what he or she is trying to accomplish with the patient. For example, many people are brought to the emergency room against their will by the police. They often have the fantasy that the psychiatrist is working for the criminal justice system and has the power to incarcerate them. The clinician should identify him- or herself as an employee of the hospital and should briefly describe the evaluation process. The emergency interview may be highly stressful. The doctor should inquire as to the comfort of each patient and should offer his or her appreciation for how long the patient has been waiting. Psychotic patients, other very disturbed patients, and children may need to be told that it is permissible to ask questions and make requests of the staff. Generally speaking, psychiatric patients are not particularly violent. An act of violence in the psychiatric emergency room is usually committed by a person who feels, for whatever reason, threatened. Listening attentively to patients, with an ear toward appreciating their fright and pain, is the single best way to make them feel safe.

Prior to and concomitant with the ongoing determination of the patient's degree of safety, the psychiatrist should be performing a self-assessment of the same issue. He or she must be in the proper frame of mind to take on the responsibility of the emergency evaluation. The psychiatrist should remain alert to possible countertransference reactions evoked by working closely with the patient and aware of his or her own concerns regarding safety. Listening attentively to him- or herself—to the conscious and unconscious derivatives of fantasies that the psychiatrist brings to the clinical situation and that are sparked by the patient's issues and affects—is the best way for the psychiatrist to maintain a position of safety and to work effectively and appropriately with the patient.

For the safety of the individual and of the emergency room population as a whole, violence cannot be tolerated or condoned. The nature of emergency room work is predictably unpredictable. When verbal interventions fail or are contraindicated, the psychiatrist must be prepared to order medication or physical restraint to help a patient regain control of him- or herself. At the appropriate time, the rationale for such a decision should be explained to the patient and his or her reactions solicited. Careful attention to the possible outbreak of agitated, provocative, or otherwise disruptive behavior beyond acceptable limits is good insurance against untoward occurrences.

Differential Diagnosis

In the initial diagnostic evaluation, equal consideration must be given to the possibility of organic and functional etiology or a combination of the two. Common metabolic, endocrine, infectious, and neurological conditions may have prominent psychiatric manifestations. Acute intoxications or states of withdrawal, diabetes mellitus, acquired immunodeficiency syndrome (AIDS), and head trauma, to name just a few, may mimic psychiatric syndromes. Such conditions may be life-threatening if not identified and treated quickly. In general, the treatment of medical illness is more definitive and the prognosis better than for psychiatric disease. Just because someone "acts crazy" doesn't necessarily mean that they are. Psychiatric symptomatology is frequently dramatic and disturbing to both the clinician and the patient. Such symptomatology is often the most prominent feature of the presenting problem. The emergency room psychiatrist, in particular, must remain ever alert to the possible existence of underlying physical disease. He or she should be comfortable in working with all patients, regardless of their problems, and in working collaboratively with other medical specialists.

Some psychiatrists think of themselves as "doctors of the mind." This notion, whether born out of an intense interest in mental processes or a disinterest in—or aversion to—physical illness, is a fallacy. Advances in neuroscience confirm that the mind, brain, and body are best understood as equally important components of the individual. It is incumbent upon the psychiatrist to assess the total person in his or her diagnostic evaluation.

The same is true for those who consider themselves "doctors of the body." Some non–mental health professionals tend to downplay or ignore the complaints of patients once they have been labeled "psychiatric." Symptoms such as paranoia, somatic preoccupation, suicidality, and acute agitation are perplexing and disturbing to the clinician and the patient alike, and can make even routine medical diagnosis and treatment quite difficult. Each patient must be assessed for the possibility of physical illness masquerading as emotional illness or of physical illness and psychiatric disease presenting in combination. The agitated, uncooperative high school student with bizarre affect may be suffering from hypoglycemia and juvenile diabetes rather than from marijuana intoxication. The elderly chronic alcoholic who comes to the emergency room 4–5 times per month with slurred speech and alcohol on his breath may, today, have sustained a subdural hematoma in a fall. Indigent people, including many deinstitutionalized and homeless chronic mentally ill individuals, are the most likely to use emergency rooms for their primary medical care. Such individuals are at great risk for developing tuberculosis, nutritional deficiencies, and other easily overlooked, yet treatable, conditions. They are also more likely to be the victims of physical and sexual abuse. The psychiatrist who functions as a consultant to other branches of the emergency service or who receives patients sent from the medical emergency room after being "medically cleared" must retain a high index of suspicion for the possibility of primary and/or secondary physical illness in formulating his or her differential diagnosis.

It is often impossible to make a definitive diagnostic evaluation in the emergency room. Many psychiatric and medical conditions present with a similar clinical picture during their acute phases. The patient may be unable or unwilling to provide a history. The volume of cases, needs of more emergent patients, limited access to radiographic and other ancillary services, and the like, may limit the physician's ability to do a thorough job. The emergency psychiatrist should recognize these factors and convey his or her degree of certainty or uncertainty regarding the diagnosis to the physician assigned to continue with the patient's care and treatment. Initial impressions based on the most florid picture of the patient and his or her illness are very valuable. A thoughtful consideration of all possible diagnoses that "leaves no stone unturned" is more helpful and realistic than a "rush to judgment." Treatment planning should begin at the time of the initial evaluation and should follow logically from the diagnostic assessment. Such planning will often include recommendations for further evaluation to achieve the most definitive diagnosis or diagnoses possible. At the same time, treatment should not be delayed if the patient is in acute distress. Hallucinations can be as unbearable as a kidney stone or any other type of physical pain. The psychiatrist must be sensitive to the patient's immediate needs as well as to the longer-range goals of his or her evaluation.

Reality Testing

In conjunction with his or her concerns about safety and accurate diagnosis, the emergency room psychiatrist should make a rapid assessment of the patient's ability to tolerate reality. *Reality testing* refers not only to the presence or absence of psychotic thinking or perceptual abnormalities, but also to the degree of severity of the patient's symptoms and the disruption they may cause in his or her life. Evidence of withdrawal from external, objective reality, level of affectivity, intellectual functioning, and degree of regression are other important parameters. Judgment of the patient's tendency to regress and the conditions under which such regression tends to occur may be of crucial importance, both to the successful completion of the diagnostic examination and to the patient's compliance with treatment recommendations. A hypervigilant patient with paranoia may misperceive the physician's efforts to help as an attempt to control him or her. Such a patient may become hostile and uncooperative in giving a history. If the clinician becomes frustrated and strident, the patient may feel attacked and isolate him- or herself even further, or may lash out in self-defense. Failure to appreciate a melancholic patient's sense of worthlessness and hopelessness as indicative of a severe depression may lead the psychiatrist to conclude that the patient is unmotivated for treatment and to accede to the patient's wish to be sent home. Command auditory hallucinations may tell a schizophrenic patient to downplay or deny his symptoms and to toss the prescription he receives into the garbage after exiting the emergency room. The psychiatrist should be aware that complications may arise in working with patients whose reality testing is impaired. Never assume that the patient understands or believes you. Do not assume that he or she wants your help.

The psychiatrist must be aware of the impact of his or her interactions and interventions on the patient and should conduct him- or herself in a professional way at all times. Communication with patients should be straightforward and in language they can understand. The psychiatrist's failure to consider that a lapse in empathy or other countertransference reaction might have caused the patient to regress may result in a flawed assessment of the patient's degree of pathology. For example, a clinician disappointed by her third consecutive patient demanding admission on a cold winter night may be inadvertently brusque and incorrectly assume that the patient is a malingerer feigning psychosis to gain entry into the hospital, thus misdiagnosing a borderline patient who is experiencing a predictable reaction to a rejection.

The psychiatrist must be realistic about his or her goals. An attractive, intelligent college student having her first schizophreniform episode may activate rescue fantasies in a male psychiatrist, causing him to underappreciate the patient's psychotic symptomatology and make a referral for outpatient psychotherapy instead of a more appropriate inpatient admission. Emergency psychiatrists must be realistic about themselves if they are to accurately assess a patient's sense of reality. This ability will ultimately become the clinician's most valuable diagnostic tool. The psychiatrist must be prepared to structure, modify, or even interrupt an interview to limit the potential for regression or agitation.

Potential for Violence

By clinical and legal definition, symptoms of actual or potential violence are dangerous to the patient and/or others. Suicidal ideation is the most common chief complaint made by patients coming to the psychiatric emergency room. Assessment of suicide risk is the most common reason for referral to a psychiatrist by other physicians working on an emergency service. Suicidal ideation may be part of any clinical presentation, and cuts across all diagnostic categories. All threats, gestures, and thoughts of this nature must be taken seriously until proven otherwise. Such patients should be placed under close observation. They may perceive the hospital as dangerous rather than as an asylum. They should be given the option of asking for help in controlling their self-destructive impulses before safeguards such as restraint or seclusion are ordered. The emergency psychiatrist should be thoroughly familiar with the various risk factors for suicide, including family history, presence of underlying medical illness, and psychosis, to name just a few. Most important, he or she must be adept at listening for the conscious and unconscious fantasies contained in the suicidal ideation or action. Gaining an appreciation of the patient's fantasies of suicide as a solution to his or her conflicts, and considering these against the backdrop of the patient's overall psychosocial adjustment, is the single most effective way to make an accurate evaluation of the likelihood that the patient will act on those feelings. It is also the best way to formulate interventions to help the patient to more realistically gain control of such feelings.

> Mr. J, a 45-year-old accountant, newly married for the second time, is brought to the emergency room by his wife after taking an overdose of sleeping pills in an admitted suicide attempt. He has become distraught over his wife's demand that they have a child. Mr. J has two children from his first marriage whom he loves very much, but he feels that these are enough. Although he says he understands how his

wife, now married for the first time and childless, could have such a wish, he feels confused and deceived. They had discussed the issue during their courtship and Mr. J had made clear his feelings. He saw this marriage as his opportunity to "live it up" for the first time in his life. Hardworking and financially successful, Mr. J had been shocked when his first wife sued for divorce: "She said I was never home and more interested in my clients than her and the kids." He prided himself on his reputation as an indispensable member of his firm. On the basis of the large house and other amenities he provided his family, Mr. J also saw himself as a devoted husband and father—unlike his own father, who had abandoned the patient when he was 6 years old, along with his mother and two younger siblings. Depressed after the breakup of his marriage, Mr. J began psychotherapy for the first time. After several years of treatment, he felt much better and recognized that he had been out of touch with the true needs of his family. It was around the time that his therapist announced he was retiring at the end of the coming year that Mr. J began to think of remarrying.

Mr. J took the pills on a night when his wife was away on a business trip: "I expected her to come into the house the next day and find me dead. Then she'd see how she was ruining my life." When he awoke the following morning, he became frightened and told her what he had done.

This conscious fantasy of revenge, in a man suffering from pathological narcissism with depression, overlaid several other deeper layers of wishes: a need to restore his inflated self-esteem by getting his wife to be worried about him; a desire to punish his therapist for abandoning him, as his father had done; a message to his therapist clarifying his need for further help, in hopes that the retirement would be postponed; a longing to find and be reunited with his father in heaven; guilt over his perceived oedipal victory in having succeeded in getting his mother all to himself; and hatred toward his mother for driving his father away and forcing him to become caretaker to his brother and sister. Mr. J was terrified of having to parent children for the third time in his life—a responsibility for which he felt as ill prepared now as he had when he was 6.

This clinical vignette illustrates several points of particular importance to the emergency psychiatrist. Fantasies—including suicidal fantasies—may be conscious or unconscious. They are not bound by the usual rules of logic or reality—anything is possible in fantasy. Mr. J's longing for a strong father he could love, be loved by, and identify with, was timeless. That the fantasied solution to his conflicts over being an adult and wanting to be cared for and to have fun like a child would result in his death was a reality of which he was only dimly aware. More frightening was this patient's expectation that those in his life who were currently causing—or had previously caused—him pain would now suffer. The psychiatrist must have the healthiest respect for the power of the unconscious. Superficially, this patient might be considered rather well adjusted. By asking the question "What do you think will happen if you kill yourself?" the psychiatrist can listen for the wealth of valuable information contained in the fantasy. Decisions about inpatient admission, treatment, and follow-up care can then be better informed.

The patient and his wife did not feel that inpatient admission was necessary. The psychiatrist, however, recognizing that Mr. J was functioning on a level closer to a 6-year-old child, disagreed. He communicated his concerns to the patient and his hypothesis about the patient's fantasied fear of fatherhood. Although Mr. J voiced the thought that the doctor was crazy, he passively consented to a voluntary admission and seemed quietly pleased.

Periodically, debate arises over the issue of suicide as an appropriate solution to problems such as AIDS, terminal cancer, quadriplegia, severe dementia, and other conditions with bleak prognoses. Regardless of one's philosophical and moral outlook, it is essential to recognize that it is against the law to kill oneself. Physicians are sworn to uphold the law and must clearly see their responsibility to preserve life regardless of its quality. While society is addressing these issues in such developments as the living will and proposed guidelines for physician-assisted suicide, psychiatrists remain in the difficult position of having to help patients, sometimes against both the patient's wishes and their own feelings. Psychiatrists, because of their major responsibility in the evaluation of suicide risk, must be particularly alert to their own attitudes on this subject. The psychiatrist's impression of a patient's suicidality and the manner in which the psychiatrist conveys that impression to the patient can have serious consequences.

Mr. K, a 25-year-old cocaine and heroin addict, is brought to the emergency room by the police after taking an overdose. It is his third such presentation in the past 6 weeks. After medical clearance, the psychiatrist is called to assess the patient. Mr. K boastfully describes how he flagged down a patrol car because he needed a safe place to come down from his high and wanted to avoid a drug dealer to whom he owes money. He admits to testing positive for human immunodeficiency virus (HIV) infection only after being specifically questioned about it. Mr. K cavalierly talks about knowing he will probably die from drugs long before the infection becomes fatal and then begins demanding to be released so he can steal money to satisfy his craving. The psychiatrist is disdainful of Mr. K and his lifestyle, despairing of her ability to help the patient recognize and change his maladaptive behavior, and troubled by her own misperceptions of risk in working with HIV-infected patients. She concludes that the overdose was accidental and discharges Mr. K with a recommendation that he seek rehabilitative treatment for his substance abuse. The patient, frightened and ignorant about the facts regarding the full-blown syndrome of AIDS, reacts to the physician's distant and uncaring manner as confirmation that he is terminally ill and goes out to kill himself.

Mr. L, a 75-year-old man who has been living alone since the death of his wife 2 years ago and is estranged from his children, comes to the emergency room after becoming frightened by suicidal thoughts. He has no suicidal plan and no previous psychiatric history. The doctor on duty, not in touch with his ambivalence over feeling neglectful of his own elderly parents and angry with them for making demands on his time, diagnoses a severe major depressive episode and hospitalizes Mr. L against his will. The patient later complains that he was not given a chance to explain that his reason for coming to the hospital was to get a physical examination so that he could attend an activities program at his local senior citizen center.

In addition to asking about the presence of suicidal thoughts and feelings and the fantasies about them, the psychiatrist should also ask the patient what he or she thinks needs to change in order for these thoughts and feelings to diminish. The reply to this question will help the clinician to better understand the level of distress and degree of reality testing the patient has about his or her problems; it will also guide the physician in making treatment recommendations. Often, the process of reviewing these issues with patients is therapeutic in itself: if they can become aware of the pain they are feeling and can tolerate this pain long enough to see the fallacies of their fantasied expectations, they may then be able to outline a more appropriate course of action.

Violent impulses are more difficult to control outside the structured hospital setting. Before releasing any patient, the psychiatrist should ask him- or herself the following questions: What has changed in this person's life that makes the risk of suicidal behavior less now than when he or she came to the emergency room? How likely are these changes to continue to work in the direction of a healthier adaptation? The physician's responsibility in this regard continues after discharge into the immediately foreseeable future. It is usually prudent to predict for the patient the possibility that suicidal feelings may recur and to emphasize that return to the emergency room or other treatment setting is always an option.

Society deems the psychiatrist an expert on predicting violence of all kinds. Homicide, rape, and child and spousal abuse are all on the rise. Because of the increased concern and heightened awareness about such issues, other clinicians, educators, and law enforcement officials are more likely than ever to refer cases involving a question of abuse to a psychiatrist. Victims themselves, because of widespread publicity, are somewhat more open about discussing such topics. The real and fantasied concerns about harm in such cases often result in immediate referral to the emergency room psychiatrist. While recognizing that prediction of violence is much more of an art than a science, the psychiatrist must be ready to listen for derivatives of aggressive impulses in all patients. He or she should consider the patient's potential to be a victim as well as an assailant. Risk factors for violent behavior, such as a history of having been abused as a child, are important but, as discussed in the assessment of suicide risk, the patient's fantasies are even more valuable. Whereas the physician's primary responsibility is to his or her patient, the psychiatrist is facing increasing pressure to consider the rights of potential victims and of society at large. If a patient reveals that he has planted a bomb in the local airport, it should be reported to the appropriate authorities despite the patient's demand for confidentiality. The psychiatrist must stay up to date with the pertinent state laws and local and national precedents regarding duty to warn. When in doubt, it is always best to err on the side of caution. As in the discussion of assessment of suicide risk, clinicians must be aware of their reactions to the patient, their own attitudes about the issues involved, and how they communicate with the patient regarding his or her situation.

> Mr. M, a 34-year-old civil service employee, is brought to the emergency room by police from his office after he threatened to kill his boss. He is under what he considers extreme pressure to be more productive at work, and feels that his boss is "out to get him" so he can be replaced by a younger, attractive female co-worker. By the time of the evaluation, Mr. M has composed himself and is quite ashamed of his behavior. He denies any intent to harm anyone. He has no prior history of violence and is released. The psychiatrist, annoyed with the police officer for what he feels is an inappropriate referral, is subtly dismissive of Mr. M's embarrassment. The patient leaves, feeling like a fool, and goes home to kick the dog and berate his wife for being unsympathetic.

As discussed above, violence toward others in the emergency room most often results from misperceptions by a patient about the intentions of the staff and the purpose of the evaluation. It may also occur as a reaction to intrusive, insensitive, or indifferent staff members. Finally, the impact of other frightened, volatile, or bored patients brought together at close quarters can have a "critical-mass" effect. Although the physician's primary responsibility is to the individual patient, he or she should be aware of the group dynamics at play in the emergency room and how they may affect the patient's condition. A stress management program and appropriate supervision of all staff can be very helpful in limiting the occurrence of iatrogenic violence.

Ability to Provide Self-Care

In addition to the immediate concerns for safety and management of the patient while in the emergency room, the question of self-care must be considered as part of inpatient admission criteria, initial treatment planning, and assessment of readiness for discharge. The ability to understand one's own needs and to perform the basic activities of daily living—obtaining adequate food, clothing, and shelter—is essential for survival. In some states, self-neglect is considered adequate reason for involuntary hospitalization. Although this is a gray area under the law, it is increasingly being interpreted along this line of reasoning: "Does the person know enough to come in out of the rain?"

> Mr. N, a 50-year-old man with chronic schizophrenia, lives three blocks away from the hospital. He maintains himself in a cardboard box near a hot-air vent and forages for food out of nearby garbage bins. His appearance and affect are bizarre and he has been observed on many occasions to be talking to himself. Nevertheless, Mr. N steadfastly denies any problems or psychiatric symptoms and rejects all offers of treatment and more permanent housing. Although well-meaning community work-

ers have brought him to the emergency room over the years, Mr. N has never accepted treatment voluntarily. On the two occasions in which he was held on an emergency basis, he successfully won his release by arguing that he would get help if he ever needed it. Today he is brought in by police during a snowstorm. He has a fever of 101°F. Mr. N makes his usual argument and promises he will go to the medical clinic tomorrow. It is noted that this is his second visit for the week. Review of his previous record shows that the patient was febrile then as well, and he made the same promise about treatment. After refusing an offer for voluntary treatment, Mr. N is admitted on an emergency basis. This time the judge upholds the decision.

A person's rights under the law—freedom of speech, freedom to live one's life as one chooses, and so forth—are difficult issues to reach consensus on in under any circumstances, let alone as part of an emergency room evaluation. The ability of the hospital staff to intervene on behalf of a patient to address such societal issues as adequate shelter and treatment opportunities, substance abuse, and crime is minimal. Nevertheless, the psychiatrist has some responsibility for the patient's well-being after he or she is discharged from the emergency room. This is the hottest issue of debate and scrutiny in medico-legal cases concerning emergency medicine today. It is not enough to decide that a patient's pathology does not warrant inpatient-level care; as a general guideline, the physician should consider him- or herself responsible for the well-being of the patient during "the immediately foreseeable future" after the patient leaves the emergency room. This view is analogous to the one an inpatient psychiatrist might take at the time of a patient's discharge from the psychiatric service. The psychiatrist should assess the patient's ability to understand the nature of his or her problems and need for treatment. At minimum, the psychiatrist must judge the patient's ability to follow through with outpatient treatment recommendations and capacity to adjust to difficulties if there are any delays in implementing the treatment plan (this includes such issues as obtaining adequate food and shelter). As always, patients should be given the message that the emergency room is always open and available to them if they feel the need to call or return.

Clinical Process

Most emergency psychiatric evaluations are done by nonpsychiatrists in a general medical emergency room setting. However, because of factors such as the increased incidence of violence, the greater recognition of cases of abuse, deinstitutionalization of the chronic mentally ill and emphasis on ambulatory care, and the epidemics of alcoholism and other substance abuse, specialized psychiatric emergency rooms are increasingly favored for such evaluations. Regardless of the composition of the treatment team, the importance of clear communication and lines of authority cannot be overstated. Responsibility for each patient must be assigned from the time of entry into the emergency service through discharge or transfer to another treatment setting. Immediate access to the medical emergency room and appropriate laboratory and other ancillary services is necessary because of the high incidence (5%–30%) of patients presenting with medical problems having psychiatric manifestations (Kaplan and Sadock 1993). Children and younger adolescents are best served in a pediatric setting. If there is a risk of elopement or behavioral problems, such youngsters may be sent to the more secure adult emergency psychiatry service. Patients who have been physically abused, raped, or otherwise traumatized are usually first evaluated in the medical emergency room. If psychiatric consultation is then requested, it should be done in the same place or in an ambulatory service setting. Transfer to the psychiatric emergency room may give such patients the message that they are sick or are not believable in some way, thus compounding their existing trauma and feelings of guilt or shame.

As discussed above, safety is priority number one in the emergency room. Security is best managed as a clinical issue by the clinical staff. Law enforcement agents, including hospital security guards, should be kept apart from patient waiting and treatment areas to limit the possibility of friction and provocation. They should remain on alert to assist the clinical staff, if called upon, in times of extreme emergency. Weapons have no place in the emergency room. As in any intensive care setting, the danger of physical injury and burnout is real. Inservice training for clinicians and nonclinicians to allow feelings to be ventilated and to discuss aspects of countertransference reactions evoked by acutely ill patients is highly recommended.

It is essential for the entire staff to appreciate the fragility of the patient in emotional and physical distress. Patients in crisis, even those who are strongly motivated to get help, are anxious, ambivalent, hopeful, and fearful of the experience they are about to have. They arrive at the emergency room with fantasies and expectations based on their conscious and unconscious wishes and fears. Patients may be desirous of symptomatic relief, cure, asylum, or absolution. They may be frightened that they are crazy, or will be punished, physically harmed, or stigmatized. These concerns are compounded by information patients receive from those they have contact with during the referral process, as well as by any previous experience they have had with medical and mental health professionals. This transference readiness is then modified by patients' impressions of the physical layout of the emergency service and of the atmosphere in the emergency room that day, their interactions with staff and fellow patients, their observations of the treatment of others, and so forth.

Every psychiatric emergency room has its cohort of "regulars." These patients typically develop an institutional transference with both positive and negative components that must be taken into account each time they present for evaluation. What for staff members is another day on the job may be a defining moment in the patient's life. Psychiatrists must be keenly aware of "where the patient is at" and, through their empathic stance and interventions, try to establish a working alliance. Attention to the patient's physical comfort, and acknowledgement of his or her preliminary interactions with other staff during registration and triage—including an explanation for what may seem like interminable delays and unnecessary repetition—will help diminish the patient's anxiety and enhance his or her ability to cooperate in the diagnostic assessment.

Many people are confused about their rights as patients and the responsibility the physician has in their care. The psychiatrist may need to review these issues to prevent delays in completing the evaluation and effecting a disposition. At the same time, analysis of the patient's resistance is an excellent way to more fully understand the patient's strengths, weaknesses, and characteristic coping mechanisms. The man with obsessional symptoms who insists on being given a point-by-point explanation of each step of the evaluation may not only be demonstrating his need to use intellectualization as a defense but also "clueing the psychiatrist in" to a possible underlying paranoid process. A teenage boy who asks several times about the need for a physical examination may be expressing realistic concerns about having contracted gonorrhea as well as conflicts over homosexual longings for his father. The emergency room is far from an ideal setting in which to conduct an exploration of the patient's symptoms, anxieties, and character. Nevertheless, the usual model of the psychiatric interview as providing a framework for the field of inquiry, with modification, still applies. All of the patient's behavior, reactions, and verbal and nonverbal communications from the time he or she enters the emergency room throughout his or her stay constitute data that can and should be used by the psychiatrist to make the most accurate decisions and recommendations for the patient's care.

Multilingual staff, or a hospital "language bank" listing bilingual staff or another translation service, should be readily available to the interviewing psychiatrist. Disorders of thought are difficult enough to pick up when patient and physician both speak the same language. The use of family members or friends as translators is unreliable because of the potential for deliberate or unconscious denial or distortion of the clinical picture stemming from their involvement with the patient. The patient may be understandably hesitant to reveal conflicts about someone in the room for fear of later retribution. This type of situation often results in the psychiatrist's asking a question that is followed by a heated 5-minute debate between the patient and a family member. The translated answer is then given: "He says no." Such information is of dubious value.

When working with patients whose command of English is limited, psychiatrists would be wise to offer them the option of using a translator, or at least should apologize for the fact that they do not speak the patient's native tongue. This is an excellent way to gain the patient's trust. Care should be given in all cases to speak at the patient's level of ability to understand, free of medical and psychiatric jargon. Psychiatrists must be alert to the impact of cultural issues in their assessment of patients. For example, in some Latino groups, it is considered bad manners to disagree with an authority figure. A patient with this background may appear to understand and concur with the treatment plan as outlined by the psychiatrist yet leave the emergency room without mentioning his or her intention to seek follow-up care with a neighborhood faith healer.

The limited goal of providing a timely assessment of the patient in crisis must be understood by the entire staff and communicated to the patient and his or her family. Often, "less is more": moving a patient out of the emergency room to a more appropriate diagnostic or treatment setting is better not only for that patient but also for the patient population as a whole. Medical problems, interpersonal conflicts, or the development of enhanced social supports may be better managed elsewhere in the hospital system. Keeping to a minimum the cohort of emergent patients in the area reduces the possibility of agitation or violence occurring as a group phenomenon. The staff's failure or inability to provide a focused, timely assessment may be a major disappointment and cause of anger for the patient and/or those concerned about him or her. The fantasy of complete cure and other preconceived expectations about the outcome of the emergency room visit should be addressed prior to discharge. The rationales for why the emergency psychiatrist is not going to continue to work with the patient, why the patient is not going to be admitted despite his or her demand to enter the hospital, or why involuntary commitment is indicated despite the patient's outrage should be reviewed in a straightforward and tolerant way.

Although safety is always of the highest priority, it should not unduly hamper completion of the diagnostic assessment. When verbal intervention fails or is contraindicated, medication or other forms of restraint should be ordered quickly. This is done according to the principle of maximum tranquilization with minimum sedation. The aim is to help the patient regain control of him- or herself, ease the anxiety that is causing his or her pain, and complete the diagnostic examination. Medication is usually preferable to the use of physical restraints. Patients find the experience of involuntary restraint demeaning. There is a risk of injury to all involved and observing such measures is frightening to other patients in the area.

If it is determined that the patient meets the appropriate criteria for inpatient-level care, it is preferable to use a voluntary legal status rather than an involuntary status. Allowing this option may give the patient a greater sense of control over his or her life and of participation in the treatment. This is true even for patients who are felt to be potentially dangerous. Every psychiatric patient who wants to leave the hospital must first be reevaluated with regard to the issue of dangerousness to self and/or others. The patient can always be held briefly for further evaluation or converted to an involuntary status if that is warranted. Sometimes the usual option to admit or discharge is not considered optimal. "Mini–psychotic episodes" in a borderline patient, suspected cases of toxic psychosis, and adjustment reactions to traumatic events are examples of situations that may be better managed by crisis intervention in an extended observation area. Giving patients additional time in a secure environment away from the external reality that contributed to their decompensation may allow them to achieve sufficient improvement on their own that inpatient treatment becomes a moot point. Such a practice can also give the treatment team a chance to clarify confusing issues and coordinate a plan that will enable such patients to safely leave the emergency room to continue their care in an ambulatory setting. Sparing a patient the trauma and stigma of a psychiatric admission or preserving bed space for those clearly in need are worthwhile goals to consider. Issues regarding emergency room crisis intervention are discussed in more detail below.

The emergency room diagnostic assessment and initial case formulation are often inconclusive. In such situations, definitive treatment is best deferred until the evaluation is completed on the inpatient unit or in the outpatient clinic. In cases where the diagnosis is clear or when response to previous treatment is known, there is no point in delay. A man with chronic schizophrenia who has discontinued his antipsychotic medication in response to command auditory hallucinations is best served by the prompt resumption of the same treatment. Efforts to help patients in crisis feel comfortable in the emergency room should be a matter of course. Patients should be encouraged to return to the emergency room if any difficulty arises after discharge or in the future. At the same time, patients should be directed or redirected to the most appropriate treatment setting. A man who is followed in the psychopharmacology clinic comes to the emergency room complaining that he has lost his supply of medication and is fearful he will regress without it. If his condition warrants it, this patient should be given just enough medication to sustain him until he can be seen by his therapist. This response will decrease the possibility of inadvertent complicity in an episode of acting out, allow the patient and his therapist the chance to explore the issue together, and deter inappropriate use of the emergency room. Ideally, the outpatient therapist should be consulted with or notified in such cases.

Crisis Intervention

The psychiatric emergency room is best suited for the rapid initial assessment of the patient in crisis. The help patients receive is primarily focused on identifying conflicts, formulating the case, and providing sufficient symptomatic relief that more definitive treatment can then be pursued. Assessment of each patient's ego strengths and weaknesses, motivations for seeking help, superego structure and flaws, and severity of id impulse derivatives, as well as the extent of disruption in the patient's external circumstances, are part of the emergency psychiatric evaluation. This process may be therapeutic in itself if it leads to the patient's gaining insight into his or her problems and to a shifting of the patient's internal dynamic forces toward a better adaptation or by virtue of a supportive experience.

In selected cases, psychotherapeutic treatment initiated within the emergency room can and should be undertaken. A surprisingly wide array of problems can be managed by means of a short-term approach (Comstock 1983). A useful model when considering a recommendation for psychotherapy is to first address the question of analyzability. Although this treatment modality is rarely suited for the emergency room visitor, other types of expressive psychotherapy should be considered. Supportive psychotherapy remains an option if the above treatment modalities are contraindicated. Several factors are of particular importance in choosing the most appropriate treatment for a patient: the patient's past history of involvement in psychotherapy, the degree of instability in the patient's external life that could threaten the therapeutic situation, the availability of good object relationships, and the degree of secondary gain the patient derives from his or her illness. Other issues that argue in the direction of supportive treatment include a history of negative therapeutic reactions with violent or self-destructive behavior, strong masochistic trends, and significant sociopathy. The severity of such factors may rule out a recommendation for any type of psychotherapy. Chronic liars, regardless of their diagnosis, are not good candidates for psychotherapy (Kernberg 1984). The patient must be sufficiently intelligent, verbal, and willing to attend sessions. Psychiatrists must be aware of their rescue fantasies and degree of therapeutic enthusiasm in making a reasoned determination of the prognosis for therapeutic benefit and risk. Patients at risk may become better candidates for psychotherapy after a course of medication or hospitalization.

Regardless of one's theoretical orientation or technical approach, crisis intervention employing an expressive psychotherapeutic technique is generally best reserved for the relatively healthy neurotic or personality disorder patient who has reasonably stable reality testing and an ability to establish a transference neurosis. For such patients, the crisis can be conceptualized as their current conflict. If the current conflict can be related to past conflicts through the use of interpretation, permanent change with continued growth and maturation can be achieved. Resolution of the crisis will be marked by decreased symptomatology and an enhanced ability to manage similar situations in the future. By coming to understand the meaning and functions of their maladaptive reactions and learning more adaptive responses to anxiety, patients will be better able to anticipate dangers and become better problem solvers.

Supportive psychotherapy in times of crisis is best used with the more disturbed borderline or psychotic patient who has suffered an acute decompensation. The aim of treatment is a return to the patient's baseline level of functioning by eliminating factors responsible for the crisis. Medication is often employed as an adjunct. Extensive social service intervention is frequently necessary. Resolution is marked by symptomatic relief without dynamic change (Malan 1976; Sifneos 1967). The advantages of such a supportive approach compared with hospitalization include minimization of inpatient regression and rapid involvement of the patient's support system.

Crisis intervention should always be employed as part of the effort to reduce a patient's suicide risk. A supportive and caring approach on the part of the clinician may decrease the patient's sense of loneliness and despair and lead to renewed hope. Sufficient time must be set aside to explore the conscious and unconscious fantasy formation underlying the ideation. Care must be taken to avoid feelings of rejection on the part of patients, who often anticipate confirmation of their feeling that they are worthless. Patients should be asked about their ideas regarding what will help. This is often a good place to begin reality-testing the issue, educating the patient about the dynamic of anger turned against the self or internalized object representations, and formulating corrective strategies to better manage anger and disappointment. Suicidality is particularly likely to generate countertransference reactions. As discussed above, the psychiatrist must remain on guard to this possibility and take the appropriate steps to prevent any complications.

Being "On Call"

Many psychiatric emergency rooms employ clinicians who are at various stages of their formal medical education. This is certainly true for teaching hospitals, where it is common to see junior and occasionally senior residents working alongside interns, subinterns, and other medical students. There may or may not be attending supervisors present. Resident-level psychiatrists and fellows may also work as moonlighters to cover off-hour shifts. There are two educational models that explain these practices. One conceptualizes emergency room psychiatry as a discrete subspeciality with a specific body of knowledge, skills, and attitudes with which the general psychiatrist must become proficient. The other views the emergency room as a place where psychiatrists in training can become familiar with a wide range of psychopathology in its most florid presentations. They can then practice the diagnostic, treatment, administrative, and other skills learned on their regular clinical rotations. The experience of working in this setting serves as a crucible in which the neophyte clinician's psychiatric identity is forged. Regardless of the educational focus, most psychiatrists view their emergency room work as a unique part of their training. It is difficult to fully appreciate how extraordinarily rich and demanding the experience can be until one gains the perspective of time.

Several issues are particularly important to be aware of when working in the emergency room early in one's career. The fact that emergency room assignments often come at the end of the workday or workweek does not mean they should be treated with anything less than a full effort. The patient evaluated at 3:00 A.M. deserves the same care and respect as one who arrives at 3:00 P.M. Although the psychiatrist is dedicated to learning, his or her primary responsibility is to the patient. The patient's needs take priority over all other considerations—including the resident's desire to read or eat or the supervisor's wish to sleep. Involvement with the patient may be limited to one shift. This is not an excuse to avoid working "in close" to the patient to achieve an empathic understanding of such difficult issues as suicide risk or melancholic depression. Clinicians must assess the needs of patients on a case-by-case basis. Their job is not to fill as many vacant beds as possible nor to "play goalie" and block all inpatient admissions. Psychiatrists are as human as their patients—they are not expected to be perfect, and they should not expect this of themselves. They must work toward gaining a realistic assessment of their patients as well as of themselves. Clinicians must learn to recognize when they have strayed from a neutral stance and to identify what, within the patient and within themselves, has caused this to occur. In so doing, they will develop ways to use this information in the service of caring for patients, including asking for help in this effort.

Conclusion

The emergency room often serves as the gateway for the medical center's various psychiatric services. First impressions carry a great deal of weight. The care and attention shown to patients in their most vulnerable condition have important implications well beyond their stay in the emergency service. Patients' willingness to face difficult issues, to consider life changes, and to comply with treatment recommendations may be largely due to their identification with the emergency psychiatrist. Patients' reactions to other staff members and their participation in their own treatment may likewise be based on reactions they had when they first arrived at the hospital. A positive experience in the emergency room may establish an adaptive context in which subsequent steps in treatment can proceed toward a healthier outcome. A negative encounter with the emergency psychiatrist may impede or undermine future treatment. The initial therapist involved in a case should be careful not to create unrealistic or false expectations about the patient's care and prognosis; rather, he or she should convey to the patient a realistic idea of what may follow, making an effort to preserve the patient's sense of hope.

For Further Study

American Psychiatric Association: Diagnostic and Statistical Manual of Mental Disorders, 3rd Edition, Revised. Washington, DC, American Psychiatric Association, 1987

Appelbaum PS: The right to refuse treatment with antipsychotic medications: retrospect and prospect. Am J Psychiatry 145:413–419, 1988

Baldessarini RJ: Chemotherapy in Psychiatry. Boston, MA, Harvard University Press, 1985

Bellak L, Small L: Emergency Therapy and Brief Psychotherapy. New York, Grune & Stratton, 1965

Bibring E: Psychoanalysis and the dynamic psychotherapies. J Am Psychoanal Assoc 2:745–770, 1954

Blum H: The value of reconstruction in adult psychoanalysis. Int J Psychoanal 61:39–54, 1980

Brenner C: An Elementary Textbook of Psychoanalysis. New York, International Universities Press, 1973 (originally published 1955)

Davanloo H (ed): Short-Term Dynamic Psychotherapy. New York, Jason Aronson, 1980

Dubin WR: Rapid tranquilization: antipsychotics or benzodiazepines? J Clin Psychiatry 49 (suppl 12):5–11, 1988

Dubin WR, Weiss KJ: Handbook of Psychiatric Emergencies. Springhouse, PA, Springhouse Corporation, 1991

Fenichel O: Problems of Psychoanalytic Technique (monograph). Albany, NY, Psychoanalytic Quarterly, 1941

Freud A: The ego and the mechanisms of defense (1936), in The Writings of Anna Freud, Vol 2. New York, International Universities Press, 1966

Freud A: Acting out. Int J Psychoanal 49:165–170, 1968

Freud S: Some character-types met with in psychoanalytic work (1916), in The Standard Edition of the Complete Psychological Works of Sigmund Freud, Vol 14. Translated and edited by Strachey J. London, Hogarth Press, 1957, pp 309–333

Freud S: The ego and the id (1923), in The Standard Edition of the Complete Psychological Works of Sigmund Freud, Vol 19. Translated and edited by Strachey J. London, Hogarth Press, 1961, pp 3–66

Greenacre P: General problems of acting out. Psychoanal Q 19:455–467, 1950

Kanzer M: Ego alteration and acting out. Int J Psychoanal 49:431–435, 1968

Katz SE, Nardacci D, Sabatini A: Intensive Treatment of the Homeless Mentally Ill. Washington, DC, American Psychiatric Press, 1992

Koran LM, Sox HC, Marton KS, et al: Medical evaluation of psychiatric patients. Arch Gen Psychiatry 46:733–740, 1989

Modell AH: "The holding environment" and the therapeutic action of psychoanalysis. J Am Psychoanal Assoc 24:285–307, 1976

Winnicott DW: Hate in the countertransference (1949), in Collected Papers: Through Paediatrics to Psycho-Analysis. New York, Basic Books, 1958, pp 184–203

References

Comstock BS: Psychiatric Emergency Intensive Care. Psychiatr Clin North Am 6:305–315, 1983

Kaplan HI, Sadock BJ: Pocket Handbook of Emergency Psychiatric Medicine. Baltimore, MD, Williams & Wilkins, 1993

Kernberg OF: Severe Personality Disorders. New Haven, CT, Yale University Press, 1984

Malan DH: The Frontier of Brief Psychotherapy. New York, Plenum, 1976

Modell AH: "The holding environment" and the therapeutic action of psychoanalysis. J Am Psychoanal Assoc 24:285–307, 1976

Sifneos PE: Two different kinds of psychotherapy of short duration. Am J Psychiatry 123:1069, 1967

Tarachow S: An Introduction to Psychotherapy. New York, International Universities Press, 1963

Winnicott DW: The Maturational Processes and the Facilitating Environment. New York, International Universities Press, 1965

Chapter 6

The Medical Hospital

Philip R. Muskin, M.D.

This chapter presents a psychodynamic overview of the hospital setting. For the psychiatric consultant to understand how to proceed with a psychiatric consultation, it is extremely useful to understand the hospital system and the interactions between the components of this system, as well as the dynamics of physical illness. In this chapter I attempt to outline this "biopsychosocial" organization in an effort to make seemingly incomprehensible behavior and reactions of patients and staff fit into a dynamic framework of interaction. It is important to recognize that the medical setting is a complex, vibrant, and ever-evolving organization that may seem confusing, bewildering, and frightening to individuals who must interact with this system. The health care workers and students who work in hospitals adapt themselves for life in this special environment; the psychiatric consultant, of course, must do the same. Such adaptation is a process that takes years to accomplish. The other group of individuals who come into the system—patients and their families—have no time to adapt to the system and therefore experience the effects both of their illness and of the hospitalization with distress.

The physical structure of the hospital is an important factor that contributes to the stress for the patient and staff. The mecca of health care (i.e., the tertiary medical center) is typically a series of buildings connected in a variety of logical and illogical ways. Negotiating this physical plant can be a bewildering experience. As the size of the health care setting increases, patients report themselves as experiencing greater degrees of anxiety (Lucente and Fleck 1972). This anxiety is separate from, but in addition to, the anxieties concerning their health. People come to hospitals because they experience themselves as being sick, in pain, and suffering, and as needing information, care, or help. The initial expe-

---

I would like to express my thanks to Dr. Donald S. Kornfeld for his critical commentary in the preparation of this manuscript.

rience of negotiating the transportation to the hospital, the emergency room, or the admitting office contributes to the stress of the hospitalization.

Hospitals have special odors. In addition to the aromas of various disinfectants, there are others which are associated with pain, suffering, and death, as well as loss of control, shame, and sexuality. Health care workers may become habituated to the olfactory stimuli but patients and their families are greeted by this sensory stimulation, even if they are not consciously aware of this. Various parts of the hospital may have different odors. There are few circumstances of life in which one's intimate bodily functions are as exposed as when one is sick and hospitalized, with the exception of the earliest years of childhood. Although the impact of the olfactory experience has never been measured systematically, it may contribute to the stress of hospitalization and to the regressive pull that illness and hospitalization exert upon patients.

Admission to the hospital means leaving the comfort of—and relinquishing control over—one's personal environment. Not only does the patient leave home, he or she is asked to give up personal belongings. Most importantly, patients are asked to relinquish their clothing. In giving up their clothes, their belongings, and their home, individuals attain a new status, that of patient. The individual must adapt to the patient role. All patients are viewed as the same in the health care setting. The typical trappings of power, wealth, and position are lost. The individual is expected to follow a rather rigid set of rules, although those rules are often vaguely defined. When and often *what* a patient eats may no longer be under his or her control. Access to family and friends is restricted. As the severity of the medical illness increases, the patient suffers an ever-increasing loss of control, sometimes to the point of the loss of bodily functions, respiration, and even cardiac function.

The Patient

How an individual copes with the inescapable stress of hospitalization will emerge as the central focus of the psychiatric consultant's task. How the hospital structure, the personnel, and the resources of the patient (financial, social, cognitive) limit the ability of the patient to cope with the stress of hospitalization may determine whether a particular patient successfully copes with illness and a hospital stay. The interaction of these various components requires systems analysis and reflects the biopsychosocial approach to medical care (Miller 1973a).

The consultant is frequently required to separate each of these three spheres. Psychiatric consultants are often most comfortable with the "psychological" sphere, typically the psychoanalytic. Biological and sociological components of the patient and the system are ignored or given inadequate attention. For some consultants, how they view the importance of each of the components and what information they choose to collect will determine their ability to fully understand the patient and the system (Miller 1973b).

Psychological Stress

It seems reasonable to conclude that serious illness and hospitalization create a situation of psychological stress for all patients and their families (Kornfeld 1979). *Psychological stress* is anything that destabilizes a person's life. Serious illness, a sudden financial change, the illness or death of an important person, and many other expected and unexpected occurrences all cause stress. Patients vary both in their vulnerability to this stress and in their ability to adapt to the situation. How a patient adapts to stress depends on his or her previous experiences with illness and doctors, the patient's characteristic manner of coping with stress, and the particular type and severity of stress that the patient is experiencing. The genetic endowment of the individual, his or her particular character style, and the external resources of the family will also play powerful roles. The experience of an illness severe enough to require hospitalization will be modulated by the early childhood experiences of the individual. The remnants of the past, no matter how distant, will be reflected in this current life crisis. As Strain and Grossman have noted, "the vast majority of patients are able to cope and to assume the role of patient without difficulty, and this is extraordinary in itself when one considers the magnitude of these stresses" (Strain and Grossman 1975, p. 24).

Strain and Grossman (1975) have outlined seven categories of psychological stress faced by the hospitalized patient. An understanding of each of these psychological stressors is of crucial importance to the psychiatric consultant. The following section is derived from these authors' seminal book:[1]

The basic threat to narcissistic integrity. Certain unconscious beliefs are commonly held: that each of us is indestructible; that we will always be capable, independent, and self-sufficient; and that we are always in complete control of what happens to us. Illness, particularly sudden illness with hospitalization, undermines such fantasies. The infantile fantasy of omnipotent parents who ensure the child's protected, pleasurable existence is challenged by this state of sickness, pain, and suffering. The infantile fantasy of parental omnipotence can easily be transferred onto the doctor, resulting in rage that the doctor has failed to protect the patient from his or her illness. As is obvious, patients who handle this stress in such a maladaptive manner will generate in their physicians reactive feelings that can disrupt the doctor/patient alliance.

Fear of strangers. It is remarkable that we expect patients, upon entering the hospital, to put themselves, and even their survival, into the hands of complete strangers. Such a situation reawakens early fears about strangers. These fears cannot interfere with permitting access to one's body, bodily fluids, intimate information about one's past experiences, present experiences, and the like. Instead, an

---

[1] Strain JJ, Grossman S: *Psychological Care of the Medically Ill.* New York, Appleton-Century-Crofts, 1975.

expectation of basic, unquestioning trust in those assigned to their care is imposed upon patients, who have little information on which to base such confidence. This situation can be particularly problematic for individuals whose psychopathology makes trust difficult—for example, paranoid patients or those with borderline personality disorder.

Separation anxiety. As noted above, hospitalized patients are separated from the important people and things by which they define their world and, sometimes, from themselves as well. Anxiety regarding this separation may be especially acute in individuals whose capacity to adapt to new situations is limited by their cognitive abilities (patients with moderate to severe dementia) or psychological abilities (patients with severe personality disorders).

Fear of the loss of love and approval. This stress may be overt in its manifestation, as with patients who believe that their illness will render them no longer lovable. Examples might be a woman who, following mastectomy or hysterectomy, feels she will not be loved, or patients who fear that their need for nursing care and convalescence will result in the disapproval or rejection of family or friends. Patients also fear loss of love and approval from their physicians because they have become ill, because they are not recovering at a rapid enough rate, because they are in continued pain, or even because they are dying. For some patients, the very circumstance of being ill reactivates dependency conflicts from childhood and generates tremendous stress in the current situation that is both inappropriate and maladaptive.

Fear of the loss of control of developmentally achieved functions. Physical illness, and often the therapeutic measures taken to address the illness, may cause suspension of physical and mental functions that were previously under the patient's control. Occasionally, these changes are both permanent and progressive. Frequently, patients lose physical strength secondary to their illness or to bed rest. Occasionally they may lose control of bowel and/or bladder function or experience incoordination and the inability to speak articulately. Secondary to illness, medication, and sleep deprivation, they may lose the ability to adequately regulate both their emotions and their expression of those emotions. Such losses can be particularly distressing for patients. There are few circumstances of life in which adults may not have control over when they go to the bathroom. In contrast to the typically private function performed in everyday life, using a bedpan in the hospital may require the aid of one or several people. Patients whose medications (as a direct or a side effect) cause such sequelae or patients who are recovering from general anesthesia, central nervous system disturbances, or endocrine disorders can find themselves unable to regulate the expression of emotion and/or to adequately express what they think and feel to friends, family members, and physicians. These distressing circumstances can cause a decompensation in patients whose self-esteem depends on an image that can tolerate no loss of control in any sphere of life.

Fear of loss of or injury to body parts. As we know, both men and women experience castration anxiety, or the fear of losing a part of one's body. However, the phenomenon is often not as simple as the actual loss of a body part. The loss of function, alteration, or even temporary dysfunction of a body part may also be experienced as a castration threat. Whereas the underlying fantasy may connect to fears of genital injury, this concern is often deeply buried and inaccessible to the adult patient. Any loss of power or strength—regardless of its relation to a surgical procedure or to actual threat of damage or loss of a body part—potentially constitutes an intensely stressful castration threat for some patients. This broader conception of castration fears does not mean that some patients do not sexualize their injuries, treatments, or diagnostic procedures. These patients experience such events as threats to their genital integrity or sexual potency. Appropriate, compassionate, empathic, and practical interpretations of such fears may provide great relief.

> The patient, a 42-year-old woman scheduled to have a colonoscopy, spoke at length about her fear and anxiety of being damaged and anally raped. The consultant, who knew the patient well, told her that this was the least sexual procedure imaginable, that the doctors and nurses were not enjoying themselves, and that her fear of someone using her body for their own pleasure was understandable but inaccurate in this instance. Giving no details, the consultant told her, "I know what I'm talking about; I've had this procedure myself." The patient felt greatly relieved and reported her psychological comfort in going through the procedure, which she found unpleasant and somewhat painful. She was pleasantly surprised at how professional the staff were and that the procedure in no way resembled a sexual situation.

Reactivation of feelings of guilt and shame and accompanying fears of retaliation for previous transgressions. Patients often voice, but more frequently wonder, "Why has this happened to me?" Physical illness may be perceived as a punishment for prior crimes, either in deed or in thought. Occasionally, the guilt experienced by the patient relates to reality issues—for example, in an overweight patient who has a heart attack or a patient with lung cancer who was a heavy smoker. Illness can serve as a metaphor for guilt for a patient when it is viewed as confirmation or proof that he or she is a bad person.

Regression

The stresses of illness and of hospitalization as outlined by Strain and Grossman (1975) follow from the developmental stresses of childhood. The experience for the patient is a *regressive* one. The individual is placed in a situation of dependency that replicates the experience of childhood. Behavior, coping skills, and experience of and expression of emotion all take on qualities from previous stages of the person's development. Manifestations may range from the temporary loss of recent gains in psychological makeup to a behavioral style more appropriate for a young child. Regression is a common response for many people when they are ill, but is most easily observed in children. Febrile 5- or 6-year-olds may suck their thumbs or act in a clingy manner—behaviors they had abandoned some months or years previously. Although regression unfortunately evokes a negative image, it is not necessarily an undesirable response. Regression might be better thought of as a *dedifferentiation* of the individual, such that he or she is in a more plastic state, but one that is simultaneously more primitive. As such, regression provides the person more flexibility to adapt to the environment and the potential for positive change. This conception also suggests that, for some period of time, the person may function in a manner different from his or her usual one, which exerts a stress upon friends, family, and caregivers. Regression implies that the person is using defenses that are less reality oriented, based more upon unresolved conflicts from childhood, less stable, and less adaptive to the demands of the environment (Field 1979).

The regressed adult operates with a defensive structure more appropriate to someone who typically functions at a lower level of psychiatric health. The adequacy with which they negotiated the stresses and conflicts of development, and the strengths and/or deficiencies of their relationships with their parents, will play a crucial role in how adults will cope with illness and hospitalization. This, then, is the starting point for the patient. The lower the starting point, the more primitive the defensive structure to which the patient regresses. Simultaneous with this process are patients' reactions to their regression and their attempts to return to their usual level of function and control. Frequently, it is these attempts to regain control—and not the regression—that generates the request for a psychiatric consultation.

Character Styles

The character style of the patient will also influence his or her experience of illness and hospitalization. Character style does not mean character pathology; rather, it refers to the characteristic manner in which an individual experiences and behaves in the world. We all have a personality that has certain typical features. Although there are pathological concomitants to the personality types, the consultant is always alert to not overemphasize the "diagnosis" versus the patient's characterological reactions (Geringer and Stern 1986). Character style thus plays an important role for the psychiatrist in understanding a particular patient/doctor dyad as the doctor is engaged positively or negatively by the patient's character (Kahana and Bibring 1964).

A review of the seven personality types, as described by Kahana and Bibring (1964), and a conceptualization of how the anxieties characteristic of each of these types of patients should be approached, are presented in the following paragraphs.[2]

[2] The original work (Kahana RJ, Bibring GL: Personality types in medical management, in *Psychiatry and Medical Practice in a General Hospital.* Edited by Zinberg N. New York, International Uni-

People who are dependent and overdemanding (oral). These individuals seem to need special attention and have an urgency about their needs. They can be impulsive, seemingly naive, and demanding of care without limitations from their doctors. There is the potential for anger, depression, and inappropriate use of medications or drugs stemming from a low tolerance for frustration. Persons with this character style are in conflict around their fears of abandonment and their wishes for unlimited care. Illness reawakens the desire to exist in a secure, infantile state where all of their needs are provided for by another. Acute illness is perceived as the result of a failure of protection and caring by others. In dealing with such individuals, physicians need to structure their interactions to convey the intent to care for the patient as is necessary—that is, make it clear what they will do to help the patient recover. The inevitable setting of limits should be presented not as punishment for the patient's inexhaustible demands, nor as the doctor's withdrawal, but as thoughtfully considered realities.

People who are orderly and controlled (compulsive). "Knowledge is power" might best describe these people, who seek to control their anxiety by finding out as many "facts" as they can. These orderly, neat, conscientious individuals may be quite obstinate in their dealings regarding their health. In the patient role, their defenses against impulses to soil, be aggressive, or act hedonistically are threatened by their illness, thereby increasing their need to be orderly and to contain emotions, which results in ritualized or intensely formal behavior. In an effort to gain control through knowledge, such patients ask questions repeatedly. Never satisfied that they have enough information, they may become indecisive when they have to make decisions regarding their care. "Informed consent" can become a caricature with such patients. The provision of details of what the physician plans, why a procedure is required, and the science of the medical approach is reassuring to these patients. Giving adequate—but not overwhelming—detail permits these people to use intellectualization to calm their anxiety and the fear of losing control of their impulses. When practically possible, they benefit from active participation in treatment planning and in carrying out appropriate components of their treatment.

People who are dramatizing and captivating (hysterical). These patients are often charming, interesting, and pleasurably challenging. They act toward the physician in a personal and warm manner. The physician may wonder if these individuals are malingering, given the contrast of their way of relating with the fact that they claim to be ill. Their dramatic, sometimes teasing or seductive manner and their attempts to form idealized and intimate relationships with their doctors protects these patients from their fears of punishment for forbidden unconscious wishes. Illness means that they are weak, unattractive, and unloved and it is expe-

---

versities Press, 1964, pp. 108–123) is strongly recommended as important reading for the psychiatric consultant.

rienced as a threat to their masculinity or femininity. Attempts to master their fears may result in displays of their strength, power, and sexuality. Such attempts at reestablishing control typically overstimulate, frighten, anger, and distance doctors and nurses from these patients. At times, the staff's reactions, particularly to the patient's seductiveness, are an effort to control their own impulses aroused by the patient. Establishing a comfortable degree of appreciation for the patient's attractiveness and strength, while remaining aware of the possibility of their seeking intense emotional involvement, is the ideal way for the physician to treat such patients. The often-quoted clinical pearl of the physician telling the counterphobic body builder with a recent myocardial infarction that he has to be "strong enough" to lie in bed doing "specialized" finger and toe exercises, as opposed to vigorous calisthenics, is the insightful comment to the anxious patient with a hysterical character style.

People who are long-suffering and self-sacrificing (masochistic). This personality style is perplexing to medical staff, who cannot understand how unfortunate events seem to "occur" to the patient. There is often the suspicion that these individuals play some role in their misfortunes and there is often "evidence" that this is the case (though the causation is on an unconscious basis). Patients with this character style are exhibitionistic about their suffering, in contrast to their humble manner. The need to prepay for pleasure—or to pay for experienced or fantasied pleasure—fuels such patients' experience and behavior. They wish to be loved and cared for, but feel unworthy and guilty; thus, they expect to either not get what they want or to be punished for having gotten their wishes gratified. Such patients can cause great frustration in their doctors, who often find a patient seemingly worsened by news of his or her positive progress. Although these patients do not malinger or create illness, they are disheartened by the good news. Acknowledging their difficulties and suffering, and demonstrating an understanding of their "burden" works far better for these patients. Structuring recovery as a tough ordeal, or as motivated to benefit others for whom the patient feels responsible, may enable such individuals to resolve their conflicts regarding attention and care from the medical staff.

People who are guarded and querulous (paranoid). The suspicious, watchful individual who reacts to the most minimal of slights is obvious to even the least psychologically minded observer. These people overreact to any criticism and seem to expect an attack at any moment. Everything is externalized—that is, nothing is their fault. This attitude can be particularly problematic in the hospital setting, where there is much in the way of bad news, unexpected discomfort, lost laboratory results, or incorrect meals. It follows from this that such patients blame others for their illness. Their fears of being harmed intensify when they are ill, which increases their aggressive impulses. The anxiety thus stimulated is defended against by an increase in guardedness, suspiciousness, and the need to control others—principally, the doctors and nurses who are responsible for their care. These are patients for whom care needs to be taken that they not be surprised by what happens in the hospital. Particular attention should be paid to informing them of what is expected to happen at each step of the diagnostic and therapeutic process. There should be an attempt to acknowledge how these patients feel rather than a hostile confrontation of their "perceptions." Such attempts at empathy can be particularly difficult for an exhausted intern or resident. It is sometimes possible to ally with these patients and to enlist their cooperation in "putting up with" the realities of the hospital setting.

People who have a feeling of superiority (narcissistic). These people see themselves as being powerful and important, whether their station in society substantiates that feeling or not. Overtly, they may appear quite humble or modest, but this facade is seen through by others. Relating to a doctor, upon whom the patient must depend, can be a difficult task, especially if the doctor does not reinforce the patient's special status by having a special status him- or herself. Illness threatens these individuals' need to be perfect and invulnerable, and their increased grandiosity and entitlement serve as defensive maneuvers. They easily find fault with their caregivers but fear that the doctors might not be able to help them. The fantasy of these patients that they must have the "great professor" can be demoralizing for the intern or resident, who feels devalued. The tactful, not defensive, acknowledgment of one's knowledge, training, and abilities is reassuring to such patients, who can then idealize their doctor and contain their anxiety.

People who appear aloof and uninvolved (schizoid). These patients seem eccentric or odd in their behavior on the ward, uninvolved with their doctors and nurses and seemingly "too calm" regarding their illness. They do not seem easily swayed by things and appear quite independent. This external calm conceals a fragile interior that requires a withdrawal from everyday life to manage otherwise overwhelming anxiety. Whereas these individuals may function apparently well in their regular lives, and may have VIP status as a result of their accomplishments, their illness and hospitalization present a stress with which they cannot cope. This stress may result in their denial that they are ill, in spite of hard evidence to the contrary, as illness disrupts their carefully balanced system. Although the impulse to "break through" to such patients may be strong, a better management technique acknowledges their need to remain safe, with the physician and family doing a large portion of the decision making.

The Doctor

In the teaching hospital, patients are cared for by their primary care physician, often a first- or second-year resident. Every doctor has, of course, his or her own personality style, which influences how they adjust to their role as physician and to working in the medical setting. There are physicians who face each patient as a test of their personal intelligence, power, and ability. When stymied by a difficult diagnosis or faced with a disease for which no treatment is effective, they experience a personal and painful defeat that may propel them toward doing more and more, even when a more appropriate approach would be to do less. Other physicians are brilliant at making a diagnosis and reading X rays or frozen sections, but deal poorly with patients and treat them as if they were things, not people. Such physicians are comfortable with X rays, laboratory results, electrocardiogram (ECG) findings, and the like (i.e., facts). Knowledge and information has a powerful—even magical—quality, whereas the intangibles such as symptoms without physical findings, pain with no obvious trauma or lesion, or strong emotions make them less comfortable. This is in contrast to the fact that many physicians are compulsive, with the accompanying triad of doubt, guilt, and an exaggerated sense of responsibility (Gabbard 1985). They experience difficulty with taking time off for themselves or their family and feel they don't do enough, although they work extremely hard. Their unrealistic sense of responsibility results in self-recriminations for things that are not in anyone's control.

There are many important accommodations physicians must accomplish to work successfully in the medical setting. The most important task is to make the pain, the suffering, the odors, and the infliction of discomfort or pain a part of the routine of their daily existence. By making it part of their routine, doctors are protected from the emotional disquiet that engaging in these activities would otherwise arouse. These are all the aspects of illness and hospitalization that frighten, stress, and anger patients. Nothing of this medical world is routine to a patient, yet their caregivers act as if it was all just part of the job, which for them it is! "Routine bloods" are not routine to the person whose blood is routinely withdrawn for testing, nor does pain or the invasive quality of a procedure necessarily make it less or more routine or acceptable for a patient. A case in point is the magnetic resonance imaging (MRI) scan, which although perhaps one of the least invasive procedures today, is one that frightens many patients so much that they cannot undergo the procedure.

This is not to suggest that physicians should be insensitive or uncaring. However, they must endure in a setting that is stressful—a setting in which they become aware that they have only minimal control and yet carry the responsibility of being omnipotent. They must learn to split experiences that are otherwise unitary, yet not become cold and unemotional. For example, the foundation of the entire medical experience, the history and physical, requires such a disconnection. Patients would be understandably distressed if physicians reacted with arousal or disgust when they asked about intimate details of a patient's life or when they examined a patient. Yet, in everyday life, seeing or touching a person without their clothes on is expected to result in an emotional response. Medical students and physicians must learn to isolate themselves from any erotic affect, yet not become overly cold and distant. Erotic sensations noted by the physician can indicate that the patient is using seduction and sexuality in a way more intense than other patients. This kind of observation permits an understanding of the patient's defensive dynamics and allows the physician to deal with the feelings in an appropriate manner. Similarly, causing pain and suffering is consciously experienced by most people as "bad." Unless physicians can separate the necessity of sometimes causing pain from being bad, they run the risk of experiencing themselves negatively. Such self-perceptions can damage their self-image and lead to their becoming depressed. Not surprisingly, there is a high incidence of depression in house staff (Valko and Clayton 1975).

Psychiatric consultants witness astonishing behavior and attitudes in house staff. Although it is common to see exceptionally caring and compassionate interns and residents, the angry, impulsive, overtly prejudiced house officer is also not unknown. Consultation case discussions sometimes center upon the doctor, not the patient, as the person who really needs the help. Patients are occasionally treated in a way that is shocking in its apparent unconcern for their pain, well-being, or need for continued care posthospitalization. The following clinical example may help illustrate this point:

> A 32-year-old man with tuberculosis, who was also human immunodeficiency virus (HIV) seropositive, was refusing treatment. He had a long substance abuse history and was currently homeless. Although there was ample evidence that the patient's judgment was impaired and that he could not comply with necessary treatment, the resident insisted that the patient be transferred to the psychiatry department and threatened to discharge the patient to the emergency room—a violation of hospital policy and state code. No degree of explanation sufficed to change this physician's attitude. At the last moment, a senior psychiatrist spoke with the resident, who was being pushed into action by a senior member of the medical department. He outlined for the resident that he saw him jeopardizing his career with the fantasy that he would be a hero for his department, that someone would get into trouble for his actions and it was not likely to be a tenured professor and, finally, that it was understandable to dislike patients such as this one. The resident reluctantly agreed to abandon the plan only when the psychiatrist promised that he would personally oversee the task of finding an appropriate disposition for the patient.

How can such behavior be understood? The regressive pull of the hospital setting affects all who come within its walls. The experiences of feeling not in control of the situation and of feeling helpless are sources of this regressive pull for physicians. Our comfort with facts and science is of little use as we confront the scant resources available for patients, the effects of drugs and alcohol, the increasing impact of acquired immunodeficiency syndrome (AIDS), and the financial crises and cutbacks in services being faced by many hospitals. With all that medical technology offers, interns and residents become painfully aware there is little that they can actually cure. Young physicians find their anxieties about not knowing enough exacerbated by the experience that knowledge does not always suffice in our dealings with disease. Their habitual use of intellectualization does not succeed in calming their anxiety. The fantasy that others have the power and control proves ultimately disappointing as they begin to recognize that those at higher levels (e.g., the more senior physicians, the administrators, the vice-presidents, the politicians) have no more control over the health care system than they do. The experience of becoming a doctor occurs in a setting of sleep deprivation, never-ceasing work, continual interruptions (Lurie et al. 1989), and disconnection from friends, family, and partners. There is the constant fear that one's actions or inactions will result in disease or death, and the fear that one will be being exposed as inadequate. There is the real concern that an accidental needle stick could result in the physician's own death (Link et al. 1988). These fears stimulate rage and an increase in aggressive impulses, which must be dealt with by the defenses available to the doctor. The chronic fatigue, nutritional deprivation, and unrelentingly intense workload—all the components that make internships and residencies what we all remember them to be—militate against the employment of higher-level defenses.

We observe the use of four main defensive operations in this setting: *splitting* (e.g., the simultaneous wish to kill the patient while heroically trying to save his or her life), *primitive denial* (e.g., making the pronouncement "this patient is medically cleared" for a patient clearly still in need of medical attention), *projection* (e.g., admissions in most hospitals are referred to as "hits"; house staff talk of being "hurt" by patients—meaning that they are overwhelmed by the work), and *projective identification* (e.g., a consultant experiences anxiety while working with a doctor who claims that the consultant's anxiety is making him or her anxious). The overwhelming desire—if not the basic motivation—of the intern becomes "to get finished with my work and get out of the hospital"—that is, to escape.

The majority of young physicians go through this maturational stage of regression with a starting point of relative psychological health. They regress into a borderline-like personality while they work in the hospital, reverting to their normal personality when away for any length of time longer than overnight. What seems like irrational and impulsive behavior and ideation can be understood as a regression necessary to change from student to physician. Some cope poorly with the stress of the medical setting and employ more destructive defensive measures, such as drug or alcohol abuse and promiscuous sexual behavior, or are unable to complete their training. However, the vast majority of physicians go through this developmental stage successfully. The cognitive dissonance imposed upon young doctors results in an idealization of the experience such that, following internship and residency, they feel that the period was "good" for them and behave unconsciously to perpetuate the status quo, seemingly forgetful of the degree to which they suffered. These same house staff become the faculty members who train, supervise, and set the emotional tone for future house staff.

The Psychiatric Consultant

Into this setting comes the psychiatric consultant with the request to evaluate "depression" or "competency to sign out against medical advice (AMA)." Prior to their assignment to the consultation-liaison service, these physicians have undergone a training experience different from that of their nonpsychiatric colleagues. By postgraduate year 3 (PGY-3) or 4 (PGY-4), psychiatric residents have been instructed in the technique of listening to one's emotions as a guide. They have, in supervision, faced their reactions to patients' rage, irrationality, seductiveness, depression, psychosis, and the like. They have lived the orderly life of the psychiatrist, each hour scheduled with patients, meetings, supervision, lunch, or personal psychotherapy or psychoanalysis. Psychiatry is a rather private endeavor: patients are seen behind closed doors, their charts are often kept in special files in hospitals, there are no "walk-rounds" to discuss cases, and patients themselves wish their psychiatric treatment to remain a secret. This environment is quite different from that of the hospital medical ward, where privacy is an illusion, charts are open, patients' beds are enclosed with curtains, not walls, and family, nurses, and physicians are waiting nearby to hear the psychiatric opinion—even the comings and goings of the psychiatrist are charted in the nurses' notes ("Psych with pat. 13:05 until 13:12. Pat. comfortable, offers no complaints"). The psychiatric consultant's once-orderly life becomes unpredictable, as in the hospital one never knows when the next consultation will be requested or when a page will disturb an activity. Accustomed to wearing business clothes, consultants now don the garb of the medical setting, white coats, and are exposed to all the same stimuli as their nonpsychiatric colleagues. How often is a therapy session conducted with the patient in pajamas, with blood infusing or a dialysis treatment ongoing, with the patient's breathing controlled by a device, or with the patient requesting help off the bedpan? The strict boundaries of the psychiatric situation become less defined, if not absent altogether. Some psychiatric residents react with anxiety; others react with fear, withdrawal, or aggression (Mendelson and Meyer 1961; Perry and Viederman 1981a). How a particular resident copes depends on that individual's personality style, his or her ability to tolerate regression, how well he or she traversed the developmental stage of the internship, and the dynamics of why he or she chose psychiatry as a specialty.

One response is to feel inadequate, as though one has little to offer compared with the "real doctors" caring for the patient (Perry and Viederman 1981b). Those students who chose psychiatry to avoid the traumatic aspects of medical practice will experience the return to the bedside with a loss of self-esteem and a reliving of the anxiety of internship. They have opted for psychiatry as a result of their feelings of inadequacy rather than through a positive choice. These psychiatrists seem unaware of their own skills, of the depth of their knowledge base regarding human behavior and psychopathology, and of their expertise in psychopharmacology. They cannot acknowledge that it is probable that they know more medicine than do the interns who call them for consultation. Some residents deal with these feelings of inadequacy by adopting an active, sometimes aggressive stance, taking over the case both medically and psychiatrically. Neither extreme is successful, as the physician who requests the consultation devalues and ignores the fearful consultant and is angered by and becomes oppositional with the aggressive one.

Psychiatric residents are often frightened by the regression they observe in their patients and mistakenly assume that traditional psychotherapeutic techniques are inappropriate in the medical setting. This is certainly not the case, however; many medically ill patients respond quite favorably to psychotherapy. One important difference is that such patients tire quickly and cannot tolerate the full time of an outpatient psychotherapy session. The regression of their medical illness may place them in a unique position to come to an in-depth understanding of themselves that would take considerably longer if they were not in the hospital. Psychotherapy can be very exciting and beneficial when the consultant is aware of its potential (Blacher 1984; Viederman and Perry 1980).

It is remarkable how little has changed since the beginning of consultation-liaison psychiatry as a formal service in hospitals (Lipowsky 1967a, 1967b, 1967c). New consultants find themselves needing both to prove their value and to assuage the fear that psychiatrists can read minds—and thus can expose the anxiety, rage, guilt and other intense emotions that consultees experience. In part, the need to repeat work done by previous consultants is the result of the constant turnover of house staff; the psychiatric consultant meets with new physicians each year. It also speaks to the intensity of physicians' experience of working in the medical setting.

Many excellent texts focus on the details of psychiatric consultation in the medical setting; these constitute important reading for the psychiatric consultant (Cassem 1991; Hales and Yudofsky 1987; Houpt and Brodie 1986; Kornfeld and Finkel 1982; Stoudemire and Fogel 1987). The systems approach to psychiatric consultation deserves special attention. To make sense of the bewildering world of the hospital, the psychiatric consultant must become a systems expert, looking at three domains for each individual: the biological, the psychological, and the sociological. Consultation psychiatrists are always "biopsychosocial" in their approach. A systems approach focuses on the interaction between each of these domains and the resultant expression of that interaction. It takes into account each domain's dispositional qualities or tendencies—for example, expressing emotions with physical symptoms rather than psychically (biological), being chronically unhappy and looking at everything with a depressive cast (psychological), or coming from a single-parent home with a parent who was alcoholic (sociological). By exploring each of these domains, the consultant can understand the patient in terms of *why now, why this way, what led to this,* and *what can be done to influence it?* Each of us has biases that favor one domain or the other and that will affect not only how we understand the data we collect, but also *which* data we choose to collect. A systems approach requires that the consultant pay attention to each domain in order to proceed with assessment.

In giving a history, patients typically describe life events such as a divorce, a graduation from college, or a job promotion. Situations in the hospital (e.g., when a patient is labeled suicidal, attempts to hit a nurse, or requests to sign out AMA) may also be conceptualized in the same manner as life events. A divorce does not happen in a single moment; rather, many events lead up to it. Even the finalization of a divorce includes meeting with lawyers, signing the papers, going home after the meeting, and so forth. What we call *events* are really a condensation of *processes* that began some time before—hours, days, even years before the event (Albert and Kornfeld 1973; Miller 1973a). Without understanding the process that leads up to the patient's request to sign out of the hospital against medical advice, it is not possible to arrive at a strategy for finding a way for the patient to stay in the hospital—or, if necessary, to leave and not be harmed. Is the patient experiencing pain that has been undermedicated, and has the decision to sign out come from anger at being made to suffer? Is there evidence of increasing agitation, inability to sleep, strange behavior, or comments that suggest that the signing out is part of a psychotic process? By using a systems approach, the consultant can identify which domain to emphasize, where the stresses and strains are in each of the domains, and how they have interacted to result in the current situation. Stresses and strains in the hospital system will be reflected by the most dependent member of the system, and that is the patient. Consultants recognize that they start at a disadvantage, because the "problem" has been formulated not by the patient, but by someone else—the physician, the nurse, or the social worker. That individual's biases will influence how they conceptualize the problem. A clinical example will help clarify this approach:

> A young woman with rheumatic heart disease was requesting to sign out AMA. She had been admitted with congestive heart failure, which had been treated with medication. She insisted on signing out and going to another hospital—one considered by the house staff and faculty to be less able to care for her disorder. The patient was adamant about the fact that she was not liked, that the staff was prejudiced toward her, and that she would get better care at the other hospital. Her "competency" was questioned and the concern that she was either psychotic/paranoid or depressed/suicidal was raised.
>
> A review of her history, interviews with the various physicians involved, discussions with the nurses, and the interview with the patient revealed that there was considerable controversy about how she should be managed. The cardiologists favored medications for as long as she was maintained adequately. The surgeons wanted to operate on her now, while she was well. Each group wrote competing notes and competed with her for a decision. The patient came from disadvantaged circumstances and a home where angry feelings were not verbalized but immediately acted upon—when her father was angry at her mother, he simply left. She could not understand why, if the doctors liked her, they did not tell her what was the "best" path to take. Their disagreement was perceived by her to mean she was not liked, which made her angry. Her decision to go to a hospital where they told her what to do, without giving her options, was a way to reestablish herself as someone whom the doctors liked.
>
> The system could not be changed for this patient, because the various physicians could not agree and could not let go. She was considerably relieved when she was told she could go to the other hospital and that her records would be forwarded, but she was welcome to return if she changed her mind. Her anxiety reduced, her angry demeanor changed and she thanked everyone for their concern.

The strain in the system for this patient arose outside of her, but within the sociological domain. The stress induced by her physicians' disagreement was an intolerable experience for her. Since stresses and strains in a system may act at some distance from the patient (i.e., may not be included in the typical information collected in the psychiatric interview), the consultant needs to investigate all of the domains. Although it is likely one domain will take prominence for a patient, ignoring the others leads to an incomplete job or an "unresolvable" consultation.

Psychiatric consultants have the opportunity to view the hospital, the patients, and the staff not from the outside, but as participant observers. Their clinical endeavors require an active component that is based on a psychodynamic understanding of the setting. This does not mean a "wild analysis" of patients and staff, but a depth of perception often greater than that available in office psychotherapy. It also requires a structure to support the consultant; the rounds, conferences, supervision, and availability of senior consultants is crucial for the operation of a consultation service. Similar to the structure of an inpatient psychiatry service that treats severe character disorders (Rosnick 1987), the intense emotional atmosphere of the hospital setting is well suited for teaching psychiatry in the broadest sense and a place where the consultant can accomplish significant psychological gains in work with patients (Viederman and Perry 1980).

The term *consultation-liaison* does not adequately describe the activity outlined above. It once seemed appropriate to separate the *consultation* (seeing the patient, reviewing the medical record, making recommendations, and instituting therapy) from *liaison* activities (meeting with nurses, house staff, and other physicians). There was then, and is today, no real separation between these activities. Psychiatric consultants' forming working relationships with nonpsychiatric consultees and other professionals was once called the liaison component. A consultation conducted without discussion of the patient with all of the staff involved is a poorly done consultation, not one lacking in liaison activity. Opportunities to educate colleagues have always been a crucial part of the consultation process. Liaison activities are one component of the psychiatrist's ability to work in the medical setting, but if the psychiatrist were not also seeing patients in consultation, there would be little value in the so-called liaison work. The name is familiar, and it is easier to say "C/L" than offer a long-winded explanation. Although the name may date back to an antiquated conceptualization of the psychiatric role in the medical setting, the modern approach should not be ignored.

Conclusion

The psychiatrist brings a unique "gift" to the patient that is of vital importance (Eissler 1955). This gift is the hope of understanding and the attempt to resolve the patient's problem. In order to accomplish these goals, the psychiatrist employs a specialized skill—that of listening. Listening is an active process for a psychiatrist, one that requires training and a diverse knowledge base that integrates psychodynamics, psychiatric nosology, and psychopharmacology. Hope does not ignore the fact that the patient has a life-threatening illness from which he or she is dying, or the disadvantaged social circumstances from which the patient came and will return, or any of the other harsh realities of the patient's life. Hope *does* promise the engagement of the two individuals in a process of exploration and understanding for the patient's benefit. Communicating hope is a skill that can be taught, but is often too difficult for medical/surgical house staff to master early on in their training.

I would like to close with a hypothesis concerning the essential nature of the doctor-patient relationship and its special manifestation in the medical setting for a psychiatric consultant. Why do patients talk with us, reveal to us, and face great psychic pain within themselves? Such encounters frequently occur in the context of physical discomfort and inconvenience, or in embarrassing, humiliating, and vulnerable situations. Patients regularly identify that this person in a white coat is a psychiatrist. Is it that we sit down to talk, that we do not have a stethoscope around our neck, or that we introduce ourselves? Is it how we structure the situation? Or is it an attitude with which we approach patients—that intention to understand them and what is occurring in their life at this moment? I posit here that it is more the latter, although the other factors are components in the formation of this attitude.

Understanding is the central need all patients possess in their relationship with their physicians. The genetics of this need trace back to the earliest parent-child interactions and form an unconscious expectation when an individual becomes ill and is seized by the regressive pull of the illness and hospitalization. In the early dyad, the parent learns to understand the child who cannot verbalize beyond crying (Stern 1985). The parent learns to tune into another mode of listening and thus becomes aware of messages that are new—that is, not experienced before. Observe a mother who hears her child cry and, upon entering the room, begins the interaction of understanding in her voice, body movements, actions with the child, and investigations to learn the cause of the distress. The "average expectable mother" will recognize and verbalize, "I have never heard that cry before. What's wrong?" This is not confined to mothers, since fathers can become equally adept at such listening if they spend the time. The child forms a representation of the parent that incorporates the experience of being understood and of being comforted as is appropriate to the understanding. The child who is fed when wet and uncomfortable, for example, does not have this experience. All parents and children have some miscommunication, and some parent-child relationships are deformed by the parents' inability to listen. Yet the majority seem to work quite well. It is this expectation from the earliest years of life that the patient brings to the hospital—frightened, in pain, confused, even unconscious.

Although most of the time patients feel adequately understood by their physicians throughout the process of diagnosis and therapy, they may still complain that their care makes them feel like a "number." Sometimes, however, the intensity of medical technology can push this unique function of understanding out of its central position in the care of patients. Such a situation occurs when the physician has not been able to establish and communicate an understanding of the patient. When the patient can no longer tolerate his or her feeling of not being understood, the doctor-patient relationship is disrupted, necessitating a psychiatric consultation. The psychiatric consultant recognizes the patient's conscious or unconscious wish for an omnipotent and omniscient parent. Neither depriving nor gratifying, the psychiatrist's endeavors to understand, to listen, and to help are beneficial to the physician and the patient alike. For patients in these circumstances, there is no more powerful healing art than psychiatry.

For Further Study

Bird B: Talking with Patients. Philadelphia, JB Lippincott, 1955

Cassem NH: Massachusetts General Hospital Handbook of General Hospital Psychiatry. St. Louis, MO, CV Mosby, 1991

Faguet RA, Fawzy FI, Wellisch DK: Contemporary Models in Liaison Psychiatry. New York, Spectrum, 1978

Finkel JB: Consultation-Liaison Psychiatry: Current Trends and Future Perspectives. New York, Grune & Stratton, 1983

Hales RE, Yudofsky SC: Textbook of Neuropsychiatry. Washington, DC, American Psychiatric Press, 1987

Houpt JL, Brodie HKH: Consultation-Liaison Psychiatry and Behavioral Medicine. New York, Basic Books, 1986

Kornfeld DS, Finkel JB: Psychiatric Management for Medical Practitioners. New York, Grune & Stratton, 1982

Oken D: Psychiatric Clinics of North America: Consultation-Liaison Psychiatry. Philadelphia, PA, WB Saunders, 1987

Pasnau RO: Consultation-Liaison Psychiatry. New York, Grune & Stratton, 1975

Stoudemire A, Fogel BS: Medical Psychiatric Practice, Vols 1 and 2. Washington, DC, American Psychiatric Press, 1991

Zabarenko L, Pittenger RA, Zabarenko RN: Primary Medical Practice: A Psychiatric Evaluation. St. Louis, MO, Warren H. Green, 1968

References

Albert HD, Kornfeld DS: The threat to sign out against medical advice. Ann Intern Med 79:888–891, 1973

Blacher RS: The briefest encounter: psychotherapy for medical and surgical patients. Gen Hosp Psychiatry 6:226–232, 1984

Cassem NH: Massachusetts General Hospital Handbook of General Hospital Psychiatry. St. Louis, MO, CV Mosby, 1991

Eissler KR: The Psychiatrist and the Dying Patient. New York, International Universities Press, 1955

Field HL: Defense mechanisms in psychosomatic medicine. Psychosomatics 20:690–700, 1979

Gabbard GO: The role of compulsiveness in the normal physician. JAMA 254:2926–2929, 1985

Geringer ES, Stern TA: Coping with medical illness: the impact of personality types. Psychosomatics 27:251–261, 1986

Kahana RJ, Bibring GL: Personality types in medical management, in Psychiatry and Medical Practice in a General Hospital. Edited by Zinberg N. New York, International Universities Press, 1964, pp 108–123

Kornfeld DS: The hospital environment: its impact on the patient, in Stress and Survival. Edited by Garfield CA. St. Louis, MO, CV Mosby, 1979, pp 154–164

Link NR, Feinngold AR, Charap MH et al: Concerns of medical and pediatric house officers about acquiring AIDS from their patients. Am J Public Health 78:455–459, 1988

Lipowsky ZJ: Review of consultation psychiatry and psychosomatic medicine, I: general principles. Psychosom Med 29:153–171, 1967a

Lipowsky ZJ: Review of consultation psychiatry and psychosomatic medicine, II: clinical aspects. Psychosom Med 29:201–224, 1967b

Lipowsky ZJ: Review of consultation psychiatry and psychosomatic medicine, III: theoretical issues. Psychosom Med 30:395–422, 1967c

Lucente FE, Fleck S: A study of hospitalization anxiety in 408 medical and surgical patients. Psychosom Med 34:304–312, 1972

Lurie N, Rank B, Parenti C, et al: How do house officers spend their nights? N Engl J Med 320:1673–1677, 1989

Mendelson M, Meyer E: Countertransference problems of the liaison psychiatrist. Psychiatry 138:115–122, 1961

Miller WB: Psychiatric consultation, I: a general system approach. Psychiatr Med 4:135–145, 1973a

Miller WB: Psychiatric consultation, II: conceptual and pragmatic issues of formulation. Psychiatr Med 4:251–271, 1973b

Perry SW, Viederman M: Adaptation of residents to consultation-liaison psychiatry, I: working with the physically ill. Gen Hosp Psychiatry 3:141–147, 1981a

Perry SW, Viederman M: Adaptation of residents to consultation-liaison psychiatry, II: working with the nonpsychiatric staff. Gen Hosp Psychiatry 3:149–156, 1981b

Rosnick L: Use of a long-term inpatient unit as a site for learning psychotherapy. Psychiatr Clin North Am: Intensive Hospital Treatment 10:309–323, 1987

Stern DN: The Interpersonal World of the Infant. New York, Basic Books, 1985

Stoudemire A, Fogel BS: Principles of Medical Psychiatry. New York, Grune & Stratton, 1987

Strain JJ, Grossman S: Psychological Care of the Medically Ill. New York, Appleton-Century-Crofts, 1975

Valko R, Clayton P: Depression in the internship. Diseases of the Nervous System 36:26–29, 1975

Viederman M, Perry SW: Use of a psychodynamic life narrative in the treatment of depression in the physically ill. Gen Hosp Psychiatry 3:177–185, 1980

Chapter 7

The Community Clinic

William H. Sledge, M.D.,
and Ken Marcus, M.D.

This is a time of great excitement and great challenge for those who are providing mental health services in the public sector; at the same time, many of society's most vexing problems are manifested in this area. The reduction in the nation's large state mental health hospitals' long-stay patient populations over the past quarter-century and the consequent shift in the locus of care to a community-based service system model (Lamb and Goertzel 1977), the spiraling health care costs in the context of the severe economic recession of the late 1980s and early 1990s, the decay and social disintegration of the nation's inner cities, the scourge of substance abuse, and the emergence of many unserved and underserved clinical populations (the homeless, the traumatically brain-injured, the mentally ill elderly, the mentally ill retarded, and the mentally ill criminal offending, to name only a few) have challenged mental health policy planners and clinical administrators to develop service systems that address the complex needs of these patient populations. Issues of care access, quality, and cost-effectiveness vie in dynamic tension, achieving complex yet constantly changing equilibria. Resources are insufficient to the task: hence the catchwords of the 1990s—"prioritization," "resource allocation," and "rationing."

In addition to attending to the clinical and rehabilitation needs of individuals in these populations, service systems must address a variety of other essential needs: food, clothing, shelter, spending money, recreation, work, companionship, safety, and security. Difficult decisions must be made: Who will and will not receive care? How much care will be provided and of what kind? What standards will be used for decision making? What proportion of the resource pool is to be devoted to research and prevention efforts, and what proportion to the care and treatment of those already ill? Who is to make these decisions, and by what process?

Needless to say, in this context the usefulness of a psychodynamic and psychoanalytic perspective must compete with the potential contributions of other perspectives for the time and attention of practitioners and policy makers who must confront these difficult problems in their everyday work. The purpose of this chapter is to review the characteristics of a public-sector system of psychiatric care and to demonstrate how a psychoanalytic perspective can be of substantial use to those working in such a system.

Background

There was a time when the aims and goals of psychoanalysis were clearly preeminent in determining the modalities of treatment in all of American psychiatry, including the public sector. As a point of historical interest, Freud's only American trip was to give his well-known five introductory lectures in Worcester, Massachusetts, at a state psychiatric hospital. Clinical services were organized along lines of care that resembled a private practice model, emphasizing the role of psychotherapy to the relative exclusion of psychopharmacological, behavioral, and rehabilitative treatment modalities. Psychoanalysis in the 1940s and 1950s served as a powerful paradigm for understanding human behavior and experience, just as it does today. Early attempts to apply psychoanalytic principles in the public sector centered on the treatment of those with severe mental illness or, in some instances, of those with conditions that were of special interest to society, such as juvenile delinquency (Aichorn 1948). Much was learned about psychosis and other severe mental conditions through the application of psychoanalysis or psychoanalytically derived methods to the treatment of these conditions; however, the efficacy of these treatment methods alone for patients with severe mental illness has not been great enough to ensure their continuation, at least as the primary form of treatment.

Nonetheless, a psychoanalytic framework can be of significant use in understanding and addressing other important phenomena and problems that arise in public-sector work—for example, countertransference (particularly with severely ill patients and across cultural, ethnic, and class lines); aspects of organizational dynamics, service system organization, and group phenomena; simultaneous application of adjunctive and/or multiple clinical modalities; and issues of role relations in multidisciplinary settings. Psychodynamically informed individual and group treatments do continue to constitute an essential—albeit expensive—element of the public-sector practitioner's clinical armamentaria, especially when used in conjunction with other treatment and intervention approaches. Hence, even though the use of traditional, office-based psychoanalytic psychotherapies has decreased in public-sector work—to paraphrase an oft-quoted quip—reports of its demise are greatly exaggerated. Psychoanalysis remains a substantial force and still has much to offer both as a primary treatment and as a conceptual tool in all settings in which people with mental illness are cared for by mental health professionals (Perry et al. 1987).

Psychoanalysis provides a powerful framework for understanding otherwise inexplicable symptoms and behaviors and can contribute to the development of treatment strategies even when achieving insight is not an explicit or primary goal of treatment.

Psychoanalytic Principles

In this section, we will not repeat an explication of principles noted elsewhere in this volume. Rather, we remind the reader of key concepts from psychoanalytic theory that are particularly germane for use in the public sector. Psychoanalytic principles posit that the conditions treated by psychoanalysis are disorders of mind—which is to say that they are disorders of meaning and symbol making, including the notion of the representation and structure of psychic reality, the representation of self and other, and the ability to use symbols in communication with others (Beres and Joseph 1970; Edelson 1975). Psychoanalysis is concerned with the meaning structure of the self and other(s). Meanings, wishes, intentions, fears, expectations, and motivations are the structures and contents of interest to those who practice and utilize psychoanalysis for aid in understanding the actions both of others and of themselves. The ideas of dynamic unconscious, transference and countertransference, object representations, intrapsychic conflict, symptom formation, and character development are repeatedly invoked in this chapter.

Public-Sector Psychiatry

System of Care

Increasingly it is being recognized that the needs of those with severe and persistent mental illness are best met within a coordinated system of care that provides a flexible range of services. Ideally, there should be a clear definition of whom the system is meant to serve. Resources do not permit an open admission process. Given that as much as 22% of the United States adult population is affected by mental illness (Reiger et al. 1993), costs and the political support for such costs are such that a variety of constraints and limitations are imposed, as described above.

There is a natural order of priorities regarding the provision of services within these treatment-rehabilitation-habitation systems that must be respected: food, clothing, shelter, and safety must come first; without these, treatment is not just ineffective, it is irrelevant. This point may seem self-evident, but it has been painfully learned over many years by well-intentioned clinical practitioners. Medical and psychiatric treatments come next, because control over symptoms and other manifestations of illness is not simply medically important and humane, it is a prerequisite for effective rehabilitation programs. Psychiatric rehabilitation programs and the psychotherapies (the "growth and development" modalities) follow medical control. These services provide the individual with the opportunity to develop—or perhaps to unlock—capacities and potentialities that can lead to greater personal freedom, maturity, autonomy, and self-fulfillment.

Optimally, these are flexible systems that provide individuals in need of care with *just enough* of what they need at a given point in time so as to maximize the efficient use of scarce resources as well as to maximally promote the individual's autonomy, growth, and development. This flexibility requires careful titration and management; too little results in poor care, whereas too much means that someone else who might need care will not receive it. In essence, a "holding environment" must be created in the community, with the type and intensity and combination of services appropriate to the clinical and developmental needs of a given individual at a given point in time serving as the basis of clinical decision making. Efficient use of resources means that individuals are maintained in high-intensity treatment settings no longer than is absolutely necessary. This "efficiency" presents significant problems in the area of risk management, and a psychoanalytic clinical perspective (among others) may be invaluable in formulating accurate clinical assessments and rendering useful clinical judgments, which are fundamental to the safe and effective functioning of such managed systems.

The functions of a comprehensive, integrated, continuous, and flexible array of services, adjusted to the changing needs of an individual over the course of his or her illness, may include the following: early intervention, intensive outreach and mobile crisis services, home and foster care treatment options, day hospital and respite care units, inpatient psychiatric units with varying tasks and prescribed lengths of stay, a variety of "step-down" alternatives, a range of residential options (supported apartment programs, "group homes," and the like), a spectrum of vocational and psychosocial rehabilitation programs, substance abuse treatment programs, and a variety of consumer, family, and volunteer-assisted self-help programs. The clinical modalities available in such a system may include psychopharmacology as well as brief and longer-term individual, group, and family psychotherapies using different clinical/theoretical perspectives (e.g., psychodynamic, cognitive behavioral, psychoeducation, skills training, network therapy, and behavior modification protocols). The linchpin and anchor of such a system, for the consumer, is usually the case manager or, for those individuals with greater degrees of disability, that specialized variant of the case manager—the assertive community treatment (ACT) team. It is the case manager, or the *case management function,* whose task it is to assess the needs of the individual seeking treatment and 1) to match up those needs with an appropriate array of services and treatment modalities, 2) to assume appropriate overall responsibility for the coordination and integration of these services, so that the work of integration is not left to an individual with a limited capacity for this kind of integrative task, 3) to monitor the progress of the individual within the treatment system, and 4) to make changes as appropriate.

Tasks

The functions of psychiatric and other mental health professionals can be conceptualized according to the four task areas identified by Astrachan and colleagues (1976): medical, reparative, humanistic (growth and development), and social control. A fifth task area, social welfare, was added later (B. M. Astrachan, personal communication, January 1988). Each task area carries with it a particular idea of the problems or focus of the patient as well as characteristic structures and modalities for accomplishing the work.

For *medical* tasks, the potential users are patients and the functions are differential diagnosis, treatment, and cure/amelioration of illness. The idea of disease as the target of intervention is the core feature of this perspective. In psychiatry, then, the psychoses, major affective disorders, severe anxiety disorders, and dementias/deliriums are the emphasized conditions. A core professional value is the commitment of the practitioner to the responsible care of the patient.

The *reparative* tasks (habilitation and rehabilitation) emphasize correcting a defect or enabling a person with a defect to live with or compensate for that defect. Function is the primary concern of the practitioner. Within the public mental health sector, this means addressing social as well as vocational consequences of psychiatric conditions (Anthony et al. 1972).

Humanistic (growth and development) tasks and reparative tasks in psychiatry frequently overlap in part because the defect to be corrected or adjusted to is frequently conceptualized as a defect in growth and development. The difference between these two task areas, however, resides in the emphasis on insight and self-knowledge in the growth and development function as opposed to the emphasis on education and skill building in the reparative function. In psychoanalysis, the growth and development task is carried out through the intense, intimate, yet professionalized relationship known as psychotherapy.

Social control tasks are aimed at the control of deviant (i.e., socially defined abnormal) behavior. In this functional area, law and psychiatry are more likely to come together in an effort to contain as well as cure deviant behavior. Psychoanalysis, like other efforts to understand, predict, and control such behavior, has had its share of failures in these particular areas. However, the psychoanalytic perspective remains a powerful conceptual and treatment tool for those who are attempting to deal with socially unacceptable deviance in a humane and rehabilitative fashion.

The later-added fifth task area, *social welfare,* addresses the provision of basic requirements for a dignified human existence, including but not limited to adequate housing, nutritious diet, the opportunity to live in a safe community, and the chance to try to improve one's lot by participating in social and vocational rehabilitative activities. This task area addresses poverty at an individual level. Whereas public mental health authorities are usually not responsible for the actual provision of food and shelter resources, they almost always have a major role in ensuring patient access to these resources.

Patients

The patients or consumers in a public-sector system are usually poor, have a major mental illness, and have little employment and educational experience. They are alienated from the broader culture on many dimensions.

Those with a major mental illness, such as schizophrenia, are plagued by a waxing and waning illness characterized by experiences of perceptual changes in the form of hallucinations, illusions, anxiety, paranoia, and cognitive impairments. Furthermore, there are the secondary manifestations of the illness that may be the result of attempts at adaptation to the illness. These reactions themselves can cause major difficulty in their own right. For instance, Selzer and colleagues (1989) have hypothesized that the negative symptoms of schizophrenia, such as anhedonia and lack of motivation, may be secondary reactions to the primary symptom defects of perception and thought, such as hallucinations, delusions, and boundary disturbances. In such an example, the tendency for schizophrenic patients to have small or nonexistent social networks may be a secondary reaction to the distress of being with people that so often accompanies a boundary disturbance in which the difference between inner and outer reality cannot be readily perceived.

We are conceptualizing schizophrenia as a complex of factors: *biological* in the form of genetically transmitted liabilities of perceptual and cognitive deficits, and *psychological* in the form of adaptations to the deficits of the illness. These symptoms may include the apparent amotivational states, isolation and withdrawal, as well as what are generally called secondary symptoms of irritability, depression, grandiosity, and denial. Frequently, persons with schizophrenia are disillusioned, demoralized, alienated, and angry both about their condition and about their inability to have the kind of life with meaningful relationships and a role that produces satisfaction and self-esteem (Perry et al. 1987; Selzer et al. 1989).

Patients with personality disorders are also frequent consumers of public-sector services. Frequently, these patients fall into one of two groups: those who seek treatment because of significant personal suffering (e.g., borderline personality disorder) and those who are in treatment because they cause significant suffering for others (e.g., antisocial personality disorder). Individuals in the first group are usually in treatment more or less on their own, whereas those in the second group are in treatment because they have committed acts that have led others to force or coerce them into treatment. Although the general approach to each of these groups is quite different, there are similarities in technique. Both require firm limits with a clearly structured treatment frame. Patients with borderline and narcissistic personality disorders can derive substantial benefit from a psychoanalytically derived therapeutic approach (Kernberg 1975, 1984). The coerced group can also benefit from a psychoanalytically informed approach that takes into consideration their psychological deficits of dysregulation of self-esteem and absent or disordered conscience. However, in contrast to the borderline and narcissistic groups, the conduct and antisocial disorder groups of patients require more focus on behavior and control of impulses (Shapiro 1989).

People who are poor, with limited access to occupational and educational opportunities (not to mention necessities such as food and shelter) also comprise a major element of the patient population of public-sector services. Most public-sector systems are oriented to those who are the most psychologically frail, socially marginal, and/or at risk for further dysfunction. Minority groups may be overrepresented. A significant number of consumers (as well as potential consumers) of mental health services may be homeless as well. These groups are no different from other classes of people in their hopes, fears, and aspirations. Their psychology is no different from more affluent groups, but their circumstances are such that they are preoccupied with physical as well as psychological survival, and, of course, they are alienated to a profound degree from the broader culture. Issues of self-esteem and belonging are major elements in the psychology of such groups. Attempts at adaptation to chronic alienation may simply result in deeper feelings of failure. Furthermore, patient groups with major basic deficits, such as the lack of food and shelter, frequently evoke strong countertransference feelings in those who attempt to care for them; such feelings can range from active denigration and devaluation—leading to the exclusion of these groups from the treatment pool—to an overzealous commitment that risks infantilizing and overwhelming such patients. Frequently, the reactions of providers may entail an element of withdrawal when the providers are trainees as opposed to those who have self-selected to work with public-sector patients. Therefore, the idea and experience of countertransference are conceptually important tools.

The clinician's feelings and subjective reactions to working with severely disturbed patients constitutes both a major source of difficulty and an opportunity for intervention (Altshul and Sledge 1989; Gabbard 1990; Greenson 1967; Loewald 1986; Searles 1965, 1979; Selzer et al. 1989). There are unconscious and irrational elements as well as work-oriented, social reality elements involved in the therapist's subjective response. An important contribution of the psychoanalytic perspective is the understanding of the therapist's reactions to working with such patients (Searles 1965). It has often been noted that work with schizophrenic patients is likely to involve more intense emotional reactions than clinical work with other patient groups. The mechanisms of this heightened emotional reaction involve aspects of these patients' difficulty in forming stable object relations and issues of projective identification, a process whereby the motivational state of the patient becomes represented by the environment and unwittingly becomes a part of the psychology of others relating to the patient. The therapist's experiences may be extreme and sometimes can be troubling enough to threaten the working relationship. Much of this difficulty has to do with the combination of unconscious motivations of the therapist in relation to some of the boundary problems of patients. It is extremely important for the therapist working with a schizophrenic person to be able to identify his or her reactions to the patient and to use those reactions explicitly in the work with the patient (Searles 1965).

The psychodynamic perspective can help clarify aspects of clinical decision making in treatment planning of other modalities by explicating the countertransference elements of that decision making. Levy (1977) has noted that countertransference problems in the work with schizophrenic patients can influence the decision to initiate or withhold medication. Other elements of clinical decision making can also be subject to intrusion of countertransference feelings. A psychodynamic conceptualization of the treatment that emphasizes the interaction between therapist and patient and the impact of the work on the clinician can serve as a guide to explicitly understanding some of the troubling feelings that accompany working with people with schizophrenia.

In addition to the countertransference reactions to patients based on the patient's psychological reactions toward the therapist, therapists themselves bring irrational transference reactions to their work with patients. These reactions may stem in part from fresh changes in the therapist's life (divorce, bereavement, marriage, and so forth) as well as from long-standing conflicts of a developmental or characterological nature. Therapists are more likely to be white, middle class, and well educated, so that patients who are from racial or ethnic minority groups or who are from a different socioeconomic class may present the greatest challenges to empathic understanding. Furthermore, to a patient who is alienated and disaffected for whatever reason, a therapist who has enjoyed the benefits of the dominant culture may present a similar transference challenge as well as an opportunity (Zetzel 1956).

One area of countertransference that has been explored to some degree is ethnicity and race (Bernard 1953; Calnek 1970; Favazza and Oman 1978; Fischer 1971; Griffith 1977). Calnek (1970) has provided a sensitive account of some of the countertransference perils of the black therapist/black patient match, noting that the black therapist must come to terms with the personal meaning of his or her race before being able to be of much help to black patients. Griffith (1977) has cautioned against attempting a "color blind" attitude, which can ultimately be destructive for an acknowledgment of the meaning of race and the pervasive presence of racism. His review of the literature reveals that whereas racial difference has an inhibiting effect on psychotherapy, racial congruence has a facilitating effect. At the same time, racial differences can be an occasion for fruitful exploration (Holmes 1992). Thematically, the issues can be characterized by racial dyad: *trust* for the white therapist/black patient dyad, *identification* for the black therapist/black patient dyad, and *status contradiction* for the black therapist/white patient dyad. Griffith urges clinicians to become intimately familiar with the cultures of their different-race patients.

A substantial issue in the delivery of services to public-sector groups is the capacity of the providers to be empathically responsive to those with substantially different backgrounds. In addition to differences in race, as noted above, gender and social class differences may also serve as barriers to understanding. Whereas other chapters in this volume address from a psychoanalytic perspective matters of clinician gender in the delivery of psychiatric services, it is appropriate here to mention some of the background literature on the effects of social class on psychotherapy (Albronda et al. 1964; Brill and Storrow 1960; Goin et al. 1965; Linn 1960; Shen and Murray 1981). Jones (1974) has provided an excellent review of the literature that addresses the influence of social class on psychotherapy. He notes the widespread prejudice that patients who are in lower social class groups do not want or cannot use psychotherapy and contrasts this belief with the widespread finding that such patients do want and can use psychotherapy effectively. These findings are echoed by others (Albronda et al. 1964; Goin et al. 1965). In this sense, a psychoanalytic perspective can be very valuable in helping practitioners identify and transcend barriers to empathic understanding (Shen and Murray 1981).

A danger that an overly zealous psychoanalytic approach may belie is that the typical psychoanalytically oriented psychotherapist's overvaluation of verbal productions—combined with a not-so-subtle denigration of case management and other pragmatic and action-oriented treatment approaches as "get your hands dirty" types of clinical activities—may itself constitute another form of countertransference reaction. To the extent that such a characterization of the work of the clinician in the public sector interferes with understanding and the delivery of appropriate services, it, too, constitutes a barrier to good clinical care.

Countertransference is all too often viewed as something of which the therapist admits only reluctantly. Such a view completely loses sight of the powerful effect of countertransference as a diagnostic and communication aid between the therapist and the patient. Recognizing that countertransference is an expected and natural element of the close, intimate work with patients can be a relief to the therapist and can allow the therapist to use countertransference reactions for their diagnostic and communicative value.

Clinical Applications

As noted by Astrachan and colleagues (1976), the medical and growth and development tasks have traditionally comprised the major activities of professional clinical practitioners' work. However, increasingly and of necessity, structures are being developed that attempt to integrate medical, rehabilitative, and social welfare functions. Social control functions, usually a task of special forensic units within a public-sector system, can also be part of the clinical enterprise. However, each of these task areas is associated with a particular provider orientation toward the patient and each has a particular paradigm for carrying out the clinical work. In this section we consider an integrated model of clinical services that includes all task areas. Obviously, the task area of growth and development will seem to be most closely related to the application of a psychoanalytic perspective; however, the point of this chapter is to consider ways in which psychoanalysis can be applied to other modalities and tasks in addition to the growth and development function within the work of public-sector mental health services.

Schizophrenia, schizoaffective disorder, and psychosis associated with affective disorder share the common symptoms of breaks with reality in the form of delusions, perceptual distortions such as illusions and hallucinations and, in some (if not all) instances, problems with thinking and abstraction. Using a psychoanalytic perspective, we conceptualize these problems broadly as disorders in the capacity for mental representation, by which we refer to the incapacity to form and maintain stable mental structures of memory, intentionality, and meaning in terms of both people (i.e., object representations) and things. Stable object representations allow one to evoke the experience of another person in the physical absence of the other; to distinguish stimuli emanating from within (e.g., memories) from those coming from outside (i.e., social reality); and to hold object representations constant even in the face of ambivalence and/or strong affects of love and hate.

Phenomenologically, people with persistent psychotic disorders have trouble with interpersonal relationships; they find themselves feeling exceedingly vulnerable to the vicissitudes of change and the give-and-take of an important personal relationship. Consequently, issues of trust and psychological safety are paramount; patients may be quite wary of new as well as old relationships while they may be very dependent on those whom they trust. The combination of extreme dependency and great vulnerability can lead to complex and dysfunctional relationships with important people in their lives. Patients with these disorders may have trouble coming to a shared reality with those around them. They also may have trouble experiencing the helpful intentions of another person when that person is not present or when they are angry at or in love with the helping person. Indeed, the helping person (therapist or clinician) may become the most important person in the patient's life. Dysfunctional consequences of these interpersonal problems are isolation, constriction, and extreme loneliness. Hence, the psychological work with such patients must take these vulnerabilities into consideration.

Patients with severe personality disorders represent a different set of clinical challenges (Waldinger 1987). These patients have faulty self and other representations that do not allow for the relatively smooth regulation and integration of affects, motivations, and intentions (Munich 1993). Therefore, these patients have episodes of extreme affect and, at times, aggression without the boundary disturbances of those who are psychotic. In other words, instead of becoming psychotic because they are unable to establish and maintain stable object representations along boundary lines (inside versus outside, self versus other, and so forth), personality disorder patients have trouble modulating strong affects attached to object (self and other) representations and regulating experiences of self and other value. The borderline phenomenon is one of exaggerating meaning as opposed to the psychotic phenomenon of delusion. Splitting is the characteristic defense mechanism of those with severe personality disorders.

Patients of different diagnostic groups frequently evidence problematic behaviors, the understanding of which can enhance the effectiveness of the therapists and the treatment system. These behaviors fall into two categories: those that are destructive to the patient and those that are destructive to others.

One particular set of behaviors that is problematic and self-defeating for patients involves the issue of compliance (Puryear 1993). To the extent that treatments can produce significant changes and alleviate symptoms and relieve suffering and disability, a refusal to engage in treatment constitutes a tragic loss for the patient. Noncompliance may have multiple antecedents, and it is important for the psychiatric clinician to be skilled in recognizing and dealing with the many forms of noncompliance. Frequently, noncompliance centers on taking medication, but it may also affect all aspects of the patient's participation in treatment. Noncompliance may be a manifestation of a denial of illness, a fear of losing autonomy and independence, or a fear of close contact with another person.

Whatever the origin of the noncompliance, the solution lies in close attention to the therapeutic alliance (Selzer et al. 1989), the basis of the working relationship between patient and provider. Explicit attention to this aspect of the relationship will go a long way toward dealing with noncompliance. The therapist must be attuned to the reasons why the patient is not able to comply and must attempt to provide an appropriate intervention rather than dismiss the patient as being poorly motivated.

Violence is a major issue in public-sector work, particularly when so many patients with major mental illness also have concurrent problems with substance abuse (Maier 1993; Schottenfeld 1993). Understanding the basis for violent behaviors is a necessary prerequisite to devising and establishing effective controls and limits. The same considerations apply to the high number of patients with severe mental illness who also use substances in a self-defeating, self-destructive fashion.

The clinical work with patients who have severe mental illness can be conceptualized as involving four different modes—engagement, restorative/recovery, maintenance, and adjunctive—based on the therapeutic goals. These goals are in part dependent on the stage of the illness and in part dependent on the capacities, motivations, and wishes of the patient.

Engagement mode. A major feature of the work with people with psychotic disorders and other severe mental illness is talking with them in a way that allows them to feel safe and able to be helped. The clinician must possess considerable patience and understanding of defensive functions and the patient's attempts at adaptation. Some people are gifted with an intuitive gift for this kind of understanding; the psychoanalytic perspective, however, provides a systematic conceptualization for this kind of listening and renders it more accessible to training and learning. An example of clinical work in the United Kingdom from south London may serve to illustrate this point.

> A nurse who worked as a case manager was covering the caseload of a vacationing colleague when it came to her attention that one of the patients she was covering was having difficulties. She made a home visit to the patient, a middle-aged woman

who was becoming increasingly psychotic, suspicious, and irritable. Believing (delusionally) that the case manager was someone from a social agency who was attempting to take away her social welfare benefits, the patient attacked the case manager by pulling her hair and attempting to throw her to the ground. A neighbor who was present in the patient's home at the time prevented the patient from harming the case manager. The case manager regained her composure, reprimanded the patient for what she had done, and left.

The case manager reasoned that despite this irritable, violent episode and the escalating nature of the patient's symptoms, she wanted to try again to engage the patient in some more collaborative endeavor in an effort to avoid a forced hospitalization (at this point, the patient had refused hospitalization). Her idea was that the patient had reacted in such an exaggerated manner because she was sensitized to the experience of loss as a result of the primary clinician's being away on vacation—hence, the patient's suspicious delusions of being taken advantage of. The case manager decided to deal with this issue very concretely.

The next day, accompanied by a visiting psychiatrist, she visited the patient, bringing a peace offering of cigarettes and milk. The patient, initially hostile and threatening, reacted with gratitude and appreciation to this offering and allowed the case manager and the psychiatrist to come into her house and carry out an evaluation of her needs. The evaluation, conducted in the patient's kitchen, revealed that this woman had become obsessed with the idea that her benefits had been taken away so that she would be unable to have the basics of food and shelter. The patient admitted that she had stopped taking her medication. It was suggested to her that she had become preoccupied with loss in the face of her valued primary clinician's being away and that she had confused the idea of losing him (even if for a brief time) with the idea that she was losing or had lost her benefits. It was decided, with the patient's cooperation and collaboration, that the plan would be to try to stay out of the hospital and to get back on track by taking her medications and allowing the covering case manager to help her out. The patient was able to be maintained on twice-per-day brief visits and a resumption of her medication until her regular clinician returned.

In this instance, the covering case manager understood, both intuitively and based on her knowledge of psychoanalytic principles, what it was that precipitated the crisis for this patient and was able to translate this understanding into a concrete action (bringing the cigarettes and milk) that facilitated engagement.

Establishing a therapeutic alliance with a psychotic person requires not only patience, understanding of the patient's psychology, and the opportunity for continuity over time but also a clear understanding of oneself and one's own capacities and weaknesses. Different patients have different kinds of needs for engagement. Some schizophrenic and other psychotic patients require a low-key, nonintrusive, "safe" demeanor from the clinician that may deviate from the conventional therapeutic stance. Issues of safety in regard to the wants and needs of others, which are so often experienced as intrusive, overpowering assaults by the schizophrenic patient, are extremely important to recognize in the early phases of the developing therapeutic relationship. The schizophrenic patient's wariness and rejection of help may actually represent an attempt at adapting to and controlling feelings of intense dependency.

On the other hand, some personality disorder patients require firm limit setting with fairly persistent adherence to the therapeutic framework and aggressive confrontation of self-destructive acting out (Kernberg 1975). These wide divergences of manner and stance with regard to patients demand flexibility on the part of the clinicians and are the basis for the clinical observation that some therapists do better with some kinds of patients but not as well with others. The following illustration may help bring some of these ideas to life.

> A young woman student with a psychotic, delusional disorder had the idea that one of her teachers was deeply in love with her and was about to divorce his wife and leave his family for her, despite the fact there had been no discernible expression of such an intention on his part. Her beginning, inexperienced therapist tried to argue her out of this obviously delusional idea, which left her even more convinced that her beliefs were true ("If it were not true, why would someone so important be trying to convince me otherwise?") and suspicious of her therapist ("You are in a conspiracy with the authorities, who do not want us to get married"). But she was not so suspicious that she could not tell her therapist about her beliefs. When the therapist tried a different approach of gently seeking the detailed basis of the delusional beliefs, the patient became less suspicious and more cooperative. It took some time, but after a few months of this approach, the patient began to question the reality of her convictions and to explore some of her underlying feelings of depression and low self-esteem. In this case, the therapist eventually focused on the formal problem of the representation of this fantasized love relationship and thereby assisted the patient in sorting out her experience. The supervisor of this therapy recognized the impact the attempt at supportive work was having on the patient and perceived the defensive role of the delusional belief as well as the need to establish a more effective therapeutic alliance before the delusion could be usefully addressed.

Restorative/recovery mode. Although studies on the outcome of psychoanalytic psychotherapy for schizophrenia have given a mixed picture of this modality's efficacy (Horowitz 1974; Karon and VandenBoss 1981; May 1968; McGlashan 1984; McGlashan and Keats 1989; Munich 1987; Searles 1965), there is a consensus that psychoanalytic psychotherapy alone is not effective. Indeed, some maintain that psychotherapy adds little of a positive outcome for people with schizophrenia. Compounding these debates about outcome is the widespread belief that schizophrenia is an unrelentingly deteriorating disorder. Indeed, the data (Harding et al. 1987) are intriguing and suggest that a considerable number of people with psychotic illness can substantially recover from the illness. In order to sidestep this argument, we will use the word *restore* to refer to the idea of "recovery." What we mean by *restoration* here is achievement of independence of living; attainment of meaningful, gratifying relationships; establishment of a role in which the patient feels important to someone else; and adaptation to ongoing, active symptoms—for in this notion of restoration, we include the possibility that some symptoms may be lifelong but not necessarily debilitating. We have known patients who have been able to live relatively comfortably with active symptoms. Of course, this ability to adapt to symptoms does not represent a failure but a triumph over the disabling aspects of the illness.

Part of this restorative function is the recognition, on the patient's part, of recurrent structures of motivation over time—how the past is repeated in the present, and how characteristic acts and behaviors carry certain meanings.

> For example, a 35-year-old schizophrenic physician who is able to practice effectively in an institutional setting has come to recognize that certain experiences in taking care of sick patients are especially difficult for him. He has set up his work setting so that he can get help when he is faced with these particular difficulties. He has come to understand how these difficulties relate to particular aspects of his youth. He has also come to know and recognize the early stages of psychosis and act in such a manner to prevent these states from becoming full-blown psychotic episodes.

In other words, we are suggesting that restoration carries with it the idea that the patient achieves gains in the realm of insight and self-knowledge. This insight is the basis for subsequent changes in psychological structures such as object representations. The psychoanalytic perspective, of course, emphasizes and encourages the patient's gain in insight as a particularly desired clinical outcome. Experientially based insight is the basis for creation and elaboration of psychological structures such as more differentiated object representations.

Maintenance mode. The idea of maintenance or support is not meant to be in opposition to the notion of recovery but actually another aspect of it. What we are referring to here is the explicit attempt to maintain adaptation and function rather than risking regression in the exploration of meaning or insight. In other words, the quest for self-awareness carries a risk of stress and regression. The therapeutic aim is the support of psychological structures rather than the elaboration of new structures. In people with stable boundary functions and the capacity for enduring object representations, such regression does not represent a substantial threat to the integrity of psychological functioning. However, in people with psychotic disorders and/or severe personality disorders, the risk of regression may not justify the potential benefits. In such circumstances, the therapist acts in such a way as to support a critical function such as self-esteem or reality performance by being explicitly reassuring or by giving advice, respectively (Rockland 1989). These functions may be at the expense of developing insight or self-understanding, but they are, nevertheless, based on a skilled understanding of how different aspects of mental function relate to one another. The supportive function is thus a blend of both insight and supportive knowledge inasmuch as the supportive psychotherapist must be both a skilled diagnostician and technically adept at offering support.

Adjunctive mode. A psychodynamic perspective has much to offer other forms of treatment as an adjunct to technique or understanding. For in all treatments of people with psychosis, the ongoing relationship is particularly important for a positive outcome. Psychodynamically informed practitioners working in areas such as the provision of medical services, the rehabilitation/habilitation functions, or the social control tasks are in a position to contribute to the quality of engagement and collaboration even though the desired outcome is not a growth and development goal. The psychodynamic perspective in such cases enhances the capacity of the therapist so that whatever the modality being delivered, the psychodynamically trained/informed provider is better equipped to understand some of the particular dilemmas of those with persistent psychosis. For instance, in addressing the worries a schizophrenic person may have in following through on a vocational rehabilitation referral, the psychodynamically informed case manager will be able to relate the patient's reluctance to a particular detail within the patient's life story (such as failure in previous school or vocational attempts), a fear of submission to the will of another person (and therefore of particular relevance for both past and present relationships), and/or a fear of becoming so independent that the valued relationship with the case manager will be withdrawn. In case management, rehabilitative, residential, and/or psychosocial services, this perspective is invaluable both for those providing the service and for those consulting with them. Likewise, the skillful use of medication entails some considerable understanding of psychology.

For an example of how a psychodynamic perspective can be helpful in an adjunctive relationship, consider the following:

> A 30-year-old, married, schizophrenic mother of two young children became suspicious that her previously valued and admired female case manager was plotting to have the patient hospitalized so that the case manager could have her husband and her children for herself. Rather than dealing with this idea directly and whether or not it was true, the treatment team decided to address the relationship between the patient and the case manger. As it turned out, the patient felt dangerously close to and envious of the case manager; the delusion both expressed the envy and fantasy of merger and provided a pretext for disrupting the relationship between them. When this problem was explicitly addressed along the dimensions of envy and fear of merger, the heightened suspiciousness and fear dissipated and the two were able to resume their otherwise effective working relationship. This intervention was possible because of a long-standing relationship with a therapist who had come to know something of the expression of themes of dependent longing and fragile self-esteem in this young woman.

Staff Growth and Development

Staff and personnel in any system need to grow and develop in order to maintain their vital connection to the clinical work. This growth and development function of providers is critical in any system of care for people with serious disability and dysfunction. The growth and development of providers is, in part, related to the self-knowledge that inevitably comes from the examination of countertransference responses and other affective and cognitive reactions to the work. Personnel should be provided with the necessary skills to carry out their work effectively and to continue to develop professionally. In addition to the perspective that psychoanalytic theory has to offer on all clinical states, honest self-reflection and insight is a skill as well as an attitude and value that a psychoanalytic perspective promotes and enhances.

Research

In the generation of knowledge, psychoanalysis offers a theory and a method of observing and ordering data, both of which can be a contribution to any research mission (Dahl et al. 1988). The place of psychoanalytic knowledge is obvious in studies that explore the therapeutic relationship, technique, or other aspects of psychotherapy. It is not so obvious in studies such as double-blind drug trials and other biologically oriented clinical work, particularly work that is strongly influenced by placebo and other "transference cure" phenomenon. Still less obvious is the value of psychoanalytic knowledge to such activities as mental health systems research.

Nonetheless, that value was recently demonstrated at a National Institute of Mental Health development conference. The level of analysis was the system of care, but it was judged necessary and desirable to make patient-level measures of outcome. Some participants in the conference had been struggling with the development of a scale for the measurement of social adjustment and quality of life. There was some back-and-forth discussion on technical issues, when a participant with no analytic background but who had worked long and hard on this problem blurted out that what really mattered were not the details or the facts of social adjustment but what the patient *believed* was the case. It was as if the concept of psychic reality had been rediscovered right then and there. And it had about it the force of revelation.

Psychoanalytic conceptualizations can relate psychoanalytic concepts regarding clinical phenomenon to nonpsychoanalytic phenomenon and concepts. This linking of theoretical perspectives that can give us a way of accounting phenomenally and intrapsychically for a phenomenon such as a negative therapeutic reaction and at the same time offer biological theories to help with the fuller understanding of the genesis of the phenomenon. For example, a colleague (with a psychoanalytic background) recently proposed that because many patients who have negative therapeutic reactions resemble in character structure the relentlessly suicidal patient, there may be biological similarities between patients who have repeated negative therapeutic reactions and those who are relentlessly and persistently suicidal. Such a study could contribute to the further understanding of the biological basis of character development.

Administration

Although administration is not a therapeutic endeavor, properly conceived administration addresses the requisite conditions of successful treatment and treatment systems. The successful administrator must be able to relate effectively to the psychological needs, motivations, beliefs, wishes, and characteristics of those to whom he or she administers.

A crucial skill for any administrator is the understanding of group behavior (Bion 1961; Slater 1966), particularly that of the small work group, which is the basis for so many committees, task forces, and other work-oriented administrative groups (Newton and Levinson 1973).

Administration in the public sector puts one in contact with workers and providers as well as politicians, bureaucrats, and other policy makers and managers. So often, effective work depends on a skillful understanding of the exercise of power and aggression. The administrator or leader who is uncomfortable with these considerations will not be fully effective. Psychoanalysis provides a conceptual framework for considering and working realistically, unburdened by personal irrational concerns with motivations of power, aggression, and control.

Leadership is a substantial feature of the function of an administrator (Kernberg 1978). One feature of leadership is understanding the actions of others with some confidence, particularly the irrational actions. Such understanding helps keep separate the actions that are functions of idiosyncratic character traits and those actions that stem more from social structural considerations in terms of the relationship between tasks and resources and what some might call politics. An explicit psychoanalytic perspective also aids those who hold administrative and leadership functions and helps them deal with the inevitable regressive pulls that are a part of the loneliness and frustration of such work (Kernberg 1978). Knowing what bothers one and why helps keep irritability, temper, and other tendencies to act out in check.

Values

Finally, we will say a word about a meta-clinical/meta-administrative aspect of the psychoanalytic perspective for any particular kind of human services work. The psychoanalytic perspective, after all, carries with it certain values, and these values should be also mentioned as part of the contribution and role of psychoanalysis to the clinical work in public mental health settings. We do not mean to imply, however, that only psychoanalysis supports these ideals. What we are referring to is an interest in and a valuing of certain uniquely human qualities. The psychoanalytic perspective assumes that what people do and think is meaningful and worthy of being understood (Gabbard 1990). It entails respect for and appreciation of the subjective life of individuals as well as esteem for their autonomy, dignity, and independence.

Conclusion

Psychoanalysis is not the treatment of choice for most people who are patients in the public sector of care, nor is a psychoanalytic derived treatment alone adequate for the effective treatment of most such patients. However, a psychoanalytic perspective provides an important contribution to public-sector systems because it offers

- A unique and valuable way of understanding psychosis and personality disorder.
- A conceptualization of a therapeutic frame for treating those with severe personality disorders.
- A way of understanding human relationships in general, but particularly in relation to personnel and administrative issues as well as research.
- A way of understanding one's own inner life—whether one is a provider or a manager.

Psychoanalysis as a theory offers the best present hope for being able to relate the psychological, the biological, and the sociocultural to one another in the broader biopsychosocial model to which we aspire. Psychoanalysis as a theory attempts to develop a broad understanding of the mind of a distressed individual both as a focus of ongoing research in its own right and in the form of multidisciplinary research on particular themes. The possibilities are legion and are all too often not developed.

As an influence on treatments, psychoanalysis has much to offer. The influence of psychoanalysis on all treatments is extensive and inextricably intertwined within the operant frame of modern psychiatric treatments. This is particularly true for psychological and socially based treatments. Ideas like transference, therapeutic alliance, insight, working through, interpretation, repression, the unconscious, and the like are derived from psychoanalysis and have become so integral to our field that we do not give them a second thought. Indeed, psychoanalysis has become such a part of our culture that it has been described as the only extant Western mythology.

Furthermore, the psychoanalytic perspective, as a personal means of understanding that which is unknown and difficult to bring forth in human relationships, is a tool that should be available within the public-sector setting to those who need and want it. For instance, for those who intend to spend a significant portion of their life doing intensive psychological work, it is an extremely important adjunct to professional growth to have some kind of experience, such as psychoanalysis or psychoanalytic psychotherapy, that provides the opportunity for personal growth and development.

Finally, the psychoanalytic perspective can be helpful to those who manage and lead mental health organizations. Such an understanding can contribute to the conceptual skills needed by managers to deal with the complex human relationships that exist in all organizations, but particularly those that care for severely mentally ill patients in a public-sector setting.

For Further Study

Altshul V, Sledge W: Countertransference problems, in American Psychiatric Press Review of Psychiatry, Vol 8. Edited by Tasman A, Hales RE, Frances AJ. Washington, DC, American Psychiatric Press, 1989, pp 518–530

Anthony W, Buell GJ, Sharratt S, et al: Efficacy of psychiatric rehabilitation. Psychol Bull 78:447–456, 1972

Astrachan BM, Levinson DJ, Adler DA: The impact of national health insurance on the tasks and practice of psychiatry. Arch Gen Psychiatry 33:785–794, 1976

Beres D, Joseph E: The concept of mental representation in psychoanalysis. Int J Psychoanal 51:1–9, 1970

Bernard VW: Psychoanalysis and members of minority groups. J Am Psychoanal Assoc 1:256–267, 1953

Bion WR: Experience in Groups. New York: Basic Books, 1961

Dahl H, Kächele H, Thomä H (eds): Psychoanalytic Process Research Strategies. Berlin, Springer-Verlag, 1988

Favazza AR, Oman M: Overview: foundations of cultural psychiatry. Am J Psychiatry 135:293–301, 1978

Fischer N: An interracial analysis: transference and countertransference significance. J Am Psychoanal Assoc 19:736–745, 1971

Gabbard GO: Psychodynamic Psychiatry in Clinical Practice. Washington, DC, American Psychiatric Press, 1990

Goin MK, Yamamoto J, Silverman J: Therapy congruent with class-linked expectations. Arch Gen Psychiatry 13:133–137, 1965

Griffith MS: The influences of race on the psychotherapeutic relationship. Psychiatry 40:27–38, 1977

Harding CM, Brooks GW, Ashikaga T, et al: The Vermont Longitudinal Study of persons with severe mental illness, II: long-term outcome for subjects who retrospectively met DSM-III criteria for schizophrenia. Am J Psychiatry 144:727–735, 1987

Holmes DE: Race and transference in psychoanalysis and psychotherapy. Int J Psychoanal 73:1–11, 1992

Jones E: Social class and psychotherapy: a critical review of research. Psychiatry 37:307–319, 1974

Kernberg OF: Borderline Conditions and Pathological Narcissism. New York, Jason Aronson, 1975

Kernberg OF: Object Relations Theory and Clinical Psychoanalysis. New York, Jason Aronson, 1976

Kernberg OF: Leadership and organizational functioning: organizational regression. Int J Group Psychother 28:3–25, 1978

Kernberg OF: Severe Personality Disorders: Psychotherapeutic Strategies. New Haven, CT, Yale University Press, 1984

Lamb RH, Goertzel V: The long-term patient in the era of community treatment. Arch Gen Psychiatry 34:679–682, 1977

Loewald HW: Transference-countertransference. J Am Psychoanal Assoc 34:275–287, 1986
McGlashan TH: The Chestnut Lodge follow-up study, I: follow-up methodology and study sample. Arch Gen Psychiatry 41:573–585, 1984
Munich RL: Conceptual issues in the psychotherapy of patients with borderline personality disorder, in Clinical Challenges in Psychiatry. Edited by Sledge W, Tasman A. Washington, DC, American Psychiatric Press, 1993, pp 61–87
Munich RL: Conceptual trends and issues in the psychotherapy of schizophrenia. Am J Psychother 41:23–37, 1987
Newton P, Levinson D: The work group within the organization: a socio-psychological approach. Psychiatry 36:115–142, 1973
Perry SW, Cooper A, Micheles R: The psychodynamic formulation: its purpose, structure, and clinical application. Am J Psychiatry 144:543–550, 1987
Searles HF: Collected Papers on Schizophrenia and Related Topics. New York, International Universities Press, 1965
Selzer MA, Sullivan TB, Carsky M, et al: Working With the Person With Schizophrenia: The Treatment Alliance. New York, New York University Press, 1989
Shapiro D: Psychotherapy of the Neurotic Character. New York, Basic Books, 1989
Shen J, Murray J: Psychotherapy with the disadvantaged. Am J Psychother 35:268–274, 1981
Slater PE: Microcosm, Structural, Psychological and Religious Evolution in Groups. New York, Wiley, 1966
Stanton AH, Gunderson JG, Knapp P, et al: The Boston Psychotherapy Study. Schizophr Bull 10:520–598, 1984
Zetzel ER: Current concepts of transference. Int J Psychoanal 37:369–376, 1956

References

Aichorn A: Wayward Youth. New York, Viking, 1948
Albronda H, Dean R, Starkweather J: Social Class and Psychotherapy. Arch Gen Psychiatry 10:276–283, 1964
Altshul V, Sledge W: Countertransference problems, in American Psychiatric Press Review of Psychiatry, Vol 8. Edited by Tasman A, Hales RE, Frances AJ. Washington, DC, American Psychiatric Press, 1989, pp 518–530
Anthony W, Buell GJ, Sharratt S, et al: Efficacy of psychiatric rehabilitation. Psychol Bull 78:447–456, 1972
Astrachan BM, Levinson DJ, Adler DA: The impact of national health insurance on the tasks and practice of psychiatry. Arch Gen Psychiatry 33:785–794, 1976
Beres D, Joseph E: The concept of mental representation in psychoanalysis. Int J Psychoanal 51:1–9, 1970
Bernard VW: Psychoanalysis and members of minority groups. J Am Psychoanal Assoc 1:256–267, 1953
Bion WR: Experience in Groups. New York, Basic Books, 1961

Brill NQ, Storrow HA: Social class and psychiatric treatment. Arch Gen Psychiatry 3:340–344, 1960
Calnek M: Racial factors in the countertransference: the black therapist and the black client. Am J Orthopsychiatry 40:39–46, 1970
Dahl H, Kächele H, Thomä H (eds): Psychoanalytic Process Research Strategies. Berlin, Springer-Verlag, 1988
Edelson M: Language and Interpretation in Psychoanalysis. New Haven, CT, Yale University Press, 1975
Favazza AR, Oman M: Overview: foundations of cultural psychiatry. Am J Psychiatry 135:293–301, 1978
Fischer N: An interracial analysis: transference and countertransference significance. J Am Psychoanal Assoc 19:736–745, 1971
Gabbard GO: Psychodynamic Psychiatry in Clinical Practice. Washington, DC, American Psychiatric Press, 1990
Goin MK, Yamamoto J, Silverman J: Therapy congruent with class-linked expectations. Arch Gen Psychiatry 13:133–137, 1965
Greenson RR: The Technique and Practice of Psychoanalysis. New York, International University Press, 1967
Griffith MS: The influences of race on the psychotherapeutic relationship. Psychiatry 40:27–38, 1977
Harding CM, Brooks GW, Ashikaga T, et al: The Vermont Longitudinal Study of persons with severe mental illness, II: long-term outcome for subjects who retrospectively met DSM-III criteria for schizophrenia. Am J Psychiatry 144:727–735, 1987
Holmes DE: Race and transference in psychoanalysis and psychotherapy. Int J Psychoanal 73:1–11, 1992
Horowitz L: Clinical Prediction in Psychotherapy. New York, Jason Aronson, 1974
Jones E: Social class and psychotherapy: a critical review of research. Psychiatry 37:307–319, 1974
Karon BP, VandenBoss GR: Psychotherapy of Schizophrenia: The Treatment of Choice. New York, Jason Aronson, 1981
Kernberg OF: Borderline Conditions and Pathological Narcissism. New York, Jason Aronson, 1975
Kernberg OF: Object Relations Theory and Clinical Psychoanalysis. New York, Jason Aronson, 1976
Kernberg OF: Leadership and organizational functioning: organizational regression. Int J Group Psychother 28:3–25, 1978
Kernberg OF: Severe Personality Disorders: Psychotherapeutic Strategies. New Haven, CT, Yale University Press, 1984
Lamb RH, Goertzel V: The long-term patient in the era of community treatment. Arch Gen Psychiatry 34:679–682, 1977
Levy S: Countertransference aspects of pharmacotherapy in the treatment of schizophrenia. International Journal of Psychoanalytic Psychotherapy 6:15–30, 1977

Linn EL: The association of permission symptoms with the social background of mental patients. Arch Gen Psychiatry 3:557–562, 1960

Loewald HW: Transference-countertransference. J Am Psychoanal Assoc 34:275–287, 1986

Maier G: Working with the repetitively violent patient, in Clinical Challenges in Psychiatry. Edited by Sledge W, Tasman A. Washington, DC, American Psychiatric Press, 1993, pp 181–213

May PRA: Treatment of Schizophrenia: A Comparative Study of Five Treatment Methods. New York, Science House, 1968

McGlashan TH: The Chestnut Lodge follow-up study, I: follow-up methodology and study sample. Arch Gen Psychiatry 41:573–585, 1984

McGlashan TH, Keats CJ: Schizophrenia: Treatment Process and Outcome. Washington, DC, American Psychiatric Press, 1989

Munich RL: Conceptual trends and issues in the psychotherapy of schizophrenia. Am J Psychother 41:23–37, 1987

Munich RL: Conceptual issues in the psychotherapy of patients with borderline personality disorder, in Clinical Challenges in Psychiatry. Edited by Sledge W, Tasman A. Washington, DC, American Psychiatric Press, 1993, pp 61–87

Newton P, Levinson D: The work group within the organization: a socio-psychological approach. Psychiatry 36:115–142, 1973

Perry SW, Cooper A, Micheles R: The psychodynamic formulation: its purpose, structure, and clinical application. Am J Psychiatry 144:543–550, 1987

Puryear D: Compliance problems and their management, in Clinical Challenges in Psychiatry. Edited by Sledge W, Tasman A. Washington, DC, American Psychiatric Press, 1993, pp 215–244

Regier DA, Narrow WE, Rae DS, et al: The de facto U.S. mental and addictive disorders service system: epidemiological catchment area prospective 1-year prevalence rates of disorders and services. Arch Gen Psychiatry 50:85–94, 1993

Rockland LH: Supportive Psychotherapy. New York, Basic Books, 1989

Schottenfeld R: Psychotherapeutic approaches to dual-diagnosis patients, in Clinical Challenges in Psychiatry. Edited by Sledge W, Tasman A. Washington, DC, American Psychiatric Press, 1993, pp 5–36

Searles HF: Collected Papers on Schizophrenia and Related Topics. New York, International Universities Press, 1965

Searles HF: Countertransference and Related Topics. New York, International Universities Press, 1979

Selzer MA, Sullivan TB, Carsky M, et al: Working With the Person With Schizophrenia: The Treatment Alliance. New York, New York University Press, 1989

Shapiro D: Psychotherapy of the Neurotic Character. New York, Basic Books, 1989

Shen J, Murray J: Psychotherapy with the disadvantaged. Am J Psychother 35:268–274, 1981

Slater PE: Microcosm, Structural, Psychological and Religious Evolution in Groups. New York, Wiley, 1966

Waldinger R: Intensive psychodynamic therapy with borderline patients: an overview. Am J Psychiatry 144:267–274, 1987
Zetzel ER: Current concepts of transference. Int J Psychoanal 37:369–376, 1956

CHAPTER 8

The Managed Care Setting

Sidney H. Weissman, M.D.

Since the time of Hippocrates, the practice of medicine has been based on the sanctity of the relationship between patient and healer. The principal concern of the healer has always been the best interest of his or her patient. For centuries this basic tenant of medical practice went unchallenged. Yet in the medical world of the 1990s, a term—or, more precisely, a set of interventions—has arisen that seems to threaten this core relationship: "managed care." Managed care allows for the intrusion of unnamed third parties to oversee and intervene in the relationship between healer and patient. The basis of this intrusion in the United States today is a desire to contain the cost of medical care. The American Medical Association (1994) defines managed care as

> systems or techniques generally used by third party payors or their agents to affect access to and control payment for health care services. (p. 274)

Techniques to implement managed care include

> (a) Prior, concurrent, and retrospective review of the medical necessity and appropriateness of services and or site of services. (b) Financial incentives or disincentives related to the use of specific providers, services, or service sites. (c) Controlled access to and coordination of services by a case manager. (d) Payor efforts to identify treatment alternatives and modify benefit restrictions for high-cost patients (high-cost case management). (American Medical Association 1994, p. 274)

In the minds of many psychiatrists, managed care has come to represent the downfall of the ability of psychiatrists to treat their patients based on the clinical competence of the practitioner and needs of the patients.

I would submit that what has changed today is not the intrusion on the doctor-patient relationship brought about by managed care, but rather the clarity with which economic realities govern psychiatric and medical practice. Economic factors have always been a major force affecting the quality of care and life. It has been said that the rich and the poor have an equal right to sleep on the Paris subway grates; however, in general, the rich choose not to do so. In 1900, it was likewise the case that the rich and the poor had equal access to the deplorable state hospitals of America. The rich chose not to use them, electing instead to seek aid in private sanatoria.

For a brief period between the 1960s and the early 1980s, we in the United States behaved as if we had unlimited resources for health care. Psychoanalytic treatment in the 1950s was restricted, because of its expense, to a small number of patients. With extended health insurance coverage in the 1960s and 1970s, this treatment became accessible to an expanded patient population. Intensive psychotherapy based on psychoanalytic principles became the standard form of psychiatric treatment in many circles. Fueled by this increased insurance support, the psychiatrist of the 1960s and 1970s had no shortage of patients and few, if any, visible outside controls on his or her practice. It should be noted, however, that unlike private patients of the 1950s, who paid for treatment out of pocket, most patients in the 1960s and 1970s received significant or majority support from third parties. The American society's priorities and its sense of unlimited resources to commit to health care for individuals who could not afford to pay for treatment out of pocket made health care available to most. Managed care in the 1970s was laissez-faire. Third-party payers elected to ask few questions about the need for the care of their insurees, but this was management of care just the same. Because of escalating costs and declining economic resources available for health care in the 1980s, society, through its health care programs, elected to actively review and—"where indicated"—limit insurance (public) portions of health care expenses. These activities are currently performed in many ways. For psychiatrists, such intrusions serve as conscious reminders that they do not work just for their patients.

Psychiatric residents or newly graduated practitioners may be aghast at the thought that they will not be able to work solely for the best interests of their patients. In fact, residents have already worked in a system of managed care throughout their residency training. Choices of clinical experiences are made for the resident based on the economic survival of the residency or on what would be the "best" educational experience for the resident. No one could seriously believe that it is in the best interest of a patient to be treated by a resident for 1–2 weeks on an inpatient unit, then be transferred to another resident for further treatment in the outpatient department, and finally be transferred some months later to still another resident. Can it really be in the best interest of the patient of a candidate at a psychoanalytic institute to be told, after a trial of analysis, that he or she is not "analyzable" but needs psychotherapy and must seek treatment elsewhere? All of these scenarios are unfortunately true and not uncommon. All are also typical of managed care. The goal in these situations is not a direct economic limit on health care expenses but rather the "maintenance" of educational goals that are not spelled out to the patient. The critical issue is that the "best" interest of the patient is, or may be, subordinated to another goal.

Managed care, when its goal is the maintenance of educational programs and departments of psychiatry, is perhaps more dangerous from the patient's perspective than managed care when its sole purpose is the containment of costs. Of course, we know that it is hard to ensure that patients receive the best, most cost-effective care when we are by no means always clear of the parameters that affect treatment outcome. But it could be argued that when economics drive mental health care decision making, patient care should at least be a passenger. When educational programs drive the system, the needs of the department of psychiatry and its students should likewise be considered passengers. Patients' needs may not be on board the process. Modern psychiatrists must be prepared to practice with the knowledge that society, through third-party intermediaries, will have a role in their treatment decisions. If they accept this premise, they can develop strategies to arm themselves with an understanding of psychotherapy such that they are able to at least neutralize some of the potential negative impact of society's intrusion into the consulting room.

It is in looking for guidance in this area that we find assistance from Freud:

> The . . . point that must be decided at the beginning of the treatment is the one of money . . . money is . . . the medium for self preservation and for obtaining power . . . money matters are treated by civilized people in the same way as sexual matters—with the same inconsistency, prudishness and hypocrisy. The analyst is therefore determined from the first not to fall in with this attitude, but in his dealings with his patients, treat money matters with the same matter-of-course frankness to which he wishes to educate them in things relating to sexual life. (Freud 1913/1963, p. 131)

If we apply Freud's dictum to patients in managed care programs when we commence treatment, we will review with patients the specifics of how their managed care program will or might affect their treatment. We will from the beginning clarify the patient's share of the fee as compared with that of the health maintenance organization (HMO) or insurance company, and we will discuss how we will communicate with the third party regarding the patient's treatment. These communications will become basic elements of the treatment. By defining the psychiatrist's role and the patient's role, both psychiatrist and patient understand one another and can then jointly decide how they will deal with the intrusion of the third party.

Thus far, I have addressed the conscious activities that psychiatrists can undertake in addressing with their patients the unique problems of financially driven managed care programs. One of the major contributions of psychoanalysis to understanding human behavior was the discovery that, in addition to conscious motivation, we are also governed by unconscious forces that affect our behavior. Because of the intensity of managed care intrusions on both the patient and the psychiatrist, both are prone to destructive transference reactions. In the next section, I review some of the special problems that the managed care situation creates for the patient as well as those it creates for the psychiatrist when he or she functions in a private practice setting.

The Omnipotent Psychiatrist (Physician) Transference

In this situation, the patient with managed care health benefits knows the limitations of the managed care coverage. The patient "assumes," however, without stating his assumption, that the psychiatrist will ensure the funding of the patient's particular treatment by controlling the managed care company. This assumption is unconscious on the part of the patient. If the psychiatrist, without being aware of the unconscious role the patient has created for her, accepts the role and assumes responsibility for obtaining funding for the patient's treatment, then the third party, if it limits the therapy, is seen as the villain by the psychiatrist, and the psychiatrist is seen as the villain by the patient. If the treatment is stopped, the patient leaves therapy feeling cheated because the doctor did not "arrange" funding for his treatment. The doctor is seen as inadequate by the patient for not obtaining what the patient felt he was due. The doctor, if not aware of the patient's transference, does not examine with the patient his unreasonable transference expectations. The psychiatrist deflects any blame from herself and colludes with the patient to focus and blame the insurance company for the breakdown of the treatment. This collusion deflects the patient and the psychiatrist from examining the patient's unreal expectations and allows both parties to avoid addressing the patient's rage at the psychiatrist and, more importantly, the patient's grandiose expectations. Such actions keep the patient from effectively using the limited psychotherapy experience.

Of course, numerous situations exist in which the psychiatrist must act as an informed advocate for the patient in explaining to the managed care company why the patient needs extended care. Here I am addressing only the potential transference distortions regarding the psychiatrist's responsibilities. The psychiatrist must differentiate realistic responsibilities from transference distortions in developing treatment plans in managed care situations.

The Omnipotent Patient Countertransference

In this next situation, the patient assures the psychiatrist that she will be able to obtain additional sessions of treatment because of her special role in her company or her special knowledge of the managed care provider. Sometimes, the physician is told by the patient, however, that the various managed care forms must be completed in a special way or the patient will not be able to obtain the needed coverage. The psychiatrist goes along with the patient's request or assurance of coverage. Treatment continues for some time after the initially approved number of sessions until the patient and the doctor are advised that the coverage will not be extended. The patient either blames the doctor for not completing the forms properly or reassures the doctor that she can overturn the denial of further benefits. The psychiatrist either feels that the patient misrepresented the extent of her coverage or accepts the patient's assurance that she will obtain the additional coverage. Careful review, in these cases, usually reveals that the psychiatrist did not adequately examine with the patient the extent of coverage and its limitations. The psychiatrist may have developed an unrealistic expectation or countertransference that led to his not examining the patient's assurances of special standing or reasons for completing forms in the "special way."

When the psychiatrist's understanding is distorted by countertransference, he fails to focus on the doctor-patient issues that might have created the problem, instead choosing to view the problem as existing outside the treatment setting and in the managed care company. Critical issues as to how the patient sees the world are avoided by both psychiatrist and patient. By carefully reviewing insurance coverage and following guidelines, the psychiatrist can avoid this trap. If the psychiatrist feels that breaking the rules of the managed care company is justified, then a careful review of the circumstances of the case is critical. Additionally, through self-analysis, a review of all of the psychiatrist's personal reactions to the patient is essential.

The Omnipotent or Uninformed Managed Care Company

In this situation, the doctor and the patient have effectively reviewed the parameters of the patient's treatment and it indeed is progressing appropriately and meets criteria for continuation. At the next review, however, the outside review by the managed care company is performed by a reviewer not knowledgeable in the treatment approach being offered and used. This new reviewer advises the therapist and the patient that the therapy is inappropriate and that the company cannot continue to fund the treatment. Unfortunately, this scenario occurs all too often and is probably the one that brings the most criticism to the managed care process. It should be noted that this type of denial represents neither the managed care company's carrying out a mandate for the cost-effective treatment of patients nor a strategy for the effective use of a nation's resource for the health care of its citizens. Rather, such denials frequently constitute an attempt by an entrepreneurial company to maximize its profits under the guise of a greater good. Many readers, at this point, will applaud this exposure of managed care companies' motives but will wish to know what the practitioner can do in such situations. Unfortunately, no text can be written to instruct another physician how to practice in a complex economic situation; rather, what each of us must do is understand the complex forces that impact upon our practices so that we can make the most informed response to a complex issue. In this discussion, therefore, I will not address the ethical breakdown affecting the managed care company; I will focus instead on the complex forces that operate within the psychiatrist.

Situations such as these force psychiatrists to ponder their responsibility to their patients as well as to examine the economics of their practices. If the treatment is justified and the managed care company says it is not, does the psychiatrist continue to see the patient and appeal the initial ruling, or does she terminate the patient? It is easy to say that medical ethics dictate that the psychiatrist continue to see the patient. But what if the psychiatrist practices in an area where the standards or principles of care are under assault, and has many patients whose financial support for care was withdrawn? Prudence would dictate that such a psychiatrist consult with her colleagues to assure herself that her clinical judgment is appropriate. But what if those colleagues are having the same difficulties? Can they be objective? And what does the psychiatrist do after her colleagues assure her that her treatment plans are reasonable and appropriate?

If we return to Freud, appropriate reimbursement is essential for the psychiatrist's needs. In these situations, psychiatrists must be clear as to the limits of their power or authority. They must monitor their own inner dynamics. They must deal with their own rage and concern about their patients' being treated unfairly and their professional judgments being dismissed. Psychiatrists must also address their feelings of helplessness as they realize that they may be powerless in such situations. They must be careful neither to act out their rage in a way that is damaging to the patient nor to displace that rage onto the patient. The decision of whether or not to continue to see a patient until an insurance dispute is resolved cannot be answered by anyone but the treating psychiatrist, on a case-by-case basis. Psychiatrists may become involved in activities of professional societies addressing the issue of managed care, but such activities alone will not help in dealing either with the specific issue of a given patient and that patient's unique pain or with other special ethical and professional concerns. An introspective posture based on the principles of self-analysis derived from psychoanalysis can assist the psychiatrist in making choices in these situations.

The Harassing Managed Care Company

In this situation, the patient has a severe chronic mental illness—for example, manic depressive disorder or schizophrenia. Any review of the patient's history reveals the extent and chronicity of the disease. In many such cases, the patient and the doctor have developed a relationship that enables the patient to stay out of the hospital. Instead of facilitating the psychiatrist's developing and maintaining a treatment plan for extended visits to support the patient, however, the managed care company authorizes two to three additional visits for the patient and tells the psychiatrist to continue to reapply after every third session. Such behavior by a managed care company can only be seen as harassing. Given that the severity of the patient's illness is clear, the additional reports only add redundant administrative time and cost to the treatment.

Because completing the managed care forms is not a reimbursable service, the care of such severely ill patients begins to require increasing amounts of time for which the psychiatrist is not compensated. The psychiatrist might suddenly begin to feel that the patient is not making any progress. The psychiatrist's anger toward the managed care company and its behavior, which neither the psychiatrist nor the patient can control, may be displaced onto the patient. In these situations, the patient may not receive the same careful care that he or she has received in the past. The patient's condition might deteriorate and, of course, this decline can be communicated to the managed care company to support the need for more sessions. In the worst case, the patient might need to be hospitalized. If aware of his feelings, the treating psychiatrist might even consider transferring the patient to another doctor, recognizing that his anger about how the patient has been treated might have contributed to the patient's need for hospitalization and might possibly interfere with further care.

In this situation, the psychiatrist's necessary actions are, in fact, clear. He must complete the forms while remaining aware of his affective response to that process. Self-analysis is mandatory and essential to ensure that the psychiatrist does not inadvertently withdraw from the patient. Depending on the section of the country where one practices, portions of this scenario can be everyday occurrences.

In any event, the psychiatrist, by knowing his response to being abused, can assure himself that he will not unknowingly displace his rage onto the patient. Effective response to managed care abuse must come elsewhere—in the legal or political arena.

The Unhelpful Patient

One of the realities of managed care is the need to complete a large number of forms. In order to make these systems work, it is essential that the patient be a part of the process and, where indicated, complete his or her share of the required forms. Inevitably, some patients feel that this task is the responsibility of the doctor or some unknown other; they have paid the insurance company, or their employer has, and this has discharged them from further responsibility. Even though the procedures may be cumbersome and difficult to follow, some are still the responsibility of the patient. Of course, if a patient has a chronic illness that interferes with his or her ability to address these administrative responsibilities, the psychiatrist is responsible for providing extra assistance. But these are exceptions. To return to Freud's comments, addressing the patient's payment for services is part of the psychiatrist-patient contract. If the patient does not cooperate, the psychiatrist does not get paid. The responsibility for completing certain forms is the patient's, not the doctor's or the insurance company's. If some patients attempt to transfer responsibility, this behavior becomes an area for psychotherapeutic exploration. If the patient is unwilling to cooperate in the "managing" of managed care and cannot participate in exploring the issue of why he or she has this difficulty in therapy, then the psychiatrist does not have a patient. Commiserating with the patient on the paperwork that he or she faces avoids dealing with the patient's unreasonable sense of entitlement and evades therapy. If therapy is to succeed, the patient must be advised that if appropriate action is not taken, the therapy will stop after a certain date.

In this situation the psychiatrist must of course complete all of the forms for which he or she is responsible. Doing so places the burden for payment for the psychiatrist's subsequent services squarely on the patient. Failure to act clearly and quickly will, first, support the patient's sense of entitlement; second, it will result in the psychiatrist's not being paid for his or her professional services, which may eventually lead to the psychiatrist's angrily terminating therapy with the patient.

Special Government Health Care Programs and Their Unique Impacts on Practitioners

Medicare

The largest managed care system with which psychiatrists contend is Medicare. Medicare provides health insurance coverage for retired individuals or, under certain circumstances, for individuals of any age who have a chronic illness. Through federal legislation, the amount and mechanism of payment for services are prescribed.

For some psychiatrists, Medicare is of little concern because they have few patients covered by this system. For others whose patients include many chronically ill or geriatric individuals, Medicare covers the vast majority of their practice. The primary problem experienced by most psychiatrists in dealing with Medicare is the low rate of reimbursement for each "unit of service." Many—if not most—psychiatrists feel that the system is economically unfair. My concern here is with how this problem affects psychiatric practice and whether there are special latent issues that either the psychiatrist or the Medicare patient brings to the treatment situation.

The government has made the administration of this system the total responsibility of the physician. The psychiatrist need learn only the patient's social security number to assume responsibility for administrative management of the patient's care. The psychiatrist must complete and send to Medicare all billing forms. In principle, the administrative management of a Medicare patient may be easy. The real issue is one of reimbursement: Medicare reimbursement for a standard 45-minute psychotherapy hour is drastically lower than that provided by virtually all private payors. For economic survival, the psychiatrist may treat in intensive psychotherapy only a few Medicare patients at a time. As previously noted, this area is not an issue for those practitioners with few Medicare or elderly patients. It is, however, a serious issue for the psychiatrist specializing in geriatric psychiatry.

The Medicare level of payment implicitly encourages the use of pharmacological therapies in a patient population most vulnerable to the side effects of these agents. If a psychiatrist elects to treat a Medicare patient, he or she must be careful not to allow the choice of treatment to be determined for economic rather than clinical reasons. As noted earlier, by using self-analysis and outside consultation, psychiatrists can, if in doubt, assure themselves that their treatment recommendations fit the needs of a given patient. This approach, however, does not work if most of their patients are on Medicare. Psychiatrists might not be aware that they routinely overmedicate many of their patients; if this is the case, a total review of their practice and practice patterns is what is needed to assess Medicare's impact on patient care. Methods of payment such as Medicare unfortunately and unfairly place the financial burden of caring for a segment of the population on the psychiatrist. Again, political action is the route for redress of such grievances.

Medicaid

Medicaid is another federally mandated managed care system. It is administered separately by each state. Payment for service varies among states. Eligibility for Medicaid is usually restricted to individuals with limited economic resources. The Medicaid level of reimbursement is, for most services, far below that of Medicare. For this reason, many—if not a majority of—psychiatrists decline to treat Medicaid patients as outpatients. A larger number will see Medicaid patients as inpatients because of the more favorable fee structure in this setting.

In the United States, physicians in private practice are free to treat or to decline to treat patients in their private practices. Returning again to Freud, each psychiatrist must establish his or her own standard of fees and his or her own standard for the income he or she wishes to earn. This is a complex decision based on the economics of the community as well as on a vast array of unique issues for each psychiatrist. Using a model of self-analysis, each practitioner can arrive at the best informed decision for him- or herself. However, when it comes to the treatment of the poor, a given practitioner's self-informed decision and set of actions may not respond to a set of societal needs. How does a responsible psychiatrist—or any physician, for that matter—address this question? If all practitioners declined to treat individuals on Medicaid, how would these members of our society obtain appropriate psychiatric care? Can a psychoanalytic understanding of behavior assist us in responding to this patient group and its medical problems? Psychoanalysis can assist us in understanding both our patients and our own motivations. With this understanding of the needs of patient and practitioner, we can proceed to develop models of treatment and reimbursement that respond to both groups. Unfortunately, society is, in most states, not prepared to supply the economic resources required to provide health care for the poor or to meet the needs of the practitioner. It is possible that future health care reforms will better provide for the needs of populations currently underserved; however, until society acts, the physician must be aware of society's attempts to displace its responsibilities onto the practitioner.

Society's artificially low Medicaid fees create conflicts for psychiatrists. For example, as previously noted, some practitioners will treat Medicaid patients when they need hospitalization; however, when these patients are discharged, these practitioners transfer the patients' care to a clinic or state facility. Although such treatment is, at times, clearly appropriate, at other times the psychiatrist takes economic advantage of one part of the payment system. It is the psychiatrist's responsibility to sustain the patient's treatment as the setting changes. Because of the economic disparities in treating Medicaid patients, it is not surprising that practitioners would limit the number of such patients. But once a psychiatrist begins a treatment, knowing the economic restraints in advance, he or she is responsible for sustaining it. The psychiatrist can with equal honesty decline at the outset. But to withdraw in the middle of treatment is to evade responsibility and to abandon the patient.

Thus far, my discussion has addressed intrusions into the doctor-patient relationship when the doctor functions in a private practice setting. The American Medical Association's definition of managed care implicitly addresses care provided in private practice, yet many psychiatrists practice in salaried settings. Such settings include—to name a few—the following: state mental health systems, community clinics, veterans administration centers, staff model HMOs, university health centers, and the armed forces.

In each of these settings, an organization has expressly stated responsibilities or policies that may support or interfere with the doctor-patient relationship and/or with the doctor's working exclusively for the best interest of a given patient. For example, the university health service psychiatrist is frequently in such a situation. A student presents with an acute depressive episode. The psychiatrist learns that underlying an acute stressor is character pathology for which the student could be helped by psychotherapy. The student has inadequate financial resources to fund essential psychotherapy outside the university health service. If the health service psychiatrist "follows" the patient after treating the acute crisis, he or she would be less available to other students in a crisis. If the psychiatrist does not "follow" the patient, the student may have a recurrence and may not remain in school. The sensitive psychiatrist in such a situation feels that he or she has been placed in a no-win bind. Someone—either someone the psychiatrist knows (the patient) or someone unidentified (another student at risk)—will not or may not receive essential care. Just as we could not specifically advise the psychiatrist how to deal with the managed care company, we cannot tell the university health service psychiatrist how to deal with a specific student patient. Again, however, the psychiatrist must be clear as to his or her responsibilities and must specify, at the beginning of clinical work with the patient, which parameters will intrude on, or limit, the student's treatment. As in any managed care setting, the patient must be made aware of these issues.

Perhaps, at this time, a new, more comprehensive definition of managed care is appropriate:

> The intrusion of unnamed third parties in the relationship between healer and patient, when a societal imperative (e.g., cost containment, national defense, education, conservation of resource, control of an infectious disease, report of abusive behavior) is mandated by society as in the society's best interest. This intrusion may take many forms. It may include prior review of care or the establishment of preset standards of care amongst many regulatory approaches.

To return to Freud, regardless of the form the management of care takes, it must be made explicit so that both doctor and patient are aware of any external powers that govern their work. In the case of the student, the doctor and student would then be able to develop a joint treatment plan at the commencement of their work together. The caveats previously noted for patients seen in private practice apply equally in all of the salaried settings. The primary issue in psychiatric treatment is not who pays but how doctor and patient establish an appropriate treatment plan cognizant of the overt economic realities that govern the treatment. Even when the psychiatrist and the patient are both clear as to these overt issues, the psychiatrist must continue to be vigilant that transference or countertransference distortions do not impair the treatment.

Conclusion

Managed care—not the recent major advances in biological psychiatry and the new psychoanalytic models—may prove to have the greatest impact on the practice of psychiatry in the last decade of the 20th century. Managed care, unless understood and "managed," threatens to interfere with the relationship that has linked doctor and patient since the ancient Greeks—a relationship that has survived thousands of years and has established the ethical framework in which we practice. Managed care is society's intrusion into medicine, which in the United States, deals for the most part with how society wishes to expend its wealth for medical care. By understanding the origins of managed care, the practitioner can better appreciate why he or she may feel powerless. Managed care is an example of the classic confrontation of the rights and responsibilities of the individual versus those of society. In a democracy, this confrontation is a never-ending one.

Managed care—or, more correctly stated, society's explicit role in health care—brings additional responsibilities to the psychiatrist. The power of psychoanalysis for the contemporary psychiatrist lies not only in its value in understanding patients but also in its role in assisting the psychiatrist to contend with the contradictory demands of society, patients, and self. Understanding these forces operating on the psychiatrist's psyche is where psychoanalysis may be of most help to contemporary psychiatrists. In this environment, psychiatrists must be clear that they are always working for the best interest of their patients while honestly assessing their own needs and responsibilities. It is here that Freud sets the tone. Psychiatrists are physicians who earn a living to support themselves and their families by treating the behavioral ills of others. Psychotherapists are not physicians single-handedly responsible for correcting the injustices of society.

We can be sure that debates on how society's resources are to be used for health care will continue. New and unprecedented methods for intruding upon the doctor-patient relationship will develop. As managed care evolves, it will place new pressures on the doctor-patient relationship.

Psychoanalysis, as the science of human behavior with a particular focus on the meanings and motivations of behavior, has a unique role in informing and advising us about how to deal with these stresses on the doctor-patient relationship.

References

American Medical Association: Policy 285.998, AMA Policy Compendium. Chicago, IL, Compendium 1994

Freud S: The Standard Edition of the Complete Psychological Works of Sigmund Freud, Vol 13. Translated and edited by Strachey J. London, Hogarth Press, 1963

Chapter 9

The Outpatient Psychotherapy Clinic

Thomas Wolman, M.D.

In the past, the psychiatric clinic offered a protective enclave in which third-year psychiatry residents could learn the art of psychotherapy. Then, the clinic was nothing more than a loose association of individual practitioners who pooled their resources and shared their minimal administrative load. The atmosphere was strictly laissez-faire; like Winnicott's (1962) "good enough" mother, the clinic remained in the background as an unobtrusive, supportive presence. Its main training function was that of mediator, matching residents with prospective patients and supervisors and distributing classroom and office space.

Nowadays, we look back on the old clinics with nostalgia. The clinic of today bears little resemblance to its predecessors. Indeed, the very presence of a book chapter on this topic testifies to the change in the way clinics function. This change reflects the move toward managed health care and the resulting institutionalization of medical services. Lest anyone think that the conduct of psychotherapy is immune from such pressures, consider the following advice from a recent issue of *Psychiatric News:* "Solo fee-for-service practice is jeopardized, and psychiatrists should prepare to reorganize their practices to do more medication management and less time-dependent psychotherapy" (R. Shellow, chair of the American Psychiatric Association's Joint Commission on Government Relations, quoted in "New Practice Patterns Said To Be Necessary for Economic Survival," August 6, 1993, p. 1).

The effects of institutionalization may be seen most clearly in an environment like that in the former West Germany, where national health insurance covered the cost of psychotherapy and psychoanalysis for most citizens. Four components of that system are becoming universally applied to psychiatric clinics: 1) the requirement of a specific medical diagnosis before analytic therapy can be considered, 2) formal treatment plans and treatment plan updates, 3) an independent peer assessor who periodically evaluates the progress of treatment, and 4) a limit of the duration of the therapy to 300 hours.

Some West German analysts (Thomä and Kächele 1987) believed that analytic therapy can be successfully conducted in a managed environment provided that the therapist take special care to explore the patient's reactions to these four components. However, other West German analysts had their doubts. Goldacker-Pohlmann (1993), for example, expresses concern about the exclusion of nonmedical therapists, the devaluation of quality-of-life issues in favor of symptomatic improvement, and the fixed time limit. She also reports a disquieting movement in recent years to encourage short-term ego support therapy to the exclusion of more intensive exploratory work.

In this chapter I take the position that institutionalization operates as an active, dynamic "agency" in the therapeutic situation whose effects are insidious, inescapable, and unconscious. I will reveal its presence behind most therapeutic transactions as a covert third party with a mind of its own, and will attempt to unravel the consequences of this changed configuration on the learning of psychodynamic therapy. Three types of effects will be addressed: the tendency toward therapy by prescription, dislocations in time and space arrangements, and the multiple effects of third-party transactions. I conclude the chapter by briefly commenting on the change in perspective necessary to confront and solve these problems.

Does such close attention to what are in fact extraneous factors divert the resident from his or her main task of mastering the art of psychotherapy? In response to this question I will argue that a careful consideration of just such details actually enhances therapeutic understanding. In the first place, the problems of institutionalization tend to draw attention to the often neglected practical arrangements of scheduling, fees, office layout, and confidentiality. In the second place, these problems tend to operate outside the awareness of clinic personnel and frequently against their stated intentions. And in the third place, the clearing away of institutional impediments introduces the technique of handling resistances. Residents discover resistances in the process of exposing the clinic's covert, disruptive, and undermining influence. They are thus exposed to the "unconscious" at the very outset of treatment.

The Tendency to Prescribe Psychoanalytic Treatment

The prospect of psychodynamic therapy raises a number of questions in the minds of both therapist and patient: Is such therapy the best treatment? Can success or failure be predicted on the basis of diagnosis? Can the treatment be "aimed" at a particular symptom or group of symptoms? What are the goals of therapy for this particular patient? How long will the treatment last?

Freud addressed these questions in his paper "On Beginning the Treatment" (1913/1958):

> The analyst is certainly able to do a great deal, but he cannot determine beforehand exactly what results he will effect. He sets in motion a process, that of the resolving of existing repressions. He can supervise this process, further it, remove obstacles in its way, and he can undoubtedly vitiate much of it. But on the whole, once begun, it goes its own way and does not allow either the direction it takes or the order in which it picks up its points to be *prescribed* for it. (p. 130 [italics mine])

In this quotation, Freud uses the word *prescribed* in the sense of "written beforehand" or "established in advance." He wished to define the analytic stance as one that does *not* presuppose the aims of treatment. The wish to prescribe analysis is, then, comparable to the typical resistance of bringing in a carefully prepared agenda to the analytic session. According to this quotation, it is questionable whether analysis ought even to be conceived of as having an "agenda" separable into a series of discrete steps carried out in a known order.

The interdiction against "prescribing" applies also to the recommendation to undertake an analysis. At a certain point in his practice (between 1904 and 1912), Freud ceased to view this decision as the outcome of a preliminary inquiry, substituting instead a brief period of "trial analysis." Except for its shorter duration, trial analysis differs in no essential way from analysis proper. Unlike other preliminary inquiries, however, its length remains indeterminate. Freud's position was simply that *the decision to undertake an analytic treatment must itself arise from a preliminary psychoanalytic exploration.* For Freud, "no other preliminary examination is possible" (1913/1958, p. 124).

Assessment

In this sense, psychodynamic therapy begins with the assessment. It is helpful if residents working in a clinic learn to incorporate an experience of "trial therapy" into the initial evaluation—a modification that may seem like putting the cart before the horse, given residents' psychiatric orientation. However, trial therapy gains credibility when used as a test of the original diagnostic impression. Trial therapy may help some patients in severe crisis to reconstitute, resulting in an adjustment of the diagnosis to the neurotic range. The same therapeutic setting may, in other patients, precipitate a regression suggestive of a borderline diagnosis. Finally, a complete absence of response may suggest antisocial or schizoid personality disorder.

Such an approach to diagnosis runs counter to the procedures of the psychiatric clinic. Like that of any institution, the modus operandi of the clinic is the division of labor. In particular, the gatekeeping and evaluation functions are usually kept separate from the treatment functions. A patient is subjected to a detailed inquiry, given a diagnosis, and provided with a specific prescription for treatment. This prescription usually specifies the type of therapy (supportive versus exploratory), the frequency of sessions, and the fee. Whatever its obvious benefits, such an evaluation by itself is exactly what Freud believed was futile in deciding the issue of therapy.

It is therefore important that residents be taught to form their own judgments and to explore all treatment options thoroughly with their patients. It must be remembered that residents often enter the clinic setting with the same bias as the clinic procedure—namely, that the decision to undertake psychodynamic therapy can be made outside the context of the therapeutic relationship. Therefore, a resident may be inclined to treat the "prescription for therapy" as a green light to proceed with exploratory work, and sometimes to lift his or her initial interpretations right out of the initial formulation. Six months down the road, the resident may be surprised and unprepared for what seems like an insurmountable resistance in the patient. After discussion of the case, however, the resident sees that the so-called resistance simply means that the patient has not yet entered into an agreement to undergo therapy. In other language, one might say that the therapeutic pact or alliance is unformed. The patient has not so much rejected therapy as rejected the *prescription for therapy.* Alternatively, the patient's ready acceptance of the prescription may have removed the possibility of voicing deep ambivalence about the entire process. Indeed, the patient may have unconsciously interpreted the prescription for therapy as a *proscription* or *interdiction* of therapy.

Analysts encounter this same unconscious reversal whenever they hear the words "I have a great analytic case for you!" Not uncommonly, the very opposite is true.

> One such patient, Ms. O, was referred for analysis in just this way. Analysis was begun and continued for quite a while with the analyst in ignorance of the patient's true feelings about the referral process. The patient's chief resistance during the opening phase took the form of constant demands for "prescriptions" from the analyst—lists of things she should do. Ms. O's preoccupation with these "prescriptions" distracted her from the work of analysis. Moreover, her need for "generic" prescriptions—ones that would apply to anyone with her problem—tended to place the analyst in the role of "generic" physician. If the analyst was helpful, it was only because he was doing his job, something he would do just as well for anybody else. Needless to say, such a viewpoint relegated the analyst to a position of impotence and the patient to one of resigned passivity.
>
> Many months later, a recounting of the initial circumstances of Ms. O's referral for analysis shed new light on her "resistance." The referral had come from a clinician who was seeing Ms. O's boyfriend in therapy. The boyfriend had confided to his therapist that he wished to break up with Ms. O. It was thought that, in the light of Ms. O's evident emotional distress, the best solution was a referral of Ms. O for analysis. On retelling, it became clear that Ms. O had experienced this referral as a rejection. She saw herself as the object of a trade from one man to another. Moreover, she was being forced to settle for second best—and worse, to accept a man who was *obliged* to care for her in place of the man who loved her for herself.

> Ms. O thus saw the referral for analysis as lacking the element of free choice. As noted, the analyst was, in her view, duty-bound to accept her as a patient, in the same way as her mother had been duty-bound to care for her as a child. She herself had chosen neither the analyst nor the analysis. Analysis had been prescribed for her in advance, and had been presented to her as the only alternative. Given her distraught emotional state at the time of the referral, Ms. O felt she had no other choice but to accept it—or, more exactly, she accepted it with the idea of ultimately freeing herself of it—like any prisoner. Sadly, she did not so much seek liberation *by* analysis as *from* analysis.

It may be necessary, as this vignette suggests, to place parentheses around any definite prescription for therapy, and even to redo the assessment from scratch. Most patients will accept such a repetition when it is prefaced with words such as "I need to hear it from you directly," or "I need to form my own opinions firsthand." It is even quite within the Freudian guidelines to begin the assessment without having read the written evaluation. Such a tactic helps the resident to avoid the preformed bias of the initial evaluation. Later, the two versions can be compared. Most therapists find that patients give a far more complete history when it is addressed to someone with whom they are going to be working, and who has already established some credibility in their eyes—and, by the same token, they are more likely to verbalize their reservations and hesitations about entering therapy.

If questions sufficient to delay the decision to proceed are raised about a patient's readiness for therapy, a period of extended evaluation may be indicated. An extended evaluation can last anywhere from 5 to 15 sessions. This transitional phase is indeed a kind of trial therapy, as Freud suggests, with the one difference that the decision of whether to commit to therapy is left open. Certainly, this period affords the therapist a chance to further test the patient's capacity for therapy. As for the patient, extended evaluation allows him or her to experience the conditions of therapy firsthand. On the basis of such knowledge, therapist and patient may agree to continue the arrangement. However, the aim of this phase is not simply recruitment of the patient, but rather *the enlistment of the patient's participation in the decision.* Therefore, the therapist should rate it a success when a patient rejects therapy, especially when that rejection is based on the patient's realization that therapy can never meet his or her expectations or resolve his or her ambivalence.

Documentation

Nothing epitomizes the literal prescription for therapy so much as the patient consent form, now a standard document in some psychiatric clinics. Although the wording of this form is somewhat extreme, it provides a good example of the potential effects of institutionalization on clinic policy. One such form states that the patient is obliged to accept "any and all treatments that the Doctor may deem advisable, including psychotherapy" *in advance.* In essence, this statement amounts to a unilateral decision made outside the therapeutic context; furthermore, it defines a decision to decline therapy as a breach of contract. Certainly, the consent form can be presented to the patient with qualifications and exhortations not to take it quite literally, but such words cannot totally erase the binding nature of the agreement.

As an illustration of the significance of the consent form, consider the following:

> Mr. P, a 33-year-old man, presented for treatment because of doubts about whether to get married. This man had long ago severed his roots in the country of his birth and now lived the life of a global vagabond. In the course of his wanderings, he had tried numerous jobs and had relationships with hundreds of women. At the time of his referral, Mr. P was simultaneously "engaged" to two women. This prospective clinic patient told his story with considerable candor, but when presented with the consent form, he balked and refused to sign it. As he put it, he had never made a serious commitment in his life—this was his problem. By not signing, Mr. P felt he was only being honest, because countless times throughout his life he had failed to deliver on his promises.

There is a tendency to view all clinic documentation as written prescriptions for treatment. This expectation can be mitigated by introducing the patient to the helpful effects of *retelling* his or her story. Freud, for example, was in the habit of asking patients to tell him their dreams a second or even a third time. In the same way, the history always finds its place as a retelling of the patient's life story. In this regard, Freud (1913/1958) acknowledged that many patients will begin the treatment with an account of their whole life story, but added that "a consecutive narrative should never be expected and nothing should be done to encourage it. Every detail of the story will have to be related afresh, and only with this repetition will additional matter appear, enabling the significant connections which are unknown to the patient to be traced" (p. 136).

In writing down the history, one should proceed pretty much as if one were taking process notes for a session or recording a lengthy dream. The final "document" will then highlight those items—dreams, childhood memories, traumata—that obtrude in the otherwise smooth flow of the story, as well as the so-called para-amnesias that cover gaps in the story. This first sketch of the history will thus be as useful for what it leaves out as for what it emphasizes or overemphasizes. Later comparisons with different versions of the same history will reveal significant deletions, changes of emphasis, or reversals of chronology.

The written formulation, usually based on the history, can never be more than a "trial interpretation." In fact, it may be of value to share all or part of this conjecture with the patient, and to hear how he or she responds to it. In the same vein, it is useful to elicit and record the patient's own first interpretation of his or her life history. This interpretation may turn out to contain more than a grain of truth; in any case, it contributes to one of the aims of analytic therapy—namely, the *making* of history, in the full sense of that term. Part of this process would then consist of noting and recording the questions arising out of a consideration of the history by both patient and therapist. Such a list of questions provides a more secure guide to the work of therapy than any predetermined explanation of the patient's psychodynamics.

This list can also serve in place of a treatment plan. In most psychiatric clinics, the therapist is given the latitude to individualize the treatment plan as he or she sees fit. Like a treatment plan, questions address themselves to the future, and like a treatment plan, they can be referred to again and again throughout the treatment. But unlike the treatment plan, questions leave open the direction from which the answer will come. Thus, instead of the typical statement of aim ("I will find a job"), the corresponding question might be "What do I really want to do?" This kind of revised treatment plan can also serve as an adjunct to the resident's supervision of the case, as it does in West Germany (Thomä and Kächele 1987), where analytic treatment plans are reviewed by outside assessors.

Most psychiatric clinic records are top-heavy, with the bulk of the documentation at the beginning, less in the middle, and practically nothing at the end. In fact, some clinics appear to have very few actual terminations, so that one is more likely to see a transfer note than a closing note. When a closing note is present, it is often perfunctory and sketchy. Yet, according to Freud (1912/1958), the proper place for the complete summary and formulation of a case is in the closing note. Preferably, this report should be written some time after the case has terminated to allow for temporal perspective. This case writeup now gives the resident the opportunity to set down what he or she has learned about the case, what new material has been uncovered, how he or she understands it, and what questions still remain open. When training directors require formal case reports (a not-uncommon practice), they are implicitly validating this idea of an expanded "postscript."

Managing Dislocations in Time and Space

Another area in which clinic procedure is liable to clash with analytic principles is in the handling of time and space. From the clinic's perspective, time and space are viewed as interchangeable commodities; hence, the quantity of space-time that a patient receives matters more than its specific location. On the other hand, the analytic arrangement (Freud 1913/1958) is based on the leasing of a specific time slot in the analyst's working day. A patient is not seen for just any hour, but specifically for the 1:00–2:00 hour or the 4:00–5:00 hour, for example. The same principle applies to office space: a given patient is always seen in the same office.

The following scenario illustrates the dislocation of time that can result from such a conflict of interests:

> The patient, Ms. Q, was a young college student working her way through college as a waitress. She was caught up in the problems of love and work characteristic of young adulthood. As a part-time student with two part-time jobs and several part-time boyfriends, Ms. Q's main conflict centered on whether to commit herself to a project "full-time." The resident, subject to many of the same time pressures as his patient, identified with her "part-time" status. In the first months of treatment, he and the patient renegotiated a different appointment time each week, hoping thereby to accommodate both of their hectic schedules. However, their sincere efforts to make the meeting times more convenient backfired. Having to keep so many different appointment times in mind led to missed appointments on both sides—and when an appointment was missed, neither party knew when to meet next. Such a built-in trap opened up a golden opportunity for the resistance: suddenly, Ms. Q's occasional latenesses and missed sessions became magnified tenfold.

Another ambiguity concerns whether the patient should be charged for missed sessions. The rule that patients are always responsible for their hours is only tenable when those hours are fixed and constant, according to the principle of the leased time slot. Patients may complain bitterly about having to pay for a missed session when they have a good excuse, not realizing that the lease arrangement always guarantees their *place* in the treatment, even when they are absent. The moment the time slot becomes variable, for whatever reason, the arrangement becomes void. From the analytic standpoint, this means that the missed sessions constitute an *interruption* in the treatment, exactly as if the treatment were suspended briefly and then started anew. Freud (1913/1958) actually treated lengthy absences from treatment in just this way: he suspended the treatment for a period, during which he felt free to fill the hour with another patient. Then, when the patient returned, the two of them would renegotiate another hour.

In the clinic, working space may be subject to the same variability as time slots. If one time slot is as good as another, then one office is also as good as another. Space limitations and the consequent necessity of sharing offices naturally contribute to this policy. When all the offices are occupied—a not-uncommon situation—therapists will scramble for any available location as if they were playing "musical chairs." In the time frame of a year, residents will end up meeting some of their patients in more than one office. Sometimes the change will occur at erratic intervals; at other times, it will take place on a regular schedule. The space problem also leads to the frequent reshuffling and reassigning of offices. Hence, a resident may start out in one "permanent" office and after a year be relocated to another.

In some ways, changing offices has the same effect on patients as changing time slots. It may induce a state of mild disorientation or of obsessive doubt about the correct address. If the new office is in a different building from the old, patients can get lost on the way to the session. And in some patients, the sense of disorientation conceals a deeper question about *whom* they are addressing. A new office may raise questions in patients' minds about the very identity of their therapist—and not just in deeply disturbed patients. Even after the disorientation has dissipated, patient and therapist are reminded of the question of identity by the very fact that the two offices are not the same.

This issue is brought into sharp relief whenever a patient is being seen in two offices that differ greatly. Consider the following example:

> The patient, Ms. R, met with her therapist twice a week in a plushly carpeted, well-appointed office and once a week in a bare, institutional-looking office. Normally unobtrusive, the therapeutic setting became for the patient the main focus of her associations. Ms. R especially concentrated on the *walls* of the two offices, one set of which was covered with hangings and the other of which was completely vacant and white. These walls quickly became associated with starkly contrasting images of the therapist.

Even a healthy ego has difficulty reconciling such opposites. When the ego is prone to defensive "splitting," as in this patient, it will find it difficult to prevent the opposites from splitting apart. Then, every change of offices will seem like a change of therapist—and, therefore, a breach of trust, necessitating temporary withdrawal.

Just as patients notice qualitative differences in offices, they also notice differences in time slots—for example, those between nighttime and daytime, or between the beginning and the middle of a session. In the latter instance, patients may treat the beginning and/or the end of the session as a social interchange with the doctor. "In this way," wrote Freud (1913/1958), "they divide the treatment in their own view into an official portion, in which they mostly behave in a very inhibited manner, and an informal 'friendly' portion, in which they speak really freely and say all sorts of things which they themselves do not regard as being part of the treatment" (p. 139). Freud cautioned that any such "partition" must not be allowed to stand, lest it permanently undermine the therapeutic process.

As shown in the above vignette, all such differences introduce an element of discontinuity into the therapeutic process. By *discontinuity,* I mean a breakdown in the inherent "hanging together" of the therapeutic setting that is analogous to the "partition" mentioned above. The resistance can magnify a discontinuity into a disruption, using it like a wedge to split therapy in two and then pitting the two halves against each other. Hence, what starts out as a tiny chink in the wall may eventually bring down the foundation.

As if anticipating this problem, residents in a clinic usually agree upon the norm of meeting with their psychotherapy patients once per week. At first glance, this arrangement seems an ideal compromise: the residents' time is divided evenly among all their patients, allowing them to accommodate their heavy caseloads; the fixed time allows patients regular access to the doctor without making excessive demands on the doctor's time and resources; and the once-weekly session provides continuity. Everyone is happy. Many patients begin therapy with enthusiasm and some appear to thrive in this arrangement for months and even years.

But what remains hidden is the 7-day interruption between sessions. It is easier to see the glass as half-full than as half-empty. The once-per-week format, in fact, creates a "partition" between the day of the session and the rest of the week. Experiencing the session as an encapsulated island in the middle of the week makes it quite easy for patients to talk freely, because they can disassociate these thoughts from the rest of their lives. Besides, the 7-day hiatus allows plenty of time for the accumulation of "events," which provide a ready-made agenda. And for their part, residents tend to treat the hiatus as "dead time" during which nothing happens. Against this background of "dead time," residents tend to view the end of a session as a kind of "deadline," thereby creating an atmosphere of haste and forcing them to make premature interpretations.

These covert difficulties will often reveal themselves when a once-per-week format changes to a twice-per-week or a three-times-per-week one. The previously loquacious patient now becomes almost mute. Without the "partition," this patient is forced to confront his or her resistance for the first time. On the other hand, residents often note that they feel more relaxed knowing they have time to work through the resistance. In a new version of an old truism, one might say that treatment really begins when both the patient *and* the therapist run out of things to say.

Variability of time and space also introduces the idea that therapy is temporary or transient. When these changes occur at the beginning of therapy, the patient may think of them as a "temporary arrangement" that will end as soon as a more permanent venue is decided upon. But if the makeshift arrangement continues indefinitely, how can the patient avoid thinking that the therapy itself is temporary? These changes have the same effect on the therapist. When a group of residents was asked how they felt about sharing offices, their answer was unanimous: it made them feel transient, like they were just passing through. Hence, they were more likely to accept such offices "as is," making little effort to transform them into their own work settings. This attitude fosters the belief that one office is just like another—and that the therapist is just as temporary as the shaky chair, the frayed upholstery, or the faded rug.

Termination

The most definitive time variable—the one that most exemplifies the effect of discontinuity—is the practice of fixed terminations. Fixed terminations are problematic precisely because they are "fixed," not because they lead to shorter treatments. It is quite possible for a therapy to remain brief without the termination date's being fixed. All that is required is a *negotiated* termination occurring as part of the therapeutic process and within the context of the therapeutic relationship.

Frequently, fixed terminations occur, not out of any special intent, but as a result of the inevitable turnover of residents in the clinic. With few exceptions, this condition limits the maximum time over which a resident can see a patient to 2 years. Patients who are picked up in the fourth year are limited to 1 year or less. The clinic tries to maintain continuity for such patients by periodically transferring many of them to new residents; however, as I will argue in the following section, this policy does not eliminate the problematic effects of forced termination.

The effects of forced termination are most visible during the termination phase. Knowing they must inevitably lose their therapist, many patients react to termination with an increase in their defenses and a "flight into health." They may minimize their continuing conflicts, deny their anger and sadness, and exploit their newfound independence. Their message is clear: "I really don't need you anymore—I can take care of myself." Other patients deal with anticipated loss by developing a new, possibly severe exacerbation of their symptoms. In cases like these, the emphasis is placed exclusively on the transfer to a new therapist. Such patients seem to be saying, "I am not really losing a therapist; I am just so sick that I need a new, more capable therapist to take care of me."

Residents unwittingly add to the patient's problems during termination because they themselves are undergoing a similar termination from the residency program. Preoccupied with their own feelings and defenses over the loss of friends and valued mentors, and having to rely on their own independence, residents may be as unwilling to deal with such issues as their patients. Indeed, it is not uncommon for a supervisor to notice a resident ignoring his or her patient's overtures to begin talking about termination. It is still possible to ameliorate the patient's reluctance when the resident shows his or her emotional readiness to deal with loss. The worst possible scenario involves the *collusion* of resident and patient to mutually avoid talking about termination.

I want to emphasize, however, that the effects of forced termination are not limited to the "termination phase." The collusion spoken of just now may develop as soon as both parties become *aware* of the fixed termination, even if the date is a year away. The knowledge that therapy cannot last beyond a certain date acts to limit the emotional investment of both therapist and patient (Freud 1937/1964). But the effect can seem paradoxical: On the one hand, the patient might think, "I can afford to be more open about some things, knowing I will escape before they amount to anything." On the other hand, he or she might think, "There are certain other things I can never tell because therapy might be over before I can work them through." This, in fact, was what Ms. O admitted to her therapist toward the end of her analysis. Even though there was no fixed termination date, her conviction that analysis was prescribed implied a fixed termination date. So what was the point in getting too deeply immersed in something when the analyst was, by definition, only a temporary fill-in?

Residents who are aware of the consequences of forced termination are in a position to mitigate some of these effects. First, they understand that the time to begin exploring the significance of termination is at the beginning of therapy, not at the very end. The time to listen for reactions to termination is when the patient first learns about the time limit, even when the actual date is not yet specified. Second, residents may use the anticipated termination as an opportunity to explore their own conflicts about separation from their training programs. Third, they can raise the issue of a termination date while there is still enough time to vigorously work through the anticipated loss. And fourth, residents can, within certain limits, allow the working-through process to determine the actual termination date.

The Transference and Third-Party Relationships

In his technical writings, Freud (1913/1958) advised his patients to "treat the analysis as a matter between [themselves] and [their] physician, and to exclude everyone else from sharing in it, no matter how closely bound to [them] or how inquisitive they may be" (p. 136). Many of Freud's recommendations in "On Beginning the Treatment" concern the handling of such third parties. For example, the analyst who has a friend or relative in common with his or her patient "must be prepared for it to cost [him or her] that friendship." The patient too, must forgo discussing the analysis with an intimate friend, lest this communication take the place of analysis itself. Freud remarked that the first test of this fundamental rule occurs when "something intimate about a *third person* comes up in [the patient's] mind for the first time" (p. 135 [italics mine]). Even other physicians must be considered "third parties." Previous treatment by another physician creates certain disadvantages for the therapy, such as a preformed transference that must be laboriously uncovered at the beginning of the analysis. Freud specifically cautioned against the concurrent treatment with another physician on the grounds that "patients withdraw their interest from analysis as soon as they are shown more than one path that promises to lead them to health" (p. 137).

Third parties are nowhere more obtrusive than in a busy psychiatric clinic. Before their visit, patients will have been evaluated by another doctor and possibly a social worker. On arriving at the clinic, they are greeted by the receptionist and perhaps accosted by the billing clerk. Seated in the waiting room, they are surrounded by other patients, some of whom share the same therapist. Patients may have come with spouses or children who are seeing another therapist. Once inside the office, they may be bombarded by ringing phones, buzzing intercoms, unexpected knocks on the door, the hum of recording equipment, or the resident's beeper going off. And when soundproofing is inadequate, they have the murmur of other voices to contend with.

Who is this busybody who keeps interrupting, who will not rest until it has found its way into the very heart of therapy? Who else but the clinic itself qua intrusive agency. No single individual intends any mischief, yet it almost seems as if some divisive force were operating unconsciously and despite the good intentions of all concerned. One would interpret such behavior in a patient as the child positioning itself between the parents so as to prevent them from having sexual intercourse. In this case, however, the "excluded third party" is an institution—or rather, that institution's unconscious aims and agenda.

The clinic gets its foot in the door of the consulting room through the instrument of the "fee" and the mechanism of third-party payment. In using the phrase *third-party payment,* I refer not just to insurance companies but, more specifically, to the clinic's status as payee for all fees. Thus, in every case of analytically oriented therapy conducted in the clinic, the fee goes to a third party—the clinic—and not to the resident. This fact is important because *every financial transaction creates a relationship between the parties.* Hence, third-party payment establishes a relationship between the patient and the third party that competes with the patient's relationship with the therapist. The therapist is excluded from the third-party relationship except to the extent that he or she is perceived as an "agent" of the third party.

The resident is often not privy to the criteria for setting the fee, the insurance coverage, or even the amount of that fee. This clinic policy excludes the resident from the financial transaction at the outset. Even if he or she were to insist upon receiving the checks him- or herself, the resident could not completely avoid being perceived by the patient as a "functionary" of the clinic. The critical question in this regard is this: Can patients be totally candid with residents about their finances, knowing that their fees could be raised on the basis of such disclosures? Many residents have seen what happens when one of their subsidy patients is "bumped" to a higher fee category. Not infrequently, the formerly enthusiastic patient decides to terminate. Equally disillusioning is when long-standing therapy patients ask residents to "lie" on their insurance or Medicaid forms.

The following vignette illustrates a related effect of third-party interactions:

> Mr. S, a podiatry student in his early 20s, sought treatment for symptoms of anxiety. Because of his student status, his father, a prosperous dentist, was paying for the treatment. In the beginning, there was little discussion about how the fees were to be paid. Mr. S adopted a passive, nonparticipatory role. During most sessions, he just sat there like a lump, waiting for something to happen. When he did talk, he complained loudly about his lack of progress and the therapist's inability or refusal to do something helpful. Mr. S exhibited the same attitude outside sessions, feeling unable to make decisions and confused about what he wanted to do with himself.
>
> After many months of therapy, the issue of the fee was raised. At first, Mr. S appeared uninterested, but with some encouragement, he admitted that there was something not right about it. He said that he felt like a go-between—as if the real relationship were between his father and the therapist. Mr. S had been seeing himself *(my inference)* as a passive object—literally, as *an object of exchange between his father and the therapist.* Therefore, he had never acted as if he were a party in the therapeutic transaction. Therapy was something happening between others, with himself as passive spectator. In effect, the patient's father—a third party—had taken his place, forcing him into the excluded position.
>
> In the wake of these disclosures, patient and therapist decided together that Mr. S would pay a "token" portion of the fee until such time as he could afford the entire fee. This change resulted in a slight improvement in therapy. But the real change

> came the following year, when the patient obtained his first job. From the very day he started paying the full fee, Mr. S was like a different person. He entered the therapy frame as if it were his own personal "investment." He talked and worked on his problems as if he really had a stake in them. Moreover, he now wanted to come twice a week, even though it would mean a greater sacrifice.

The point here is not that every patient must pay the full fee, but rather that any contribution that patients make to their own treatment—even if token—increases their level of involvement and the probability of their viewing therapy as a working partnership.

Part of the work of therapy is uncovering the third party's "hidden agenda." The patient carries these agenda in the form of unconscious directives and compulsions. In the above vignette, for example, Mr. S felt compelled to fulfill his father's wish that he complete podiatry school. If the third party is the patient's spouse, the hidden agenda might be a marital scenario in which the therapist "cures" the other spouse, gives him or her permission to divorce, or uses him or her as an ally in an ongoing marital war. Sample medical agenda include the verification of illness, the labeling of a troublesome patient as "psychiatric," and the "dumping" of a patient who has no discernible organic pathology. Whenever a patient has a court case pending, the legal agenda is almost always the same: to avoid legal penalties.

The clinic benefits from all these agenda, because one of its major aims is to recruit "bodies." I say *bodies* instead of *patients* to stress the hidden requirement to fill up the clinic's rolls, regardless of patients' individual diagnoses, readiness for treatment, or reason for seeking help. This aspect of the clinic's hidden agenda is dramatized by Mr. S, who was present in body but not in spirit. Since a body invites medical intervention rather than psychotherapeutic collaboration, another part of the clinic's agenda is also served: that of maintaining ties of identification with other medical clinics.

The common practice of transferring patients from one resident to another at the end of a term is yet another method of keeping the number of patients constant. In such situations, the patient's passive body becomes an object of transfer between one resident and another. True, this practice is done for the laudable reasons of maintaining continuity and at least ensuring the possibility of longer-term therapy. But the one thing that remains constant in these multiple transfers is the omnipresence of the clinic as third party.

The unlimited substitution of one resident for another—and there are patients who have gone through five or more residents—demonstrates that therapists are, at base, interchangeable. The so-called transference to institutions (Reider 1953) reflects, in large part, a transference to an "interchangeable therapist"—the counterpart of the interchangeable room and the interchangeable time slot. In every transfer, patients are bound to feel like an object of barter. They may even try to maximize their outcomes—that is, avoid being "downgraded" to a less-experienced therapist. But many patients must feel without much autonomy and as if their participation is minimal. They will therefore come to rely on the clinic as a surrogate parent. Although patients vary in the extent to which they assume a passive position, even very psychologically minded patients may experience a degree of institutional transference.

In the typical "countertransfer" reaction, the resident feels like an object of comparison with the patient's previous therapist. Some will behave as if they have something to prove with their new patient; others will find themselves withdrawing in the shadow of an idealized predecessor. Residents are thrown off track regardless of which way the comparison goes. If they are vilified, they feel ineffectual; if they are greeted like a savior, they inevitably feel guilty, as if they are annihilating the former therapist and all his or her work.

In this, as in all other intrusions of the clinic, the obstacle can be overcome if residents are open to exploring the emotional impact of the recent transfer. Their first task, as Freud suggested, is to finish the task of termination. In word as well as in deed, residents need to recognize that the object of the patient's transference is still the former therapist and not themselves. Indeed, the process of helping the patient to bring this unresolved transference into the foreground will help *establish* a new transference to the current therapist. If, on the other hand, residents ignore this preliminary labor and attempt to merely supplant the old therapist, they will in fact reinforce the patient's idea that residents are interchangeable. Their implied message is something like this: "Let's go on as if nothing has changed—as if it doesn't matter who is sitting in the therapist's chair."

Conclusion

In all the problems discussed in this chapter, the conflict between psychoanalytic and institutional modalities reflects the intrapsychic struggle with the psychodynamic perspective. In the minds of some residents, the clinic takes on the censoring, prohibiting function of the superego directed against the implied sexual intimacy of the therapeutic partnership. Insofar as the clinic's presence evokes conflicts in the resident, it will constitute a specific blind spot or countertransference. Residents' difficulties with these issues will vary in proportion to their own ambivalence concerning the psychodynamic perspective. Exploring these difficulties can certainly help residents to assume more fully the mantle of analytically oriented therapist, and thereby to resolve some of the identity diffusion associated with training in psychiatry.

Once this task is undertaken, the solution to the problems of institutionalization is simple: The resident assumes the therapeutic role right from the start and never allows this role to be co-opted or delegated by anyone else. The analytic orientation allows the resident to keep matters open in the face of institutional pressures for closure on several fronts. Hence, in the face of the temptation to prescribe analytic treatment, the resident "keeps the file open"; in the face of scheduling pressures, he or she "keeps the time slot open"; and in the face of third parties, he or she "keeps the door open." The resident responds to each of these pressures, not by capitulating, but by reassuming an intrapsychic focus once again, and starting anew.

Regardless of where they find themselves—after the assessment, in the middle of an interruption, dislocated in space-time, occupying the third-party position, or engaged in a transfer—residents can always find their way again at the beginning. The resident has to be willing to look at the patient's material with a fresh eye. This attitude on the part of residents is actually a rediscovery of Freud's (1913/1958) original conception of the analytic method. In recommending a daily analytic session, Freud's intention was not to count 1, 2, 3, . . . , but to make each succeeding session a repetition of the one before. Hence, each new session does not take off from the one before, but starts the process all over again as if it were the first in the series. The analytic attitude of *evenly hovering attention* (Freud 1912/1958) in fact demands that one approach each new session free of expectations and presuppositions.

In this sense, all analytic practitioners are "beginners." Whereas residents are learning these lessons for the first time, more experienced analysts are relearning them as they, too, encounter increasing institutionalization both without and within psychoanalysis. Since 1984, the psychoanalytic community has had to confront such institutional issues as documentation for insurers, a major lawsuit, the controversy over delinkage of membership and certification, the problems of outside accreditation, and the new influence of the International Psychoanalytic Association on American soil (Bulletin of the American Psychoanalytic Association 1992). The clinical problems described in this chapter may perhaps serve as a "natural experiment" for analysts who are already finding this issue hard to avoid.

For Further Study

Freud S: Recommendations to physicians practicing psycho-analysis (1912), in The Standard Edition of the Complete Psychological Works of Sigmund Freud, Vol 12. Translated and edited by Strachey J. London, Hogarth Press, 1958, pp 109–120

Freud S: On beginning the treatment (further recommendations on the technique of psycho-analysis I) (1913), in The Standard Edition of the Complete Psychological Works of Sigmund Freud, Vol 12. Translated and edited by Strachey J. London, Hogarth Press, 1958, pp 121–144

Freud S: Analysis terminable and interminable (1937), in The Standard Edition of the Complete Psychological Works of Sigmund Freud, Vol 23. Translated and edited by Strachey J. London, Hogarth Press, 1964, pp 209–253

Reider N: A type of transference to institutions. Bull Menninger Clin 17:58–63, 1953

Thomä H, Kächele H: Psycho-Analytic Practice, Vol 1: Principles. Berlin, Springer-Verlag, 1987

Winnicott DW: Metapsychological and clinical aspects of regression within the psycho-analytical set-up, in Through Paediatrics to Psycho-Analysis. London, Hogarth Press, 1978, pp 278–294

References

Bulletin of the American Psychoanalytic Association 40:607 (no author or title), 1992

Freud S: Recommendations to physicians practicing psycho-analysis (1912), in The Standard Edition of the Complete Psychological Works of Sigmund Freud, Vol 12. Translated and edited by Strachey J. London, Hogarth Press, 1958, pp 109–120

Freud S: On beginning the treatment (further recommendations on the technique of psycho-analysis I) (1913), in The Standard Edition of the Complete Psychological Works of Sigmund Freud, Vol 12. Translated and edited by Strachey J. London, Hogarth Press, 1958, pp 121–144

Freud S: Analysis terminable and interminable (1937), in The Standard Edition of the Complete Psychological Works of Sigmund Freud, Vol 23. Translated and edited by Strachey J. London, Hogarth Press, 1964, pp 209–253

Goldacker-Pohlmann U: The influence of the health insurance system on psychoanalytic training in Germany. International Psychoanalysis (Summer 1993)

New practice patterns said to be necessary for economic survival. Psychiatric News 28:1, 4, August 6, 1993

Reider N: A type of transference to institutions. Bull Menninger Clin 17:58–63, 1953

Thomä H, Kächele H: Psycho-Analytic Practice, Vol 1: Principles. Berlin, Springer-Verlag, 1987

Winnicott DW: Ego integration in child development, in The Maturational Processes and the Facilitating Environment. New York, International Universities Press, 1962, pp 56–63

Section III

Clinical Syndromes

Harvey J. Schwartz, M.D.,
Section Editor

Chapter 10

The Psychotic Patient

Richard L. Munich, M.D.

Current Psychodynamic Perspectives and Differential Dynamic Diagnosis

Psychodynamically oriented theorists and clinicians have always had an uneasy relationship with psychotic patients. In addition to changing his mind about the psychological roots of psychosis, Freud did not believe his therapy could be effective with patients suffering from psychosis because of their inability to form a recognizable transference. Although many practitioners have challenged Freud's views and have used psychoanalytic theory to understand and treat the disturbance, especially in providing support for patients in the throes of an acute or chronic psychosis, the recent neuroscientific advances in conceptualizing the etiology and facilitating the amelioration of psychotic states require a periodic reassessment of the role and status of psychodynamic concepts and practice in this area (Grotstein 1989).

Meanwhile, it is the person whose mentation and function are painfully disordered in the midst of psychosis who ambivalently requests our psychosocial assistance, who struggles to restore or enhance community integration and tenure, and whose life goals may be facilitated by psychiatric rehabilitation. Principles related to the dynamic unconscious are helpful in organizing an interpersonal approach to these issues as well as in assessing the impact of various environmental and developmental demands upon and adaptive style and character of the person with a psychosis. It is the aim of this chapter to outline the development and demonstrate the relevance of a psychodynamic point of view in understanding various aspects of the psychotic condition.

I would like to thank John Grimaldi, M.D., and Sonia Kulchycky, M.D., for their help in the preparation of this chapter.

What are the critical features of a psychosis? In contrast with individuals with a neurosis, those with a psychosis first and foremost have *an alteration in their capacity to test reality*—both consensually validated external reality and the internal world of thoughts and feelings. In the case of external reality, the psychotic person is unable to evaluate his or her perceptions accurately or to make correct inferences about them. Judgments about psychic reality, the internal world of conscious and unconscious self and object representations, thoughts and affects, wishes, impulses, and fantasies are also affected, as well as the capacity to distinguish between internal and external reality. Neurotic individuals know, for example, that a daydream is just that, even when experienced powerfully, whereas psychotic persons may not only believe a daydream is true but also feel compelled to act upon it.

Altered reality testing is intimately connected with *a regression in the spheres of thinking and of self–object representation and differentiation.* The regression in thinking—otherwise known as a *thought disorder*—is to a level that is less organized and differentiated; for example, the rules of logic may be suspended, parts may stand for the whole, associational pathways may become loose and fragmented or blocked completely, and perception and memory may be distorted. In psychodynamic terms, secondary process has been replaced with primary process—thinking is now governed by the pressures of basic drives, a lack of organization, and a loss of capacity both for delay and for orderly discharge.

A person may exhibit various aspects of a thought disorder without being considered psychotic. However, when that person begins to cope with the regression by changing reality to fit his or her thinking—as occurs in thought broadcasting (hallucinations), false or distorted thoughts (delusions), or thought insertion (ideas of reference), also known as *restitutional symptoms*—then he or she is considered psychotic. As with symptoms in the neurotic individual, restitutional symptoms represent both the result of a regression to a prior point of fixation or trauma and the effort to resolve or to make a compromise with the inciting conflict and move on. In other words, such symptoms have often been seen as dynamically meaningful. Disordered thinking probably accounts for much of the language disturbance seen in psychotic states. Such disturbances include tangentiality, circumstantiality, word salad, neologisms, and alterations in the rate and flow of speech. In chronic states, there is an absolute poverty of speech.

In *the regression of self–object differentiation* associated with psychosis, conscious and unconscious mental images of the self and of important objects in the individual's life may become less coherent or fragmented and the differentiation of these self and object representations may become blurred or fused—or, like the disturbance in thinking, invested with primary process or drive material. The dedifferentiation of these internalized representations usually has a profound dysfunctional impact on the individual's adaptive and functional capacity, as in social withdrawal, bizarre or idiosyncratic behaviors, amotivational states, and catatonia. Restitutional symptoms, disturbed language and associations, and severe maladaptive behaviors are the most common presenting features of a person in an acute psychotic state. A person who is chronically or persistently psychotic may have all of these features but reveal them only in an extended interview, during a complicated social interaction, or when asked to perform a task.

From the therapeutic perspective, it is important to note that considerable controversy exists as to what extent the basic personality organization of the psychotic individual is affected by regression. The most widely held view is that the greater the regression, the greater the dedifferentiation in self and object representations and, thus, the greater the final effect on identity and personality as a whole. Certainly, the fear of fragmentation or loss of self, or loss of coherence of the self-concept, is a prominent aspect of the experience of a person with a psychosis. Others hold that even in highly regressed patients, the personality remains essentially intact and, depending on its configuration, can have both facilitating and inhibiting influences on the treatment, the treatment alliance, and the course of the illness (Terkelsen et al. 1991).

There are many pathways to the problems with reality testing and its associated regression in thinking and self–object differentiation. These pathways range from toxic states secondary to the ingestion of psychotomimetics, to deficiency, neoplastic, and infectious diseases, and to trauma and postpartum hormonal alterations. Psychosis is usually associated with the various forms of schizophrenia but may also be a consequence of major affective, schizoaffective, or delusional disorders. Transient psychotic states have been reported in otherwise intact persons who are undergoing sensory deprivation or severe stress, as well as in persons with severe borderline, schizotypal, or paranoid personality disorder. Disturbances both in the individual's orientation to reality (as in perceptual distortions, defects in attention, primitive and infantile object relations, and the use of transitional objects) and in the individual's sense of reality (as in depersonalization and heightened states of perception and self-observation) can be important precursors to a loss of capacity to test reality. It has been postulated by psychoanalysts and neurobiologists that the psychosis associated with schizophrenia comes about when social and developmental demands outstrip the organism's biochemical and neuroanatomical capacity to cope. In all likelihood, this capacity has been shaped by genetic, psychological, and environmental factors (Liberman and Corrigan 1992; Robbins 1992).

Finally, an important conceptual problem and a controversial pathway to psychosis is whether altered reality testing and regression in thinking and behavior are, as in neurosis, rooted in unconscious conflict, except more intense, more severe, and more regressed; or whether these disturbances represent something altogether different, with a different etiology and, therefore, unrelated to conflict (London 1973; Wexler 1971). Another way of putting this distinction is that, in the first position, neurosis and psychosis exist on a continuum, with their differences being essentially quantitative; the opposite position, of course, holds that there is a qualitative difference between the two. If psychosis is—like neurosis—rooted in conflict, then the alterations in reality testing and the regression in thinking come about as a defense against the anxiety associated with libidinal and aggressive drives, particularly those related to the oedipal constellation. This was the position Freud held in 1894 (Freud 1894/1961).

Later, however, Freud (1911/1958) believed that there was a qualitative difference between psychosis and neurosis—that the psychotic individual had withdrawn his or her interest or investment (cathexis) from the outside world and retreated inward, and therefore was unable to evaluate reality, think purposively, or make an investment in the outside world. In this view, also thought of as the *deficiency theory,* the inability to form or maintain attachments is considered primary—a basic defect of ego functioning—rather than defensive: hence the term *narcissistic neurosis.* Although this view was very much a dynamic construct in the beginning, advances derived from modern genetic, neuroanatomical, and biochemical studies lend some credence to the idea that when psychoanalysts refer to basic and primary deficiencies or deficits in the individual's capacity to cathect an object, they are also talking about—as Freud predicted, and in line with some of the pathways alluded to earlier—actual molecular and neuronal defects in subcortical tissue, enlarged ventricles, decreased dopamine receptors, altered eye-tracking mechanisms, slow reaction times, and whatever neurophysiological problems lead to the inability to maintain attentional sets.

Historical Review[1]

The history of the psychodynamic point of view of psychosis is congruent with developments in psychoanalysis in general. It moves, therefore, from drive theory to the structural theory and then to object relations and interpersonal and self psychological perspectives. One of Freud's (1894/1961) earliest ideas on the subject was that the ego dealt with an unbearable idea or fantasy by a "flight into psychosis" (p. 59). At that time, he characterized this flight as "the expression of a pathological disposition" (p. 59)—perhaps his first allusion to the deficit model. A little later, Abraham (1908/1927) wrote of the regression seen in *dementia praecox,* which involved withdrawal of libido from the external world back to the self, a loss of the object, and functioning at the autoerotic or narcissistic stage of psychosexual development.

In the Schreber case, Freud (1911/1958) used Abraham's formulation as groundwork for the early dynamic point of view of delusions, not only as a consequence of regression but also as a restitutive effort to maintain a failing sense of reality. Freud postulated that the process of regression and delusion formation was triggered in the patient by his efforts to ward off a homosexual wishful fantasy ("I love him"), first by withdrawing interest in the object of such a wish ("I hate him"), and then by defensively projecting the wish onto the object

[1]The form and content of this section owes much to the work of John Frosch (1983, 1990).

("He hates me"), thus experiencing himself as the object of persecution. Although the early stage of psychic development is reflected in the extreme self-centered, grandiose, and narcissistic aspect of the patient's construction, the alternating effort to withdraw from and restore contact with the object may also be seen. As noted, Freud at this point thought that disturbances with the object took place because of an intrinsic flaw in the ego. Interest in this flaw led early dynamic theorists to postulate trauma during the oral stage of psychosexual development as especially meaningful in the etiology of the psychoses. As we shall see, trauma or disturbance at this early stage, especially involving the infant's first objects, informs virtually every theory of psychosis.

With some modifications, Abraham's and Freud's early conception has remained the centerpiece of the psychodynamic view of the psychoses, with delusions in the paranoid individual and severe regressions in the schizophrenic individual being regarded as efforts to manage or get rid of the conflict by altering reality. Hartmann (1951) felt that the withdrawal and restitution was a continuous, alternating process, and Nunberg (1951) construed the restitution as a move toward recovery. Of great importance to therapeutic work is the debate about whether or not the object is given up completely, whether what appears in delusional form is an archaic or part object, and whether it is representations of objects or objects themselves that are withdrawn from. Freeman (1973) hypothesized that self-representation and self–nonself differentiation are more affected, leading secondarily to an overvaluation of objects. Meanwhile, many highly creative efforts were made to relate the withdrawal from objects to the content of delusions (e.g., of the end of the world [Katan 1949; Klein 1946; Macalpine and Hunter 1953] or of the influencing machine [Tausk 1919/1948]), stereotypies, hypochondrias, and somatic delusions (Fenichel 1945; Ferenczi 1927; Schilder 1951).

With the publication of "The Ego and the Id" (1923/1961), Freud introduced the structural theory in which the ego and its defense operations take precedence over the drives and their vicissitudes. In the dynamics of the person with a psychosis, we now see the important shift—from withdrawal of libido and a deficit in the ego's capacity to cathect an object to a version of psychosis based on conflict within the ego, dedifferentiation of the ego–id and ego–superego structural divisions, and repersonification of the superego, which theoretically had been consolidated and internalized by resolution of the Oedipus complex.

Signal anxiety is the mover of the structural system. In a chapter entitled "The Nature and Danger of the Conflict," John Frosch (1983) outlined the specific contributions to anxiety in the psychotic process as opposed to more neurotic processes. Using birth as a prototypical emergency situation, he described "the feeling of helplessness and an inability to cope with an overwhelming situation" as a kind of basic anxiety. Fundamental to the psychotic process is this basic anxiety in response to the "sensed possibility of disintegration and dissolution of [the] self, . . . i.e., psychic and emotional death" (p. 205). Psychoanalysts of all theoretical persuasions have identified versions of this basic anxiety, relating it to a collapse of the self system; the dissolution of psychic structure;

the fear of disintegration, fragmentation, and engulfment; and the dedifferentiation of ego boundaries and self–nonself and self–object structures. The intensity of the anxiety in each of these psychic scenarios is heightened by the belief that the process is irreversible, that libidinal and aggressive demands cannot be controlled—and, harking back to Freud's comment about the ego's relation to the external world, by the fear that reality is lost altogether (Bak 1954).

Arlow and Brenner (1969) proposed a revision of the psychopathology of the psychoses that reflected Freud's shift from withdrawal from the object to conflict within the ego, emphasizing that the differences between the psychoses and the neuroses are quantitative. According to Buckley (1988), "[Arlow and Brenner] conceded that instinctual regression tends to be more pronounced and severe in the psychoses, that conflicts over aggression are more frequent, and that disturbances of ego and superego functioning are much more severe than in the neuroses" (p. 2). In other words, the symptoms of psychosis are compromise formations between anxiety and defense, just as are seen in neurotic symptoms, distortions of character, and severe inhibitions.

While we are on the topic of the structural theory, it may be useful to mention the predominant defenses used by the person with a psychosis. In contrast to the higher-level defenses of repression, displacement, and reaction formation used by the neurotic patient, the defensive mechanisms employed by the patient with a psychosis are more archaic and include the regressive dedifferentiation mentioned above, introjective and projective techniques, projective identification, fragmentation, splitting, and massive denial (Jacobsen 1967). Splitting and projective identification are more commonly seen in patients with borderline personality organization, but obviously are relevant when such patients experience psychotic states and/or regressions. Similarly, denial exists on a continuum, from negation in the neurotic patient to the denial of reality in the patient with a psychosis—in fact, psychotic levels of denial are inconsistent with reality testing. Thus, in 1924, Freud wrote that "neurosis is the result of a conflict between the ego and its id, whereas psychosis is the analogous outcome of a similar disturbance in the relations between the ego and the external world" (Freud 1924/1961, p. 149). Of course, denial may operate in relation to psychic reality as well, assisting the process of repression but also playing a role in the symptoms of depersonalization and derealization and, finally, in a diminished appreciation of the boundary between internal and external realities.

Margaret Mahler's (1960) view of psychosis centered on the failure of the ego's perceptual-integrative function, which leads in the child with a psychosis to primitive ego levels and primitive object relations. In addition, the child uses massive denial, condensation, and dedifferentiation to defend itself against a threatening and usually disturbed human environment. These processes are superimposed on a phasic, developmental schema in the infant that begins with a symbiotic stage, the essential feature of which is "hallucinating or delusional, somatopsychic omnipotent fusion with the representation of the mother and, in particular, the delusion of a common boundary of the two actually and physically separate individuals" (Mahler 1968, p. 9). The symbiotic phase is central for childhood psychosis but clearly has congruence with adult forms of psychosis as well.

Edith Jacobson (1954, 1967) used the concept of psychotic identification to describe the state of deterioration and fusion of self–nonself images and ego–superego structures. She linked the level of regression in these systems to manic-depressive and schizophrenic illness, the former representing a less severe state in which a conflict exists between the superego and the self-representation and the latter representing a fusion between these self and object images within the now-failing ego-id.

The roles of incorporation, introjection and identification, and processes of internalization in the psychotic process provide a useful transition from the structural to the object relational point of view. Object relations are, after all, an important ingredient of external reality. Conceived of by the structuralists as an operation of the ego, internalization, derived from the organism's interplay with external objects, is critical to the formation of psychic structures. From the developmental perspective, increasingly larger and more abstract aspects of significant others are assimilated into and become part of the ego, superego, and ego-ideal of the maturing individual. Stable, integrated identifications are the end point of this process. It is clear that a psychotic process represents a reversal of assimilation such that what might be an introject, a transitional object, or a fantasied companion in a young child becomes the core of delusion in a decompensating adult. This "disidentification" is close to what has been referred to earlier as the dedifferentiation of self and object relations—a concept obviously central to a psychodynamic understanding of psychosis.

Object relations theory, most articulately represented by the British Object Relations School, began with the work of Melanie Klein. Rather than focusing on the structural deteriorations, object relations theory is more concerned with the deterioration of the representational world in the mind of an individual in the midst of the psychotic process. As is well known, Klein (1946) postulated oedipal dynamics as beginning at a much earlier age in infantile development, thus condensing many of the aggressive and destructive impulses into a stage corresponding to what structural theorists would identify as preoedipal, or the age or fixation point to which the patient with an incipient psychosis regresses. A more concise way of expressing this idea is via the paranoid-schizoid position and its accompanying defensive mechanism, projective identification. In this schema, a situation involving oral, anal, or even genital frustration initiates a sequence in which the infant experiences a complex mixture of helplessness, aggression, and anxiety. This experience is, according to Klein, accompanied by elaborate fantasies about the infant's relationship to its mother's body. To preserve the integrity of the self, the toxic affects are split off from the self and projected onto the depriving object, which comes to be viewed as dangerous and persecutory. As the infant reintrojects those projected bad parts, the conditions for paranoid and schizoid anxieties are established. If these anxieties are not managed or worked through—if the good and bad parts are not integrated (i.e., if the infant does not move from the paranoid-schizoid to what Klein described as the depressive position)—then psychotic processes in the adult will ensue. These processes can have the same content as the infantile anxieties and associated fantasies described above.

Whereas Klein herself attempted a version of the original Freudian prestructural drive position, her followers, especially Fairbairn (1941), postulated and focused on object-seeking activity from the beginning of infantile life. Gratifying and rejecting experiences with the object become the foundation for the personality, and their integration the basis for mature representational structures. For Fairbairn as well as for Winnicott (1945), the interruption of these object ties—either by separation activity or by virtue of problems in the facilitating environment—lead to schizoid withdrawal and fears of ego fragmentation and loss of self—all elements present in previous descriptions of the psychotic state. The object relations theorists after Klein, including Guntrip (1969), Bion (1957), and Balint (1979), located the etiological factor for the psychoses in disturbances in the maternal holding environment—or, as Sutherland (1980) characterized it, a lack of fit between the infant's needs and the mother's response. It is interesting to note this theory's congruence with early drive theories of trauma at the oral phase of development as well as with some of the basic features of psychosis in other theories. The British theorists wrote extensively of their psychoanalytic work with psychotic patients (Bion 1957; Rosenfeld 1965, 1987; Segal 1950).

In the United States, the therapists most active in working with psychotic patients were those in the Interpersonal School, founded in the Washington-Baltimore area by Harry Stack Sullivan (1962) and his most notable followers Fromm-Reichmann (1950), Will (1961), Hill (1964), and Searles (1959). Whereas for the object relations theorists the line between psychosis and neurosis was indistinct, for members of the Interpersonal School it was the line between the normal and the pathological that was unclear. Much like the members of the British School, these therapists postulated that the key to the individual with a psychosis lies within the primary nurturing relationship, the fear of its loss, and an extreme anxiety closely resembling the nothingness and the dissolution of self described earlier in this review with respect to the developing child.

Finally, Pollack (1989) argued, from the self psychological point of view, that Kohut's (1971, 1977) experience-near concept of the primacy of the self—in particular, the self's development and its vicissitudes of fragmentation and cohesion, as well as the legitimacy of selfobject needs in all human relationships—can be applied to psychotic and schizophrenic experience. In other words, the psychotic experience may best be understood as "the expression of threats to the cohesive intactness of the self . . . [and] the loss of self-objects" (Pollack 1989, p. 317) that could compensate for the missing or fragmented structures. Early dysfunctional childhood experiences in the form of empathic failures figure prominently in the adaptation of self psychology to the psychodynamics of psychosis. The historical trends in the understanding and treatment of the psychoses are represented in Figure 10–1.

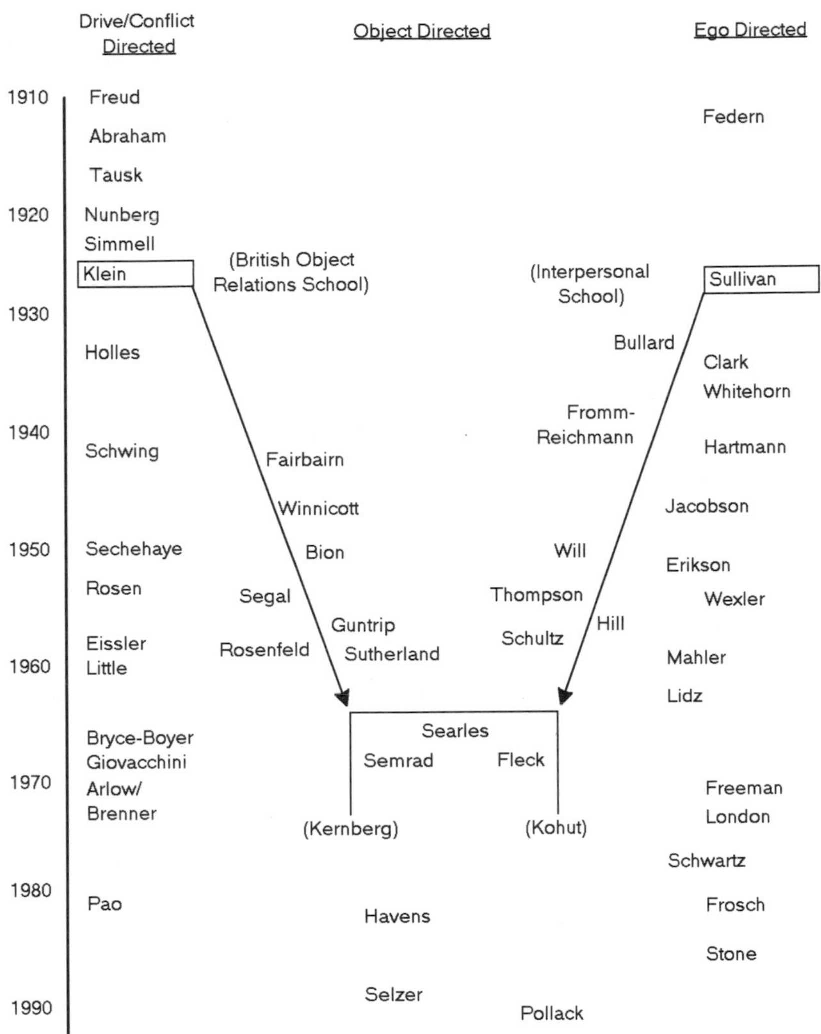

Figure 10–1. Major theoretical/clinical trends in psychodynamics of psychosis.
Source. Compiled from Frosch 1983, Kernberg 1976, Munich 1987, Pao 1979, and Rosenfeld 1969.

Case Example

At the time of his tenth psychiatric hospital admission, Dr. T was a 36-year-old, never-married, Jewish man with a diagnosis of schizophrenia, paranoid type. He had obtained his medical degree 8 years previously but had never practiced. Records indicated that Dr. T had been virtually psychotic for at least 12 years prior to this admission. His hospitalizations, which had begun 8 years before, were primarily for acute decompensation characterized by pronounced paranoia, incoherent and rambling speech, grandiose thoughts about his intelligence, obsessional religious rumination and preoccupations, writing religious material on the walls of or flooding his apartment, and delusions that he was being pursued by security police, the FBI, or Nazis. He believed that he was especially vulnerable to the malice of others, and "afflicted because he was a fatherless child." At his last position 3 years before admission, he was not offered a continuation because his performance was considered marginal and his judgment poor. Referred for a combination of extended milieu treatment and medication stabilization, as well as to work through the obvious and profound issues related to the early loss of his father, the patient stated on admission that he did not know why he was at the hospital.

Dr. T was the second child born to his 27-year-old mother and 38-year-old father and was the product of an uncomplicated full-term pregnancy, labor, and delivery. He reached all developmental milestones either early or on schedule and was considered "a good child who never cried." His early memories focused primarily on his relationship with his father, whom he described as warmer, more sensitive, and possibly "needier" than his mother. Regarding early peer relations, he stated that although he had had many playmates, he preferred reading or studying rather than playing games or participating in sports. When the patient was 5 years old, his father died suddenly at the age of 44 of a myocardial infarction. Nothing is known about the mourning process; rather, the patient's recall of the next few years conveyed a sense of increased closeness with his mother, a wish to bring his father back to her by becoming a doctor himself, and high academic achievement. There were no discipline problems, and although his mother's remarriage 3 years after his father's death was a severe blow, Dr. T continued to function well and was his grammar and junior high school valedictorian. He described his stepfather as having tricked his mother into marrying a poorly educated man, inferior to his biological father. Dr. T left home at the age of 16 to attend an Ivy League college, where his claim of many close friends is contradicted by his report that he never attended classes and spent most weekends at home with his mother. It was toward the end of college that the patient first sought psychiatric help at the university health service for what he describes as "panic attacks." This contact was apparently brief, and he did not again come to psychiatric attention until 1 year after graduation from medical school.

The patient graduated *magna cum laude* from college and the following fall began his medical studies. As in college, he mainly relied on reading and independent research rather than on attending classes to get him through the basic science years. Dr. T completed his medical training in 4 years despite severe conflicts with house staff, and successfully obtained an internship in internal medicine. In the late fall, he resigned this position because of "hassles" with his resident about time off for religious holidays, and returned to his home town. After several months, Dr. T resumed residency training at a program closer to home but again resigned for unclear reasons after approximately 2 months. He was referred for psychiatric consultation early on in these conflicts, was first hospitalized when he was found psychotic on a street corner, and over the next 8 years had several hospitalizations of varying lengths related in part to medication noncompliance. Between the time of his first resignation and the present hospitalization, Dr. T had applied and been turned down for several training positions. He explained these multiple and repeated rejections by stating that the program directors must have known they could not offer someone of his exceptional talents and abilities adequate training; by blaming others, such as his stepfather, for getting in the way of his being able to proceed with the application process; or by citing other factors such as antisemitism.

While Dr. T was in the referring hospital, his mother died at the age of 61 from thyroid cancer. Born in Germany into a middle-class Orthodox Jewish family, she and two sisters were the only members of her family who survived tenure in a concentration camp, perhaps as a result of taking care of one of the camp officer's families. She was described by the patient as an intelligent woman who had to settle for jobs below her capabilities in order to support the family during her husband's training and after his death. Previous records indicated that she had an enmeshed relationship with her son and believed, as she had with her husband, that she should sacrifice her life so that he could become a physician, perhaps in hopes of restoring the economic and social status the family had enjoyed in Europe. The patient's father was born in Poland, and he met his wife in Germany following the war. At the time of his death, he was functioning as an internist and attempting to complete a residency in surgery, having graduated from medical school in Europe before the war. The patient's older brother was alleged by the patient's stepfather to have recently had a psychotic breakdown.

Dr. T's physical exam was unremarkable, revealing a genial and sociable man who was mildly overweight with longish hair and a shaggy beard. His clothes were usually clean but rumpled. On mental status, he was able to engage in social conversation with other patients and staff and participated in a wide variety of activities, albeit with a pervasive empty, bland, and suspicious demeanor. Evidence for delusional thinking and paranoid hostility varied widely, depending on the situation. Dr. T tended to become most guarded and defensive when confronted about his status as a psychiatric patient or when discharge was addressed. He held tenaciously to the delusional belief that it was not possible for him to have a psychiatric illness because he was a fatherless child and the scripture explicitly states that such persons are exempt from illnesses of all kinds. He had a concrete and highly personalized interpretation of the Bible, spent much of his time copying it over word for word, and claimed to live his life by its laws. Otherwise, his speech and thought were coherent, goal-directed, and organized. He denied having any auditory or visual hallucinations or suicidal or homicidal ideation. His intelligence was in the above-average range, but his judgment and insight were minimal. Positive prognostic features included Dr. T's high premorbid level of functioning, his lack of deterioration, and his intelligence. These were balanced by the length of his illness, his lack of a social network and personal connections, and his inability to obtain and keep a job.

During the first several months of Dr. T's hospital stay, he continued to deny vigorously any psychiatric or emotional disturbance, rigidly maintaining that the doctors who had recommended transfer were themselves psychiatrically disturbed and for reasons of professional jealousy had "railroaded" him into extended hospital treatment. With each serious discussion of discharge planning, however, he became progressively depressed, disorganized, and delusional. At the same time that he never missed taking his medication, he insisted that it be discontinued because he was not psychiatrically ill. Although he participated in various activities on the unit, his attachments remained superficial and his attitude one of hostile compliance. In fact, an intense contempt and sarcasm suffused all his relationships and was implicit in his delusional organization.

In the hope that if Dr. T were more acutely symptomatic, he might be more likely to recognize and accept the severity of his illness, all psychotropic medications were discontinued. In preparation for this, a list of possible symptoms was formulated with the patient, with the agreement that, if these symptoms were to occur, he would agree to restart the medication. Over the course of a 4-month period, Dr. T became more agitated and floridly psychotic. His religious ruminations intensified, and he began writing biblical passages on his walls. He required restriction to his room because of hostile and sadistic behavior toward some patients; despite those problems, however, it became easier to recognize the suffering, terror, and helplessness he was enduring. His therapist became aware of Dr. T's intense need for and ambivalence about attachment, and this understanding allowed him to empathize more fully with Dr. T. The patient's desperation gradually propelled him more toward others, and he appeared to develop more meaningful attachments to selected staff members and patients. These attachments were facilitated by his coming to the realization that his sarcasm and contempt not only kept him from actual closeness but also prevented him from experiencing his need for others.

Because Dr. T's ruminative symptoms and bizarre behaviors made reintegration into the milieu nearly impossible, he was restarted on neuroleptic medication, this time at a higher dose. At this point, his hostility and threatening behavior markedly diminished; he slowly reintegrated into the treatment program and began participating in the patient government and attending a full schedule of vocational rehabilitation activities. By the time of his discharge, Dr. T had been interviewed and accepted for a volunteer position in the basic sciences laboratory at the hospital. Although he still had little insight into his illness, his denial was diminished and he was beginning to appreciate the way he affected others. The discharge plan included a halfway house, a day program that allowed for Dr. T's volunteer job, and medication maintenance and supportive psychotherapy.

Discussion

As a starting point for discussing this clinical material, an oedipal conflict is postulated as a central mechanism forming the content of the patient's psychotic regression: each time Dr. T is in a situation that approaches the consummation of his stated goals—finishing a residency, completing a task in vocational rehabilitation, or leaving the hospital—he becomes subject to overwhelming anxiety, signaling danger and simultaneously putting him in mind of his identification with, and the death of, his father. This occurs because his father died as he was about to complete his own medical studies, and the death happened at a time in Dr. T's life (age 5) when he was struggling with murderous wishes toward and consolidating his identification with his father—the latter in the service of mitigating the anxiety and guilt associated with the former. This unfortunate timing was complicated by inadequate mourning. Insofar as the father represents the values and demands of external reality against the regressive pull of the mother, the loss of the father at this time represented a further obstacle against completing tasks in the real world. And finally, the father's loss left Dr. T unprotected against an identification with his mother who, in addition to mourning the loss of her husband, was also filled with images of loss and death.

To use Freud's imagery, when an army cannot negotiate a gain, it retreats to a previous area of fortification—a kind of base camp. In situations of stress, then, such as completing a difficult task, Dr. T's ego collapses and returns to previous times of similar stress and trauma, and he functions at a less organized and differentiated level. In Dr. T's case, this level is represented by the compliant, preoedipal child obsessively ruminating over and compulsively recopying his biblical translations or the good chemistry and math student who quietly studies his way through medical school, goes home on weekends, avoids personal connections, and gets tangled up in quasi-legalistic disputes about the correct observance of holidays. One might say that the obsessional part of Dr. T's psychosis results from his regression from oedipal concerns. The delusional part—that of the invulnerable fatherless child—represents his failing ego's efforts to massively deny his desperate fears of emptiness, vulnerability, and death.

It was on the basis of such an overall formulation that Dr. T was originally sent to long-term treatment to explore and work through these issues. However, his virtual inability to absorb or internalize these elegant explanations suggested that the formulation was incorrect or irrelevant, incomplete, or ill timed. Very likely these psychodynamics exist upon the substrate of something instead of or in addition to oedipal conflict. One useful place to begin is with Dr. T's intensely ambivalent relationship with his psychotropic medication. Consuming it like a starving child, he would simultaneously complain that he was being persecuted, poisoned, humiliated, and afflicted, thus highlighting oral conflicts and aspects of his earliest object relations. This leads to Dr. T's identification with his mother, all of whose objects were destroyed in the Holocaust. His object situation most closely resembles hers, at least as we know it. There is a report from a previous hospitalization that the patient and his mother were enmeshed, but as with many patients, there are important unanswered questions. What was she like? Was she religious? Did her concentration camp experiences make her guarded and suspicious? Were there ways in which she devalued her new—and incidentally, uneducated—husband? Could this be the source of Dr. T's behavior toward his first physician employers and his later ward psychiatrists? It does sound as if the identification was catching up with him in college, and in spite of his considerable intelligence and academic achievement, Dr. T appears to have been having considerable difficulty separating from his mother. In addition, there is abundant evidence that relates to Dr. T's obvious need for a certain kind of holding environment—that is, when faced with discharge, he decompensates. When the environment is right, his style of superficial compliance and covert defiance works to defend him against his emptiness and rage. When it is threatened, however, his aggression has a disorganizing impact and puts him back into the delusional world. In the delusional world, the aggressive and destructive impulses, possibly derived from his identification with his mother and her family's murderers, can only be dealt with first religiously and then psychotically.

These formulations have included elements of and lead us to an object relations view of Dr. T's dilemma. We are aware of his long-standing and pervasive difficulty in forming and sustaining new attachments. The early introjective-projective continuum and conflict described above was replicated in his ongoing dilemma of being taken care of by versus being the caretaker of his mother, a premature internalization of the paternal physician and the maternal breadwinner roles, a fusion of these objects with his self system, and complex issues of survivorship. Inherent in each of these object relations paradigms is not only failure, aggression, persecution, and death, but also aspects of guilt and humiliation—processes acted out in the patient's religious preoccupations and delusional system. The dynamic impact of these identifications is most intense when Dr. T begins to experience interpersonal closeness; thus, he maintains distance in spite of his wish for something else. In fact, the combination of severe conflict or noncompliance with medication, help-rejecting behaviors or highly unstable therapeutic alliances, and continued enmeshment in the family or absence of a social network may represent different facets of a fundamental flaw in internalized object relations. In this case, the object relational paradigm would be founded on an intensely ambivalent relationship with early nurturing figures in which the child simultaneously needs these figures and their resources but feels deprived or attacked by them.

Finally, it should be noted that Dr. T's nonpsychotic adaptation through adolescence must be viewed through the lens of a relatively protected family environment, high intelligence, a focus on economic survival, and the nurturance of religious affiliation. This environment served to cushion the young Dr. T from acknowledging and examining the implications of his rather primitive object relations, incomplete mourning, and hopelessly unresolved oedipal dynamics. As he ventured into the world of interpersonal and adaptive expectations, however, this cushion could no longer protect him from the emergence of a process that led to a fundamental alteration in his reality. Thus, his first noted "break" with that reality came about in his first job, in which religious concerns dictated his leaving work and returning home. This withdrawal from the world symbolized his regression from adaptation—the retreat into a delusional solution and a more or less relentless psychotic process.

Summary

Knowledge of the basic elements of the dynamic formulation elaborated for Dr. T obviously did not lead to his cure—he suffers from a serious and persistent mental illness. It is hypothesized, however, that the careful and informed attention accorded to the patient's ambivalence about attachment and about accepting care from medical authority made a substantial contribution to the positive outcome of his hospitalization. This outcome went beyond symptom suppression, environmental manipulation, and discharge planning to encompass the patient's acceptance of his treatment regimen and his demonstration of considerably more adaptive behavior vis-à-vis possible employment. Acceptance of the treatment regimen was facilitated by the caregivers' appreciation of the possible meanings of imposing treatment and their tolerance for a drug-free interval, as well as by the availability of a compromise and less threatening vocational option. The supportive psychotherapy, psychotropic medication, milieu containment, and vocational rehabilitation that led to Dr. T's recompensation used psychodynamic principles not to select the treatment but rather to inform the delivery and mode of treatment. Treatment involved respect for Dr. T's self system, his areas of intact functioning, and his overall life goals. His therapist did not insist on meaning, his milieu did not insist on interaction, and his vocational counselor did not insist on his leaving medicine. All, however, took very seriously the importance of these elements in formulating their interventions and in not abandoning the patient to his delusional world.

The case of Dr. T suggests a modern conception of severe mental disturbance in which the structure of the psychosis derives from the patient's genetic predisposition, constitution, and brain, whereas its content issues from the patient's developmental environment, meaning system, and mind. From the point of view of the content and meaning of the psychosis, it seems evident that the multiplicity of factors involved in understanding Dr. T extends beyond a single theory to include drives, ego operations and failures, object relational and self system paradigms.

For Further Study

Arlow J, Brenner C: The psychopathology of the psychoses: a proposed revision. Int J Psychoanal 40:5–14, 1969

Buckley P (ed): Essential Papers on Psychosis. New York, New York University Press, 1988

Freeman T: A Psychoanalytic Study of the Psychoses. New York, International University Press, 1973

Freeman T: On Freud's theory of schizophrenia. Int J Psychoanal 58:383–388, 1977

Frosch J: Psychodynamic Psychiatry: Theory and Practice, Vol 2 (especially Chapter 9: The Psychoses). Madison, CT, International Universities Press, 1990

Frosch J: The Psychotic Process. New York, International Universities Press, 1983

Grotstein JS: A revised psychoanalytic conception of schizophrenia: an interdisciplinary update. Psychoanalytic Psychology 6:253–275, 1989

Lidz T, Fleck S, Cornelison N: Schizophrenia and the Family. New York, International Universities Press, 1965

London N: An essay on psychoanalytic theory: two theories of schizophrenia. Int J Psychoanal 54:169–194, 1973

Munich RL: Conceptual trends and issues in the psychotherapy of schizophrenia. Am J Psychother 41:23–37, 1987

Pao NP: Schizophrenia Disorders. New York, International Universities Press, 1979

Robbins M: Psychoanalytic and biological approaches to mental illness: schizophrenia. J Am Psychoanal Assoc 40:425–454, 1992

Rosenfeld H: Psychotic States: A Psychoanalytic Approach. London, Hogarth Press, 1965

Selzer MA, Sullivan TB, Carsky M, et al: Working With the Person With Schizophrenia: The Treatment Alliance. New York, New York University Press, 1989

Strauss JS, Carpenter WT: Schizophrenia. New York, Plenum, 1981

Sullivan HS: Schizophrenia as a Human Process. New York, WW Norton, 1962

References

Abraham K: The psychosexual difference between hysteria and dementia praecox (1908), in Selected Papers on Psychoanalysis. London, Hogarth Press, 1927, pp 64–79

American Psychiatric Association: Diagnostic and Statistical Manual of Mental Disorders, 3rd Edition, Revised. Washington, DC, American Psychiatric Association, 1987

Arlow J, Brenner C: The psychopathology of the psychoses: a proposed revision. Int J Psychoanal 40:5–14, 1969

Bak R: The schizophrenic defense against aggression. Int J Psychoanal 35:129–134, 1954

Balint M: The Basic Fault. New York, Brunner/Mazel, 1979

Bion WR: Differentiation of the psychotic from the non-psychotic personalities. Int J Psychoanal 38:266–275, 1957

Buckley P (ed): Essential Papers on Psychosis. New York, New York University Press, 1988

Fairbairn WR: A revised psychopathology of the psychoses and the psychoneuroses. Int J Psychoanal 22:250–279, 1941

Fenichel O: The Psychoanalytic Theory of Neurosis. New York, WW Norton, 1945

Ferenczi S: Psychoanalytic observations on tic, in Further Contributions to the Theory and Technique of Psychoanalysis. New York, Boni & Liveright, 1927, pp 142–174

Freeman T: A Psychoanalytic Study of the Psychoses. New York, International Universities Press, 1973

Freud S: The neuro-psychoses of defense (1894), in The Standard Edition of the Complete Psychological Works of Sigmund Freud, Vol 3. Translated and edited by Strachey J. London, Hogarth Press, 1961, pp 45–62

Freud S: Psycho-analytic notes on an autobiographical account of a case of paranoia (*dementia paranoides*) (1911), in The Standard Edition of the Complete Psychological Works of Sigmund Freud, Vol 12. Translated and edited by Strachey J. London, Hogarth Press, 1958, pp 3–82

Freud S: The ego and the id (1923), in The Standard Edition of the Complete Psychological Works of Sigmund Freud, Vol 19. Translated and edited by Strachey J. London, Hogarth Press, 1961, pp 3–66

Freud S: Neurosis and psychosis (1924), in The Standard Edition of the Complete Psychological Works of Sigmund Freud, Vol 19. Translated and edited by Strachey J. London, Hogarth Press, 1961, pp 149–158

Fromm-Reichmann F: Principles of Intensive Psychotherapy. Chicago, IL, University of Chicago Press, 1950

Frosch J: The Psychotic Process. New York, International Universities Press, 1983

Frosch J: The psychoses, in Psychodynamic Psychiatry: Theory and Practice, Vol 2. Madison, CT, International Universities Press, 1990, pp 383–434

Grotstein JS: A revised psychoanalytic conception of schizophrenia: an interdisciplinary update. Psychoanalytic Psychology 6:253–275, 1989

Guntrip H: Schizoid Phenomena, Object Relations and the Self. New York, International Universities Press, 1969

Hartmann H: Discussion of paper "On the development of Freud's concept of the attempt at restitution" by M. Katan (abstract). Psychoanal Q 20:505–506, 1951

Hill L: Psychotherapeutic Intervention in Schizophrenia. Chicago, IL, University of Chicago Press, 1955

Jacobson E: Contribution to the metapsychology of psychotic identifications. J Am Psychoanal Assoc 2:239–262, 1954

Jacobson E: Psychotic Conflict and Reality. New York, International Universities Press, 1967

Katan M: Schreber's delusion of the end of the world. Psychoanal Q 18:60–66, 1949

Kernberg OF: Object Relations Theory and Clinical Psychoanalysis. New York, Jason Aronson, 1976

Klein M: Notes on some schizoid mechanisms. Int J Psychoanal 27:99–110, 1946

Kohut H: The Analysis of the Self. New York, International Universities Press, 1971

Kohut H: The Restoration of the Self. New York, International Universities Press, 1977

Liberman RP, Corrigan PW: Is schizophrenia a neurological disorder? J Neuropsychiatry Clin Neurosci 4:119–124, 1992

London NJ: An essay on psychoanalytic theory: two theories of schizophrenia. Int J Psychoanal 54:169–194, 1973

Macalpine I, Hunter RA: The Schreber case: a contribution to schizophrenia, hypochondria and psychosomatic symptom-formation. Psychoanal Q 22:328–371, 1953

Mahler MS: Perceptual de-differentiation and psychotic object relationship. Int J Psychoanal 41:348–553, 1960

Mahler MS: On Human Symbiosis and the Vicissitudes of Individuation, Vol 1: Infantile Psychosis. New York, International Universities Press, 1968

Munich RL: Conceptual trends and issues in the psychotherapy of schizophrenia. Am J Psychother 41:23–37, 1987

Nunberg H: Transference and reality. Int J Psychoanal 32:1–9, 1951

Pao PN: Schizophrenic Disorders. New York, International Universities Press, 1979

Pollack WS: Schizophrenia and the self: contributions of psychoanalytic self-psychology. Schizophr Bull 15:311–322, 1989

Robbins M: Psychoanalytic and biological approaches to mental illness: schizophrenia. J Am Psychoanal Assoc 40:425–454, 1992

Rosenfeld H: Psychotic States: A Psychoanalytical Approach. London, Hogarth Press, 1965

Rosenfeld H: Impasse and Interpretation. London, Tavistock, 1987

Schilder P: Introduction to a Psychoanalytic Psychiatry. New York, International Universities Press, 1951

Searles HF: Integration and differentiation in schizophrenia. Br J Med Psychol 32:261, 1959

Segal H: Some aspects of the analysis of a schizophrenic. Int J Psychoanal 31:268–278, 1950

Sullivan HS: Schizophrenia as a Human Process. New York, WW Norton, 1962

Sutherland JD: The British object relations theorists: Balint, Winnicott, Fairbairn, Guntrip. J Am Psychoanal Assoc 28:829–860, 1980

Tausk V: On the origin of the influencing machine in schizophrenia (1919), in The Psychoanalytic Reader. Edited by Fliess R. New York, International Universities Press, 1948, pp 52–85

Terkelsen KG, Smith T, Gallagher RE, et al: Schizophrenia and Axis II (letter). Hosp Community Psychiatry 42:538, 1991

Wexler M: Schizophrenia: conflict and deficiency. Psychoanal Q 40:82–99, 1971

Will OA: Paranoid development in the concept of self: psychotherapeutic intervention. Psychiatry 24:74–86, 1961

Winnicott DW: Primitive emotional development. Int J Psychoanal 26:137–143, 1945

Chapter 11

The Self-Destructive Patient

Melvin Singer, M.D.

At best, psychotherapy with the self-destructive patient is an arduous task; at worst, it can produce in the therapist intense feelings of guilt, fear, and helplessness. In either case, the therapist is always burdened by a preoccupation and fear that the patient either will take his or her own life or will take over the therapist's life if the therapist is not careful to maintain a clear therapeutic stance and goals.

Complicating matters is the fact that inexperienced therapists (e.g., unsuspecting residents or neophyte graduates) are the ones most likely to treat these patients, since seasoned clinicians know enough to pass them on to their younger, more idealistic colleagues. As one senior journeyman once reflected, on listening to my travails, "there are patients who help you live a long life and there are those who don't; this is an example of the latter." My own experience has taught me that whereas one's rescue fantasies may entice one into treating these patients, such fantasies will certainly ruin one's chances for success unless they are understood and mastered.

Despite these potential pitfalls, it is possible to understand the psychodynamics and the methods of treatment of self-destructive patients. If this is done, the success rates can be high and the rewards many. In a significant number of such cases, one finds oneself working with a very moldable personality, waiting to be given the fertile emotional soil in which to grow. In such instances, both patient and therapist are enriched as the result of participating in a very moving human encounter.

Historical Review

Historically, interest in the self-destructive patient has been late in coming and seems to have paralleled the increasing interest in and understanding of severely impulse-ridden patients, especially borderline patients (see Crabtree 1967; Graff and Millin 1967; Grunebaum and Klerman 1967). Until some psychodynamic and psychogenetic understanding had evolved, no treatment approach was available and thus no treatment was given. During this author's training, borderline self-destructive patients were never accepted for treatment in outpatient residency training clinics because the only treatment approaches available were derived from the classic psychoanalytic model for neuroses and character disorders. Such models were utterly disastrous when applied to deprived, impulse-ridden, chaotic, and primitive personalities. Advances in psychoanalytic developmental theory, especially in the evolution of object relations and identity (self), provided the conceptual scaffolding to support new treatment approaches. The first symposium on self-mutilating patients, held at Chestnut Lodge (Rockville, Maryland) in 1969, produced an inspired series of papers (Burnham 1969; Kafka 1969; Pao 1969; Podvoll 1969). Aspects of these papers will be referred to throughout this chapter.

In this chapter I attempt to review the precipitating events, dynamics, ego and superego disturbances, problems in self and object development, and treatment approaches for self-destructive patients. A number of short clinical vignettes are provided to illustrate the problems that are encountered. But first we must start with a proper assessment of the self-destructive patient.

Differential Dynamic Diagnosis

Borderline personality disorder is the diagnosis most frequently associated with self-destructive behavior in the DSM-IV (American Psychiatric Association 1994). Moreover, many Axis I (clinical syndromes) disturbances can be comorbid with borderline disorder. Matters are further complicated by the fact that self-destructive behavior can escalate in severity, leading to suicide.

Self-destructive behavior cuts across a gamut of diagnostic categories and populations, from mentally retarded individuals to prison inmates. Up to 40% of mentally retarded patients may self-injure. A dramatic example is found in patients with Lesch-Nyhan syndrome, an X-linked enzyme deficiency disorder in which the self-injuring behavior is unremitting, even requiring restraints to interrupt the act. The self-destructive act within the mentally retarded population as a whole is characterized by its stereotypy and apparent lack of symbolism. The stereotypy is an intentional, repetitive, fixed pattern of behavior that can be rhythmical. Head banging is the most common form. On the opposite end of the continuum are prison inmates, who at times are accused of malingering as a cause of their self-injury. At other times, self-injurious behavior can sweep across a prison population secondary to the group phenomenon of contagion—a phenomenon also seen in inpatient adolescent populations (Favazza 1985; Favazza and Rosenthal 1993; S. Johns, "Self-Mutilation in the Character-Disordered Group," June 1994 [Glencairn Award Paper, Institute of Pennsylvania Hospital, unpublished]; Winchel and Stanley 1991).

However, as previously mentioned, self-destructive behavior is most commonly seen in individuals with character disorders, especially borderline personality disorder, and can range in severity from superficial, through moderate, to severe and even bizarre, as in psychotic patients. The borderline's self-destructive behavior is not stereotypic. Although it is repetitive as a means of "self-medicating," their dysphoric effects which, as mentioned, can inadvertently result at times in suicide.

Major depression, of course, involves the most common threat of suicide as the ultimate self-destructive act (Lion 1987). Revenge and self-hate dynamically join forces—complicated by the presence of biogenetic determinants—to create a psychiatric emergency. Bipolar, cyclothymic, and even manic episodes, which can readily revert to the underlying psychotically driven depression, are also ominous threats.

Schizophrenic reactions pose another serious threat for self-destructiveness. Bizarreness, command hallucinations, delusions, and loss of reality testing can deprive patients of the necessary degree of self-protectiveness and the ability to comprehend the seriousness of their actions. Fantasies of being able to fly, a wish to join God, a compelling attraction to fire, a need to escape from persecution or from psychic pain of unbearable proportions, and a sense of bursting from tension are examples of symptoms that can lead to the use of escape mechanisms that are life-threatening. Autocastration and self-enucleation can occur as a punishment for internally perceived sexual sins. These self-destructive acts are more typically sporadic and highly dramatic rather than stereotypic. Schizoaffective and pseudoneurotic schizophrenic reactions are also to be considered in the differential for Axis I. Toxic reactions from drug-induced or alcoholic psychoses as well as other organically induced psychoses can also prompt self-destructive acts.

Situational crises, such as marital discord or the loss of a lover, are psychosocial stressors (Axis IV) in the immediate present that can prompt self-destructive acts even in individuals who may not have past histories of loss of control. Such crises may pose problems whose solutions may be readily at hand; more commonly, however, these situational crises represent the most recent episode in a long series of impulsive "gestures" to regain control.

Returning to Axis II (developmental and personality disorders), in addition to borderline personality disorder, one must think of intermittent explosive disorder, passive-aggressive personality disorder, dependent personality disorder, and narcissistic personality disorder. Whenever antisocial features are joined with any of these disorders, the disturbance not only is more ominous but also requires a very difficult judgment call, given that the honesty of patients with antisocial personality disorder is always in question. Given these individuals' histories of lying, one cannot trust what they say, *especially* if they appear sincere! (Conversely, it is not reasonable to expect a patient to trust a doctor who is a stranger to him or her. Nevertheless, honesty and openness in communication are to be strived for as the most auspicious means to a propitious outcome [Kernberg 1987]). The seriousness of the situation is underscored by the sobering statistic that 8%–10% of borderline patients commit suicide in the first decade of their illness (Gunderson 1985). Narcissistic personality disorder patients with a specific constellation of characteristics that Kernberg calls *malignant narcissism with pathological grandiosity* are also seriously at risk for suicide.

In general, the highest level of personality development that contains the symptom or character neuroses does *not* include impulse-ridden self-destructive behavior. For this reason, whenever a patient presents with self-mutilating behavior—regardless of how high-functioning he or she may seem at the time—that patient must be diagnosed as having (at least presumptively) a borderline personality disorder. In this situation, the primitive aspects of the self are split off and inaccessible.

Precipitant and Self-Experience

Most often, a self-destructive act is precipitated by a frustration in the interpersonal world of the individual. Although patients will often deny that their actions are in any way connected with their immediate environment, it is easy enough to target the core need or conflict that has been activated to threaten their basic survival or security. This denial of the obvious is quite striking and serves to alert the therapist to the gravity of the problem—a gravity that mandates that—with awareness of these patients' sensitivity—the therapist must confront!

Acts of self-mutilation are usually carried out in private, at times when the patient is feeling totally alone and isolated. This isolation reinforces the lack of connection between the patient's act and the outside world that the act is meant to impact. Most often, separation and loss, personal defeat, narcissistic shame and injury to self-esteem, and uncontrollable narcissistic rage are the precipitants of such acts. These patients' glaring denial of precipitating events that are so obviously apparent, even to an untrained observer, does not represent evidence for a learning or thought disorder in the classic sense; rather, borderline patients' confusion and bewilderment as to the cause of their self-mutilation reflects their defensive use of primitive denial, splitting, and projection. One might call this defense "pseudostupidity."

Phenomenologically, an acute episode of depersonalization often accompanies the impulsive self-destructive act (see Pao 1969). Such an episode is preceded by a buildup of tension that must be relieved. A common declaration is "Something has to happen to reduce the pressure at any price!" Often, the act is carried out with a cool surgical precision and determination. Afterward a calm ensues that is associated with amnesia for the episode. This is followed by a sense of renewed vitality and restored interest in the surroundings (Podvoll

1969). The patient can again sleep and relax, and remains strangely indifferent to his or her act of self-destructiveness.

Self-destructive acts can take many forms, including drug overdoses, automobile accidents, alcoholic or eating binges, head banging, hanging, self-burning, wild promiscuity, or masochistic sexual abuse. Self-mutilation by cutting is perhaps the prototypical expression of the syndrome and, interestingly, is found predominately in young women (Burnham 1969). This syndrome's striking characteristics consist of the infliction of pain, bloodletting and flow, body mortification and disfigurement, and the capacity to instill in those close to the self-mutilator feelings of terror, guilt, helplessness, and rage and a total preoccupation with the mutilated one. A sense of uncanniness and awe surrounds those who display so much freedom from the usual forms of vanity and self-love that they can, with abandon, disfigure their faces, burn their genitals, or put needles in their sexual parts! In such unformed personalities, omnipotent control over the object is far more important than one's own physical body or even one's life. Indeed, it is characteristic of borderline patients that unless they can perceive themselves as an extension of a significant other, they have no sense of being alive anyway! These individuals have no separate "selves."

Furthermore, in these patients' regressed state, the body can be experienced as a despised external object outside the narcissistic boundaries of the self—and can be treated as such. Their pathological grandiosity sees no real consequences in death, for death actually represents a triumph over the persecutory object, internal or external, which may be represented by the therapist. Such individuals cannot grasp the significance of death, since to them it actually has none, if their life is emptied of the therapist, the only significant part of them. One such patient, during a regressed suicidal state, spoke of experiencing living as actually being in hell, and of there being a better life in death after this living death—thus, a death after death!

Crucial Dynamic Issues

An interpretation or revelation of an unacceptable fantasy or wish (e.g., homoerotic masturbation imagery, unthinkable cannibalistic need, incestuous longing) can dramatically interrupt the impulsive self-destructive behavior. The act itself symbolically represents a displaced version of both the wish's transgression and its retribution. Bringing the wish to conscious awareness, and then receiving forgiveness through the softening of superego pressures as a result of the therapist's tolerance and acceptance, allows for a realignment of intrapsychic forces and then a working through. Thus, a resolution through resignation, restitution, and repentance occurs. Although the patient's self-destructive act is specifically calculated to restore—in grand dramatic fashion—the lost object relationship, it actually, in the long run, has the opposite effect. Abandonment is unconsciously sought out of guilt and the wish to suffer, following the repetition compulsion. Patients with these narcissistic-masochistic character disorders have been called "grievance collectors" (see Cooper 1986). Interpretation of this ultimate masochistic wish to drive the object away as punishment for the patients' own excessively destructive and unquenchable needs is essential for resolution.

Concurrently, patients must be made aware that their externalized conflicts and enactments have an internal unconscious counterpart in the conflict between their wishes and their perception of these wishes as reprehensible. As long as patients keep their external world polarized and their conflicts projected, split off, and denied, they avoid the anxiety of exploring and confronting what is within. Their attempted solution is resolved not adaptively from within, but outside, hidden behind closed doors and through magic. The agonizing confrontation of the splits and alliances within is the only way to avoid paranoid anxieties and defiant behaviors.

Shielding patients from their conflicts can only lead to their becoming a collection of identifications rather than authentic selves. Such treatment constitutes a moralistic control of deviancy rather than an opportunity for growth. The therapist must also do more than react to self-mutilation or starvation. The treatment must be so structured that patients can see that they are not being punished for their attacks on their bodies as acts of defiance or for neglecting their needs. The multiple meanings for these self-destructive acts must be addressed (these meanings will be discussed in detail below). Likewise, the shift to assuming responsibility for their own lives and acts may be possible only after the patient has acquired a reason to live and a sense of the possibility of a future without pain and torment. Initially, therefore, the burden of responsibility for creating a hopeful treatment setting rests on the shoulders of the therapy team.

For conceptual clarity, the treatment of these self-destructive patients can be divided into a discussion of seven specific elements of the problem. These areas and the recommended techniques for dealing with them are detailed below.

The Impulsive Act

As was mentioned, the self-destructive act usually occurs when the individual is in an altered or dissociated state. This state is accompanied by a sense of urgency as well as a high level of tension and excitement. By definition, there is a lack of trial action in secondary process thinking—no time is spent in reflection—so that a realistic judgment regarding the consequences of the action is not possible. Instead of reflection, one sees the patient exhibit a primitive stimulus-response model for life, a failure of delay, and a preponderance of primary process thinking. In short, an undue reliance on the magic of the self-destructive action is used as a tension regulator and modulator of affects. These individuals must be provided with new models of identification through internalization that offer intermediary steps between stimulus and response. Such steps include psychic elaboration in thinking, conscious fantasy, imagery, imagination, and play—mental activities that can bind the pressures by rechanneling them into the realm of words, secondary process thinking, reality assessment and, ultimately, sublimations. Failure of the patient's early environment is usually what prevents the internalization of ego identifications for self-soothing and tension control. These mechanisms lift the ego from action to trial action in thinking and are learned during the crucial phase-specific periods of early childhood.

The Destructive Urge

As mentioned, the prototype of the self-destructive urge is self-mutilation or mortification of the flesh—whether by cutting, scalding, burning, bingeing, head banging, or bloodletting. However, the urge can also be directed against the entire body instead of only a symbolic part—as in auto accidents—or toward conscious erotic excitement—as in perversions of bondage and degradation.

The self-destructive act is highly personal, symbolic, and overdetermined. It stems from interpersonal and intrapsychic sources that are synonymous at this primitive level of functioning. The purpose of the act is to discharge an unbearable buildup of tension, primarily rage, which may be consciously undefined. The self-mutilation represents the only means available to relieve the pressure. Immediately preceding such discharge events, feelings of pain and anger are aroused to the level of narcissistic rage, but no adequate coping mechanisms are available to even acknowledge that these affects exist, let alone to let them out.

One patient described the experience of finally understanding that her desperate act of cutting was the only means she had available to her to relieve her pain, anger, and anguish. If she attempted to verbalize or act out her feelings at home, her mother would counter with a more convincing verbal blow of devastating proportions to her self-esteem and convictions, or her father would counterattack with such vicious physical abuse as to give her, as she put it, "real cause to be angry." Thus, all alloplastic discharge channels were barred; only autoplastic channels against herself were open. In a poignantly ironic sense, self-mutilation evokes a response, makes others hear, and manipulates them through guilt and fear—truly an act of desperation and a solution of despair.

The above explanation utilizes an interpersonal dynamic model. This model provides meaning to the psychic material first presented by the patient, which is the most available and immediate, and follows the therapeutic rule of analyzing from surface to depth—that is, the "onion-peel" process. Deeper layers of meaning originating from ego, superego, ego ideal, identity, and drive sources may also provide psychic data that may be necessary to engage and analyze the patient—a process requiring knowledge and skills that can span the entire gamut of psychotherapy.

The self-mutilative act is often designed to regain control over the lost object through guilt, fear, and despair. Pathological grandiosity and malignant narcissism (Kernberg 1987) may be operative as well. In this situation, the patient consciously achieves a sense of triumph over the therapist or the lost love object through the power of the act, unconsciously fulfilling the grandiose aim of power over life and even death. Furthermore, there is perverse pleasure in suffering to gain omnipotent control. The patient's self-esteem is perversely increased and his or her pathological grandiosity affirmed by the self-destructive act.

This type of patient is particularly prone to the danger of suicide when his or her malignant narcissism is too threatened by defeat, shame, failure, or loss. Similarly, the coincidence of antisocial or severe depressive or manic features and borderline characteristics further increases the danger of the self-destructive act's extending to the extreme of suicide.

Narcissistic rage secondary to a personal experience of injury through perceived rejection, defeat, or shame invokes a boundless desire for revenge. The unique characteristic that differentiates such rage from other forms of aggression is the unrelenting desire to undo the harm and right the wrong, regardless of the price or length of time required to (see Kohut 1972). Narcissistic rage draws into use all the cognitive capacities at its disposal. As in paranoid states, these cognitive capacities, ironically, are not involved in the regression but are put into the service of the rage, with access to all its powers. Furthermore, the power of narcissistic rage is magnified by the summation of forces of the injured archaic grandiose self and by the disappointment felt when the idealized object fails to realize these archaic claims. Here, passive victimization is turned into active revenge in an identification with the aggressor.

Ego Disturbance in Repression

The patient's experience both of being *in* and of actually *being* a pressure cooker, requiring immediate release from the buildup of tension, indicates a possible disturbance either in the stimulus barrier or in repression, as well as in tension regulation or frustration tolerance. The patient's unbearable feeling of fullness to the point of bursting, which is replaced by emptiness after the cutting, has the same concretistic quality as an overfilled balloon stretched to its limit. Once punctured with a pin, it explodes and is deflated. All its tension is gone.

Analogous situations of traumatic overstimulation without adequate discharge mechanisms may have existed in the patient's infancy or childhood, creating a fixation and then a compulsion to repeat the experience in a delayed attempt at mastery. An example might be unbearable bowel pressure from severe constipation or impaction to the point of being overwhelmed with the threat of annihilation. Relief may have been obtained through rectal exploration and removal, enema, or cathartic, causing discharge of diarrhea and flatulence and then relief. Other analogies are passive forced stuffing or active gorging of food followed by vomiting, and obstipation followed by urination. Experiences such as these that have been repressed are traumatic somatopsychic memories of being overwhelmed with stimuli. Such early experiences of stimulus overload without adequate discharge—especially when these experiences are preverbal—produce feelings of helplessness, unbearable pain, and despair. Furthermore, because these experiences are psychologically organized during periods of concrete, operational, or nonconceptual thinking, they demand magical solutions via the rules of primary process. Once repression has set in, therefore, the trauma falls under the domain of the repetition compulsion, which cannot be mastered until made conscious, interpreted, and worked through. Thus, we see here a combination of a possible weakness in repression and the repetition of the trauma.

Self System

Borderline patients commonly experienced phase-specific disturbances in the parent-child relationship before differentiation of self from object had occurred. Frequently, these disturbances were in the form of psychological and/or physical and sexual abuse and neglect. Such environmental failures produced a failure in the internalization of a cohesive self-experience, self-soothing devices, and advanced regulatory channels for tension reduction. Lack of emotional availability, empathic attunement, or mirroring are classic examples of deficit or understimulation. These patients' assaults on their own bodies seem so directly aimed at their objects, so childish and primitive, that this explanation must be seriously considered!

Furthermore, the failure of adult caregivers in the child's environment to perceive the infant in its own right, or their misperception or misuse of the child for their own narcissistic needs leaves the child's sense of self undeveloped. Greenacre (1953) called this experiential state *appersonation.* It has also been described as *appersonalization* to contrast it with depersonalization (Singer 1987), and as *depersonification* to depict the parental induction process (Rinsley 1971). Briefly, the infant's first experience of itself may be what it sees reflected back in its mother's eyes (Winnicott 1971a, 1971b). If the infant's emotional experience is not reflected back (a lack of mirroring), then a distortion occurs in the quality of the experience of the self. This distortion can be as slight as not feeling whole, centered, anchored, or complete (a mild identity disturbance or a disturbance in self-cohesion) or not feeling quite human or real or as major as a disturbance in identity (identity diffusion or loss of the sense of self) in which the borderline patient feels alive but not human, more akin to an animal or vegetable—or worse, to a nonliving thing like stone or wood. An acute catastrophic loss of an object can elicit an experience of disappearance or annihilation of the self (see Singer 1987, 1988).

Besides these examples of understimulation from lack of empathic attunement, another cause of appersonation is traumatic overstimulation from sexual abuse. Such overstimulation causes massive splitting and fragmentation of the ego, which leaves the experiential realm with a lack of self-cohesion. Multiple personality disorder and borderline personality disorder have extremely high incidences of sexual abuse (80% and 60%, respectively).

Many borderline patients also describe unbearable emptiness, numbness, deadness, or anesthesia throughout their bodies, especially the body surfaces, although not in their self-observing ego (Singer 1977a, 1977b, 1981). This regression in the body's self-experience is a regressive response to a traumatic interpersonal event and usually signifies that separation from or loss of the nurturing object occurred before full intrapsychic separation from the object was achieved. Because borderline patients function at a primitive level of differentiation (i.e., either at the transitional object or the protosymbiotic stage [Winnicott 1953]), their personal existence requires the actual physical presence of the object to retrieve the experience of their own self-images! Loss of the object incites such narcissistic rage over the loss of entitled omnipotent control that in retaliation, borderline patients intrapsychically destroy the object. In so doing, they inadvertently destroy themselves, since they are insufficiently differentiated. This leaves them feeling "dead" or acutely disappearing, gone, and empty. Then, as if by magic, the pain of the incision brings back a feeling of being alive. It reassures them of their existence—that they have an inside, blood and internal organs and parts—and dispels their fear.

Again, this description emphasizes such patients' atavistic view of themselves as existing only as extensions or reflections of the other. One useful metaphor for their self-perception is that of a developing film that has been removed from its solvent before the chemical reactions are complete, leaving only the images of shadowy, undefined figures on the film. Borderline patients will pathognomonically speak of an inability to retrieve an image not only of themselves but of their therapists after only a 3-day absence. This lack of evocative memory (Adler 1985) or perceptual object and self constancy (Burgner and Edgcumbe 1973) is compounded by these patients' inability to retain or even retrieve a memory of their therapist's loving interventions after 3 days' absence—that is, a loss of libidinal object constancy. To make matters worse, there is a generalized failure to internalize and retain *any* positive intervention without endless reinforcement—a true emotional malabsorption syndrome. The reason for this failure is that these patients' perceptual set is to expect betrayal, rejection, and torture no matter how much the object appears "good." Kind treatment is always viewed with suspicion—as a trick. Evil is masquerading behind good, waiting until one finally trusts before striking. This is the ultimate treachery! Thus, nothing positive can be internalized. This failure to internalize any positive experience should be viewed as both an ego deformation and a compromise formation between forbidden wish and punishment.

First, the good image is lost. It is then replaced by the bad. The good image is no longer retrievable. What is retrievable is what is immediately perceivable and that is usually the treacherous face of the negative object. The idealized good object is forever out of reach. Every interpretation of a negative misperception of treachery within the transference, in the context of a positive interactional field, replaces—memory by memory—each negative object representation with a positive one. That is why positive experiences can do nothing without concomitant interpretation of the negative.

Narcissistic Disturbances

Another important dimension to be understood in self-destructive patients is their regression to narcissism. Here the drives—libidinal and aggressive—and their objects have to a significant degree turned inward. A withdrawal from the world of other persons back into the self has taken place. In this state, by symbolic substitution, bodily parts come to represent the objects of the patient's external world, past and present. The theater of the world is now the theater of the body, and organ parts become the players in a self-contained hypochondriacal system. The observing self can stand outside as an indifferent spectator and watch the destructive interaction, giving it an eerie, surreal, and uncanny twist. To the disembodied observing ego, it is of little import what the slaughter is that is being wrought. The body is viewed as a not-me part, the proxy for the ambivalent object, whose mutilation can manipulatively create havoc in the real external counterpart. Remember, the body itself can be viewed as external to the primitive self. This allows the individual to inflict pain on the body as a persecuting object. "If thy eye offend thee, pluck it out," directs the Biblical injunction. Neatly cutting the soft skin of the wrist, or scarring the beautiful face that means so much to the other, not only injures the only thing the objects care so much about but also terrifies, horrifies, and fills them with remorse, rendering them totally within the patient's control. Many borderline patients experience bodily preoccupations and pains between periods of cutting that further reveal their potential for narcissistic hypochondriacal withdrawal.

Superego Issues

Another level of understanding of the self-destructive act pertains to its value as repentance or absolution from sin. The mortification of the flesh has been prescribed and practiced for centuries, and is the center of many religious rituals. It represents a means of absolving the soul of the passions of the flesh. Cleansing the spirit of all carnal evil by bloodletting or mutilation has been assigned divine, transcendent, and Godlike purification value in these frenzied rites. Podvoll (1969) beautifully quotes St. John of the Cross, who described the soul's ascendance "in perfect liberty to union with the beloved" only when "desires be lulled to sleep by the mortification of sensuality" (p. 219). In more recent times, St. Theresa, who is called the "Little Flower," preached that the greater the pain, the greater the glory of God! Of course, it has long been known that adolescents curb their storms of pubertal passion by flights into asceticism. Paradoxically, "Satan's religions" invert this process, linking mortification of the flesh with sexual orgies, and sexual ecstasy with transcendence and unity with the devil.

As it did for the martyrs, bloodletting acts for borderline patients as a purging of the evil spirits within. It serves as a cathartic; release from the sins of diabolical passion and rage is expressed by the flow of red blood. The myth of Dracula, in a reversal of roles, can also be seen as an expression of the magical supernatural powers attributed to blood and its contents. By sucking the blood of his victims, Dracula acquires their life forces as well as power and control over them. The reverse occurs in borderline patients, who are releasing their own evil spirits and the spirits' power over them through bloodletting.

Conscious Fantasy Elaboration

Borderline individuals do not consider the real-life consequences of their action orientation to life, which is associated with denial and splitting. Educational measures are necessary. They must be taught to think through, step by step, the effects of their actions on themselves, their careers, and their families. Preconceptions, myths, and childish notions will be exposed, such as the maudlin sentimentality of observing from above their loved ones mourning their loss at their funerals. Misconceptions will be corrected, such as recognizing that the attempted suicide may not bring their loved ones "to their senses," but rather may, through miscalculation, leave the patients themselves paralyzed or brain damaged. Many borderline patients have conscious visions of death that are closely linked to womb fantasies. Thus, they frequently depict their conception of death in such words as "peace," "sleeping," and "floating." Confronting this wishful fantasy of nirvana with the stark alternate possibility of nothingness for eternity can have a chilling deterrent effect, even if only temporarily.

Treatment Approaches

Principles of treatment must include techniques to 1) establish a therapeutic frame and set limits to contain patients' impulsivity within acceptable bounds so that treatment can proceed, and 2) provide sufficient gratification of the patients' needs, within the restraints of professional and personal ethics acceptable to the therapist, for the therapeutic contract to continue to exist. These two complementary requirements signify that the patient and therapist must agree on a therapeutic contract that allows for an "optimal level of tolerance." For patients, too much frustration of basic needs is intolerable and leads to a regression to paranoid dissociation, self-destructiveness, flight, or all of these behaviors. Similarly, therapists must be able to work in a zone of comfort so that neither their own nor their patients' morbidity or even mortality is at stake. Otherwise, it is the patient and not the therapist who directs the treatment.

The therapist must always be in control of the treatment. Hospitalization, day care, a team approach, psychopharmacological intervention, and family involvement may all be necessary expedients from moment to moment to ensure control. Of course, like all rules this one has exceptions. The patient may need to feel temporarily in control of his or her life, especially in particular areas or times (i.e., a paradoxical intervention). However, the overall direction or form of the treatment, and certainly any potential or uncertain life-and-death decisions, are the therapist's prerogative. An atmosphere of a joint venture and of mutual respect and responsibility must prevail in a setting in which, ultimately, it is the therapist who is the expert and has the final say.

Guidelines do exist. Too much gratification of infantile wishes will only awaken archaic introjects that are totally insatiable. The therapist must help the patient get a glimpse—and only a glimpse—of the fact that these voracious needs are beyond the realm of any human ability to satisfy. Thus, the therapist must establish the frame. The outer limits of the patient's actions must be defined. Obviously, no physical harm to the therapist's person or property must ever be tolerated, nor should the patient be in possession of any life-threatening weapons or pills.

The following is a typical scenario. A patient will place the therapist in a double bind by demanding that the therapist never call the police or his family if he is suicidal. If the therapist ever does this, the patient will threaten to quit. Then, after threatening suicide, he will refuse to answer his phone and will cancel his next appointment! The patient's unconsciously motivated sadism and need for omnipotent control, as well as the reenactment involved in forcing a betrayal by the therapist, must be confronted and clarified to the patient. The therapist is always appealing to the self-observing ego of the patient for a mutual alliance. The masochistic need to lose the caregiver because of unconscious guilt about excessively sadistic demands is an essential insight to interrupt the process of sabotage in the patient's life and therapy. The best indicator that the downhill slide has progressed too far and that suicide is at hand is a change in the patient's attitude toward the therapist. If the patient shows no interest in the therapist—neither care nor anger—detachment or estrangement has set in and the potential for suicide is present!

As a general rule, a therapist might tolerate some rule breaking by patients at first. But as more understanding is achieved and ego defects in judgment and control are corrected, an incremental reduction occurs in the therapist's tolerance of infractions. Patients begin to assume responsibility for themselves and for their own actions. A baseball analogy can help the therapist make this point: "Three strikes and you're out!" The first slip may be understandable, since the patient was not yet aware of the psychic significance of his or her behavior, nor did the patient have the necessary coping skills to find an alternative outlet for his or her feelings. Strike two may also be tolerated because the patient may not have had time to internalize and work through these insights. But strike three and the patient is out! The therapy is over. The therapist must mean it if he or she says it. At this crucial juncture, certain extenuating, previously unknown circumstances may come to light, bringing new insights that necessitate an exception to the rule. Working through such exceptions can strengthen the treatment approach only if the therapist retraces his or her steps back to strike two. A firm yet flexible attitude is the appropriate stance.

Another behavior common to borderline patients, both within and without the treatment setting, is what can be called the *principle of expediency.* If patients act out destructively and outrageously against another person in one direction and then, in order to avoid reprisals, act out against themselves in the opposite direction, they put their own lives on the line. Such a maneuver effectively shifts the concern and focus of attention away from their heinous crimes against their fellow human beings and onto their life-threatening destructive acts against themselves. This principle of expediency frequently manipulates the therapist as well, allowing the therapist's guilt, anxiety, and concern for the patient to gain the foreground over feelings of anger and disgust. This mechanism must be cautiously interpreted to patients because it touches on a level of savagery in themselves that they may not be ready to face.

It is also important in the treatment of borderline patients for the therapist to acknowledge his or her personal limitations. Doing so dispels patients' grandiose, paranoid idea that the therapist is omnipotent and could magically meet all their needs if he or she did not have a sadistic desire to see them suffer. Ultimately, this persecutory conviction must be seen as a projection of patients' own oral envy, greed, and rage over the therapist's powers to heal. This insight helps to open the door to increasing acceptance of patients' responsibility for their actions and life instead of reinforcing their passive, manipulative dependence on others. It also highlights their excessive investment in archaic aims of perfectionism, power, domination, and exhibitionistic needs. When the therapist is seen as having human limitations, then aspects of the grandiose self and idealized object in patients can be more readily relinquished and the more realistic, true selves and objects can be more easily acknowledged (Kohut 1972). (For an interesting case discussion regarding this topic, see Kafka 1969.)

Under no circumstances should treatment be continued unless the therapist is in control and is comfortable with the contract. No compromise of safety is justified. Therapists' tendencies to 1) enact regression-induced guilt in the countertransference, 2) play God, 3) be saviors, 4) feel that only they can help the patient, or 5) extend trust to a patient out of fear of the patient's anger or of losing the patient's love are highly dangerous. Misguided thoughts (e.g., "They'd never do this to me," "They know I care," "They care too much") are naive and overlook deep-seated and split-off hatred and sadism that are inaccessible during positive periods of relatedness. Thus, if the therapist feels that such measures as hospitalization, medication, tight observation, and strict confinement are necessary, then they *are* necessary. Anything else is dangerous, and the therapeutic relationship must take second place to concerns for life and safety.

Premature discharge of a patient in a major depression is a classic error. So is focusing on the positive and neglecting the split-off negative dimensions in order to maintain the superficially pleasant and gratifying aspects of the transference. Patients must be made aware, in no uncertain terms, that their self-destructive behavior and even their death is not the therapist's or their family's ultimate responsibility, but their own. The therapist will be sad, but he or she will get over it; his or her life will go on. Furthermore, the therapist must always alert the patient's family or responsible other to the gravity of the situation, preparing them for all eventualities. Such an action frees the therapist from indirect countertransference (Racker 1968) interferences characterized by guilt and paranoid fears of third-party reprisals. It bears repeating that a sudden change in the patient's attitude toward or attachment to the therapist, such as a change from clinging to disinterest, may signal that a decision to commit suicide has been made.

The therapist should not do or promise more than is reasonable; otherwise, unconscious death wishes will eventually arise in the therapist, reinforcing the self-destructive potential in the patient. A reenactment will then have taken place in the transference-countertransference of unconscious death wishes toward the patient that originated within the family matrix. Conversely, patients' conscious or unconscious fantasies that the therapist desperately needs them to stay alive—granting patients undue power over the therapy as well as over life and death—must be exposed and dispelled. To continue, therapists must react to self-destructive acts with more than sorrow and concern or they are denying their own counteraggression and playing into the patient's dynamics. On the other hand, empathizing with patients' universally held longings for peace, excitement, self-directed aggression, pleasure in revenge, escape from guilt, or exhilarating sense of power also has its place. In short, the therapist should empathize, confront, and contain. Finally, therapists must have the courage to end the treatment if they feel they cannot deal with the situation—that is, if the patient is escalating the treatment out of control. Hospitalization and time for the patient to obtain a new therapist, learn from the loss, and perhaps behave differently for the next treatment experience is then possible. Of course, all of the above are easier said than done.

Some "words of wisdom" from years of experience may prove helpful. Although such precepts may not be curative, they can provide encouragement and hope throughout the difficult periods of uncovering and working through. Over these years, certain observations, maxims, and truths have emerged that can serve as positive reinforcers or cognates to counter the negative thinking so prevalent in these unfortunate patients.

The first thing to remember is that most borderline patients have a deep-seated, unexpressed fear that their needs are insatiable and thus that they are ultimately unlovable. This fear is a conscious basis for their hopelessness and despair. I equate these excessive feelings of emotional hunger to those of a starving person who feels that his or her needs for nourishment are insatiable. However, experience proves that once these needs begin to be met on a more regular basis, such patients find that the needs are actually much less than they believed and even within the range of satisfaction. The driving force for the sense of insatiability was a regression to an infantile level of need and rage, instigated by rejection, frustration of need, and guilt. However, regular and consistent gratification raises the level of functioning and need to a more adaptive and reasonable point.

The second truism is that the only experience that really matters is *now.* If the patient's pain and anguish can be relieved, the past will be only a memory—one he or she could have read about. Nothing matters but now. The patient's disturbance in time, subjective and functional, is also operative here. This is a remarkable fact. Thus, in the patient's regressive state, there is only emptiness now and for eternity. Time collapses into the present. Once regression has lifted and hope is achieved, time recovers the dimensions of past, present, and future.

A final dictum is that these patients' hopelessness stems, in part, from their all-or-nothing magical thinking. The black-or-white polarization of the world is based on splitting mechanisms. If these patients are at point A, it is utterly impossible for them to contemplate reaching point Z, which is where they strive in absolute determination to be. The leap is too great. However, getting from point A to point B is possible and, even more important, getting from Y to Z is no more difficult than getting from A to B. Surgical interns can't perform open-heart surgery, but they can assist in suturing the skin on closing! If interns were expected to do the former, they'd be just as overwhelmed as borderline patients are in their grandiose, depreciatory system of thinking. Thus, the borderline individual must be educated to realize that incremental increases in functioning are possible and can lead to their achieving what seems totally improbable in moments of despair.

Case Example

In this section I present a composite portrait of a hospitalized patient representative of a number of cases that exemplify the problems discussed in the previous sections.

> The patient, Ms. U, horrified her psychiatrist and the therapeutic team by slashing her throat and then bathing her face in her blood—a true "bloodbath." Exploration of the multiple meanings of this bizarre and overwhelming suicidal self-mutilative act revealed the following.
>
> Ms. U had requested that I return to the floor to see her a second time that day, if only briefly, because she had become increasingly anxious, empty, and lonely after the therapy session. She said she wanted a hug. I was unable to return to the floor and would not have given her a hug, since the latter was too stimulating and would be breaking the rules. Also, both requests were crossing the boundaries of the prescribed therapeutic relationship. She had raised the ante too far, demanding a rejection experience in the transference-countertransference. In our previous work, she had equated rejection by me with the loss of her father by suicide when she was 4 years of age.
>
> Prior to this request that I return to the floor, Ms. U had become increasingly agitated as she was given greater freedom from her restraints over the past week. She had been on four-point restraints but now was free for 2-hour intervals to move around in her room. Talk of future plans of discharge, a new boyfriend, sex, and visiting me monthly for "refueling" were in her associations. I had not resisted her talk of her increasing separation. She perceived my silence as acquiescence. Unconsciously, she had been testing my devotion to her. Would I let her leave me? I was not going to be the father she wanted! This was to much for her to bear. The last feelings she remembered were increasing, unbearable pressure and then numbness.

> No thoughts. The cutting released the pressure, and the blood flow restored the feelings of aliveness. The immediate therapeutic work was directed toward understanding the meaning of the interpersonal event that had occurred between us. We addressed her wish, the use of omnipotent control, the insatiable demand, the forced rejection, and the symbolic expression and punishment for the rage. The ego disturbances in impulsivity and narcissism, the superego and self system disturbances, as well as issues regarding the destructive drive, were also broached.

The next psychotherapeutic task involved deeper insights into the meaning of Ms. U's cutting her throat. Her blood symbolically represented her erstwhile homosexual lover's vaginal secretions, which she longed to be reunited with and immersed in. Rather than the usual rejections by the father, a former rejection by her homosexual lover had also been rekindled in the precipitating event, which was perceived as a rejection by her therapist. This experience brought, in its wake, narcissistic longings and rage, followed by regression, fusion, and turning against the self. Thus, the self-mutilation also symbolically represented mutilation of the object and self, her own blood and the object's blood and vaginal secretions.

The next layer revealed Ms. U's wish to be immersed in amniotic fluid. Here, her bathing of her face in her own blood symbolically represented her whole body bathing in the fluids of her lover's amniotic sac. Here, self replaces object and part replaces whole. Beneath the wish for union of her own and her lover's bodies lay ultimately her longings for union with her mother of infancy. This is a classic fantasy of returning to the womb, except that it is played out under the temporary psychotic spell of massive rage and revenge.

The third layer that revealed itself was a castration wish toward her therapist, her boyfriend, her father, and herself. Here, the head and neck of her own body symbolically represented the head and neck of the three men's penises.

Thus, one single self-destructive act can be used to explore many dimensions of the mind, from deep unconscious fantasy, to ego and narcissistic disturbances, maladaptive interpersonal relatedness—and, especially, to transference-countertransference experiences.

> Another patient, Ms. V, slashed her wrist, inadvertently severing her tendons, arteries, veins, and nerves. The stimulus for this act was her feelings of increasing closeness to the therapist. On one level, she wanted to remove the hated hand that masturbated. This hand evidently represented the hated mother who hadn't given her the pleasure that her own hand did (Laufer 1982). This act also came to represent an attempt by Ms. V to firm up her boundaries, or to achieve a self-definition.

Thus, by inflicting pain at the surface, the self-destructive act delimits and defines one's shape. Furthermore, in an attempt to separate from the engulfing mother-child experience, the act of self-mutilation can paradoxically reinforce a sense of freedom from the need to cling by providing a painful masochistic separation or line of demarcation. Cutting both symbolically helps delineate separation by denying the wish for fusion and enhances fusion with the warmth and flow of the blood in a compromise formation. Thus, both sides of the conflict—the wish and its repudiation, the fear and the punishment—are enacted in grand dramatic fashion with a hysterical "La Belle Indifference" gesture.

Summary

In this chapter I have attempted to schematically review the difficulties in assessing, understanding, and treating the self-destructive patient. One must underscore the guidelines given for treatment and the need for hope. Remember that no matter how obvious an issue is to the therapist (or, if the patient is hospitalized, to the therapeutic team), it bears reiterating and clarifying to the patient because denial, splitting, and projection are pervasive first-line defense mechanisms, and the potential for rapid shifts to paranoid thinking and turning rage against the self in a narcissistic regression is ever present. Finally, the therapist must always be in control of the treatment, no matter how enticing patients' demands and arguments on their own behalf may seem.

For Further Study

Favazza AR, Rosenthal RJ: Diagnostic issues in self-mutilation. Hosp Community Psychiatry 44:134–140, 1993

Gunderson J: Borderline Personality Organization. Washington, DC, American Psychiatric Press, 1985

Kafka JS: The body as transitional object: a psychoanalytic study of a self-mutilating patient. Br J Med Psychol 42:207–212, 1969

Kernberg OF: Diagnosis and clinical management of suicidal potential in borderline patients, in The Borderline Patient: Emerging Concepts in Diagnosis, Psychodynamics, and Treatment. Edited by Grotstein J, Solomon MF, Long JA. Hillsdale, NJ, Analytic Press, 1987, pp 69–80

Lion JR: Clinical assessment of violent patients, in Clinical Treatment of the Violent Person. Edited by Roth LH. New York, Guilford, 1987, pp 1–19

Podvoll EM: Self-mutilation within a hospital setting: a study of identity and social compliance. Br J Med Psychol 42:213–221, 1969

Winchel RM, Stanley M: Self-injurious behavior: a review of the behavior and biology of self-mutilation. Am J Psychiatry 148:306–317, 1991

References

Adler G: Borderline Psychopathology and Its Treatment. New York, Jason Aronson, 1985

American Psychiatric Association: Diagnostic and Statistical Manual of Mental Disorders, 4th Edition. Washington, DC, American Psychiatric Association, 1994

Burnham RC: Symposium on impulsive self-mutilation: discussion. Br J Med Psychol 42:223–229, 1969

Burgner M, Edgcumbe R: Some problems in the conceptualization of early object relationships, II: the concept of object constancy. Psychoanal Study Child 27:315–353, 1973

Cooper AM: Narcissism, in Essential Papers on Narcissism. Edited by Morrison A. New York, University Press, 1986, pp 112–143

Crabtree L: A psychotherapeutic encounter with a self-mutilating patient. Psychiatry 30:91–100, 1967

Favazza AR: Self-mutilation and contagion: an empirical test. Am J Psychiatry 142:119–120, 1985

Favazza AR, Rosenthal RJ: Diagnostic issues in self-mutilation. Hosp Community Psychiatry 44:134–140, 1993

Graff H, Millin R: The syndrome of the wrist cutter. Am J Psychiatry 124:36–42, 1967

Greenacre P: Certain relationships between fetishism and faulty developments of the body image. Psychoanal Study Child 85:79–98, 1953

Grunebaum R, Klerman G: Wrist slashing. Am J Psychiatry 124:527–534, 1967

Gunderson J: Borderline Personality Organization. Washington, DC, American Psychiatric Press, 1985

Kafka JS: The body as transitional object: a psychoanalytic study of a self-mutilating patient. Br J Med Psychol 42:207–212, 1969

Kernberg OF: Diagnosis and clinical management of suicidal potential in borderline patients, in The Borderline Patient: Emerging Concepts in Diagnosis, Psychodynamics, and Treatment. Edited by Grotstein J, Solomon MF, Long JA. Hillsdale, NJ, Analytic Press, 1987, pp 69–80

Kohut H: Thoughts on narcissism and narcissistic rage. Psychoanal Study Child 27:360–400, 1972

Laufer ME: Female masturbation in adolescence and the development of the relationship to the body. Int J Psychoanal 63:295–302, 1982

Lion JR: Clinical assessment of violent patients, in Clinical Treatment of the Violent Person. Edited by Roth LH. New York, Guilford, 1987, pp 1–19

Pao PN: The syndrome of delicate self-cutting. Br J Med Psychol 42:199–206, 1969

Podvoll EM: Self-mutilation within a hospital setting: a study of identity and social compliance. Br J Med Psychol 42:213–221, 1969

Rinsley D: The adolescent inpatient: patterns of depersonification. Psychiatr Q 45:3–22, 1971

Racker H: Transference and Countertransference. New York, International Universities Press, 1968

Singer M: The experience of emptiness in borderline and narcissistic disorders, I: deficiency and ego defect vs dynamic defensive model. International Review of Psycho-Analysis 4:459–469, 1977a

Singer M: The experience of emptiness in borderline and narcissistic disorders, II: the struggle for a sense of self and the potential for suicide. International Review of Psycho-Analysis 4:471–479, 1977b

Singer M: Anal sadism, rapprochement and self-representation: analysis of a preverbal complaint of emptiness. Journal of the Philadelphia Association for Psychoanalysis 8:173–192, 1981

Singer M: A phenomenology of the self: appersonalization, a subcategory of borderline pathology. Psychoanalytic Inquiry 7:121–137, 1987

Singer M: Fantasy or structural defect? the borderline dilemma as viewed from analysis of an experience of nonhumanness. J Am Psychoanal Assoc 36:31–59, 1988

Winchel RM, Stanley M: Self-injurious behavior: a review of the behavior and biology of self-mutilation. Am J Psychiatry 148:306–317, 1991

Winnicott DW: Transitional objects and transitional phenomena: a study of the first not-me possession. Int J Psychoanal 34:89–97, 1953

Winnicott DW: Mirror role of mother and family in child development, in Playing and Reality. New York, Basic Books, 1971a, pp 111–118

Winnicott DW: Playing and Reality. London, Penguin Books, 1971b

Chapter 12

The Narcissistic Patient

Arnold D. Richards, M.D.,
and Arlene Kramer Richards, Ed.D.

Current Psychodynamic Perspectives

Narcissistic personality disorder was listed as a diagnostic category in neither the DSM-I (American Psychiatric Association 1952) nor the DSM-II (American Psychiatric Association 1968). It first appeared in DSM-III (American Psychiatric Association 1980) and was retained in DSM-III-R (American Psychiatric Association 1987). In both of these, the diagnostic description drew heavily on the contributions of two psychoanalysts, Otto Kernberg and Heinz Kohut, who in the early 1970s became the first to write about this condition. In the DSM-IV (American Psychiatric Association 1994), narcissistic personality disorder continues to be listed as a diagnostic category (301.81), with diagnostic features similar to those in DSM-III and DSM-III-R.

At the level of clinical description, narcissistic personality disorder is characterized by an unrealistically inflated sense of self-importance. Such patients feel they are special or unique and can be understood only by other special people. Preoccupied by "fantasies of unlimited success . . . and . . . an exhibitionistic need for constant attention and admiration," they tend to feel entitled to admiration "even without appropriate achievement" (American Psychiatric Association 1987, p. 350). Their exaggerated self-esteem is fragile, however, and grandiose feelings of superiority alternate with feelings of unworthiness and despair: "For example, a student who ordinarily expects an A and receives a grade of A– may, at that moment, express the view that he or she is thus revealed to all as a failure" (American Psychiatric Association 1980, pp. 349–350). "The person may be preoccupied with how well he or she is doing and how well he or she is regarded by others. This often takes the form of an almost exhibitionistic need for constant attention and admiration. The person may constantly fish for compliments, often with great charm. In response to criticism, he or she may react with rage, shame, or humiliation, but mask these feelings with an aura of cool indifference" (American Psychiatric Association 1987, p. 350).

Bach (1994, pp. 29–30) captured this two-sidedness of the narcissistic personality structure—grandiosity, intense ambition, and feelings of entitlement countered by insecurity, hypersensitivity, and feelings of inadequacy—by invoking the notions of "overinflated narcissistic type" and "depleted narcissistic type." Both sets of feelings are present in these patients, whose constant need for admiration renders them all but blind to the needs of others; others' assertions of their needs are, in fact, often experienced by the narcissistic individual as a personal affront. As a result of this extreme preoccupation with the self and its validation from without, feelings of empathy are either atrophied or altogether absent.

In their understanding of narcissistic personality disorder, Kohut and Kernberg differ significantly; their views on the disorder's etiology, pathogenesis, development, and treatment are often sharply at odds. For Kohut, the disorder reflects a psychological deficit due to faulty development—the result of parental failure to provide the proper interest and emotional support in the child's early years. The parents draw the child into their own concerns, repeatedly disappointing the child's need for affirmation. Repeated disappointments by the parents interfere with the child's ability to internalize appropriate feelings of self-regard or to develop self-control. The deprived child thus remains an emotional primitive, never developing a healthy sense of self.

Where Kohut sees a lack, Kernberg (1975) sees rampant, inappropriate feelings of rage and hatred (aggression) brought on by the child's internalization of disturbed relationships with others (pathological object relations). Kernberg views the narcissistic patient as the victim of exploitative and frustrating parents toward whom the child responds with rage, which in turn provokes further aggression. This is followed by projection and paranoid constellations, which are defended against by what Kernberg refers to as faulty, grandiose, and controlling behavior.

Historical Review

Although the literature on narcissism as a psychoanalytic concept is considerable and dates back to the beginning of the Freudian era, the use of *narcissistic* to indicate a category of patients is relatively recent. (Freud used the term *narcissistic neurosis* in contradistinction to *transference neurosis,* usually in the context of broad generalizations regarding analyzability; he did not in general consider it a specific diagnostic category but did refer to melancholia as a *narcissistic psychoneurosis* [Freud 1924/1961].)

It should come as no surprise that there are problematic features to the category of narcissistic personality disorder, given that the concept of narcissism from which it is derived has long suffered from ambiguity as regards both its meaning and its proper application. Freud first used the term *narcissism* in 1910 (in a footnote he added to "Three Essays on the Theory of Sexuality"), in order to account for object choice in homosexual persons, who "take themselves as their sexual objects—that is to say, they proceed from a narcissistic basis and look for a young man who resembles themselves and whom *they* may love as their mother loved *them*" (Freud 1905/1953, pp. 144–145). In the Schreber case, Freud (1911/1958) posited a stage in sexual development between autoeroticism and object love in which the subject "begins by taking himself, his own body, as his love object" (p. 60) and so unifies the sexual instincts.

By the time Freud wrote "On Narcissism: An Introduction" (1914/1957), he had been discussing the concept for some time. (He borrowed the term from Havelock Ellis. Paul Nacke had coined the term in 1899, but it was Ellis who first related it to the concept of perversion.) In this paper, Freud focused on the relation between self-love and object love (or, in the energic terminology he then favored, between libido cathecting the ego and libido cathecting objects). He postulated an initial libidinal cathexis of the ego that "fundamentally persists and is related to the object cathexis, much as the body of an amoeba is related to the pseudopodia which it puts out" (p. 75). Freud assumed a tense balance between self-love and object love: "The more the one is employed, the more the other becomes depleted" (p. 76). Thus, the ego was considered "a great reservoir of libido, from which libido is sent down to objects and which is always ready to absorb libido flowing back from objects" (p. 75). Narcissism was for Freud, as for his disciple Karl Abraham, a state of excessive self-love at the expense of object love. This imbalance is seen in its most extreme form in patients with *dementia praecox,* a dynamic state related developmentally to the infantile phase known as autoeroticism.

Although the concept of narcissism was presented initially as an extension of libido theory, it has since been lifted from this limiting framework. As Moore (1975) noted, "The concept . . . played a pivotal role in the development of the structural theory. Narcissism was a seed which germinated into ego psychology" (p. 243). Unfortunately, as he also noted, the term is often overused, for the very reason that it appears useful in describing such a variety of phenomena. It "may refer descriptively to a type of libido or its objects, to a stage of development, to a type or mode of object choice, to an attitude, to psychic systems and processes, or to a personality type which may be relatively normal to pathological, neurotic, psychotic, or borderline" (p. 244).

The problem that arises from this conceptual looseness is that theory in this area does not at present afford the therapist any clear guides in diagnosing and treating patients. This state of affairs stands in contrast to the useful diagnostic role played by such concepts as anxiety and depressive affect. But perhaps this judgment should be placed in the past tense. The classic view of narcissism, as presented first by Freud and then by his successors—including Abraham, Ferenczi, and later Hartmann, Jacobson, and Waelder—indeed did not provide a clear basis upon which to understand psychopathology. But this theoretical failing has been arguably corrected by Kohut and Kernberg; even though their theories are to some extent incompatible, each is coherent within its set of assumptions and hence may serve as a foundation for clinical theory. Freud's concept of narcissism suffered from an ambiguity regarding the relation between self and ego in his 1925 structural model, a failing Hartmann (1950/1964) tried to remedy, if not entirely with success. Kernberg himself has outlined some of the difficulties. Referring to Freud's (1931/1961) article on libidinal types, he criticized as too restrictive the attempt to classify the narcissistic character as another such type (Kernberg 1975). Kernberg noted that Fenichel (1945), one of Freud's most important systematizers, had objected to Freud's description of libidinal types, finding all such categorizations unsatisfactory: "Psychoanalysis is essentially a dynamic discipline. It evaluates given phenomena as a result of conflict. It has never considered the characteristics in terms of the actual strength of the forces operative but rather with respect to the functional relation of these forces to one another. A categorization of id person, ego person, and superego person is not a dynamic concept" (Fenichel 1945, pp. 525–526). Psychoanalytic formulations that rely primarily on the dispositions of psychic energies are, according to Fenichel, of limited clinical use.

Differential Dynamic Diagnosis

Although clinicians seem generally to agree about the kind of presenting picture they are inclined to call narcissistic, this consensus regarding phenomenology does not extend to psychodynamics. Because the two most developed and widely accepted formulations—those of Kernberg and Kohut—are either incompatible or must be taken to apply to very different patient populations, the status of narcissistic personality disorder as a clinical entity remains in doubt. It may well turn out that narcissism is encountered as a prominent feature in a variety of disorders, and that as each treatment progresses, the lineaments of the patient's specific disorder are revealed as typical of one or another of the more firmly established diagnostic categories. Whether a residue of patients would then remain for whom narcissistic personality disorder—however defined—would be the appropriate diagnosis is a question that cannot yet be answered with any certainty.

As regards treatment, Kernberg has recommended interpreting the narcissistic patient's striving for omnipotence and his or her need to idealize and denigrate the analyst. Rather than allowing these patients to project upon the analyst their feelings of exalted self-worth—or, conversely, of worthlessness—Kernberg believes that interpreting the patient's narcissistic, infantile strivings will bring to the fore the hidden rage and paranoia that lie beneath the surface of, for example, the patient's need to idealize the analyst. In such instances, the patient needs to be shown that his or her strong desire to cooperate with the analyst is a defense against deep and uncontrolled anger and a fear of being harmed. According to Kernberg (1975), the patient tries to control and devalue the analyst, to treat the analyst like an appendage and to render the analyst impotent. The task of the analyst is to interpret the patient's need to make the analyst feel deflated. If the analyst interprets this need continually, the patient will begin to express his or her rage and to reveal fears that are part of a paranoid stratum of his or her personality. Kernberg has identified the following factors as suggestive of a favorable prognosis: a capacity for depression and mourning; a transference potential for guilt in contrast to a tilt toward paranoid rage; a capacity to sublimate; an emphasis by the analyst on interpretation of the superego; and an absence of life situations granting unusual narcissistic gratifications. Keeping these factors in mind helps the therapist decide which narcissistic patients can more readily be worked with.

Despite their differing views of etiology and divergent treatment strategies, Kohut and Kernberg agree that patients with narcissistic personality disorder are extremely difficult to treat. The problem is that these patients tend to experience their symptoms as ego-syntonic—that is, as compatible with their wishes and acceptable to their egos. They fail to recognize that their need for constant reassurance and praise is extreme, and that their inability to empathize with others is a psychological deficiency. Only when the world fails to provide them with narcissistic supplies in the form of special recognition do they experience fright and despair. Whereas their presenting symptoms are often vague, their diffuse feelings of shame and unworthiness on the one hand, and of grandiose entitlement and narcissistic rage on the other, may run deep over the course of treatment.

Through much of treatment, such patients tend to persist in a persona of extreme self-sufficiency. They seem not to need other people, the analyst included, and they have great difficulty even perceiving others as separate individuals. Often, the patient exploits the therapist as a foil in order to overcome disturbances of self-constancy and self-regulation, or to shore up flagging self-esteem. For instance, the patient may achieve a temporary sense of self-sufficiency by devaluing the analyst, thereby fending off feelings not only of weakness and failure but also of rage, the latter feeling betokening the patient's inability to actualize grandiose fantasies in the real world.

Kohut, in developing his diagnostic formulations and treatment approach, introduced the term *selfobject* to capture the fact that the narcissistic patient relates to another person as if that person were functionally a part of him- or herself. According to Kohut, these patients use other people to regulate their tension states and to bolster their self-esteem; they are largely unable to relate to others in any other way or for any other purpose. Kernberg (1975) described a similar phenomenon from his own theoretical perspective, noting that narcissistic patients experience "an unusual degree of self-reference in their interactions with other people, a great need to be loved and admired by others, and a curious apparent contradiction between a very inflated concept of themselves and an inordinate need for tribute from others. Their emotional life is shallow. They experience little empathy for the feelings of others. They obtain very little enjoyment from life other than from the tributes they receive from others or from their own grandiose fantasies . . . they envy others . . . their relationships with other people are clearly exploitative and sometimes parasitic" (p. 228).

Because the narcissistically disturbed patient relates to the therapist only insofar as the latter sustains the patient's sense of self-worth, the therapist is in the paradoxical position of having to accept the patient's need for mirroring and affirmation while simultaneously attempting to help the patient to recognize that others exist in their own right, not just as selfobjects. Kohut has labeled the therapeutic solution to this paradox the "transmuting internalization." According to him, when treatment is successful, the patient is able to use the relationship with the therapist to develop a sense of self. In this context, "self" signifies a permanent psychic structure that neither dissolves nor expands unrealistically with every mood swing or minor loss.

The treatment of narcissistic patients is very difficult owing to their extreme need to control the therapist and to use the therapist to provide them with a sense of self-esteem. In particular, they will fend off efforts to help them perceive and accept the therapist as an autonomous being with feelings, wishes, and needs. Likewise, these patients will resist efforts to interpret their sense of grandiose entitlement as a defense against profound feelings of inadequacy and worthlessness. As Kohut observes, "The patient who experiences again . . . the helplessness and loss of power he felt as a child tries to regain a feeling of bliss and power by projecting onto the analyst these treasured feelings. The patient vacillates between total idealizing of the analyst and a cold rejection of him or her" (Kohut 1971, p. 67). In treatment, the patient may swing wildly between seeing the therapist as an omnipotent being whose power will energize the patient—in Kohut's terminology, an "idealized parental image"—and seeing the therapist as the ineffectual, powerless being onto whom the patient has projected a despairing sense of worthlessness. Alternatively, the patient may adopt an attitude of superiority while simultaneously revealing inordinate self-consciousness,-shame, and hypochondriacal preoccupations.

Bach (1994) underscores the essential two-sidedness of the clinical phenomenology by pointing to the countertransference issues that further complicate treatment: "Many clinicians agree that the countertransference provides the major stumbling block in treating narcissistic patients, either because we cannot tolerate the consistent disregard shown for our human rights and our very existence by the overinflated, entitled narcissist, or because we cannot tolerate the idealizations projected onto us by the insecure and depleted narcissistic patient. It may help us to remember that behind the latter's experienced inadequacy lie deeper feelings of grandiose entitlement" (p. 39). Bach adds that successful treatment, with its analysis of the patient's defenses, brings together the complementary sides of narcissistic disturbance, so that "ultimately the presenting distinctions between the two types should dissolve as a more complete human being emerges" (p. 9).

As for transference, the difficulty in establishing it with narcissistic patients was noted first by Freud, who (as has been mentioned) distinguished the "narcissistic" from the "transference" neurosis. The former was characterized by the withdrawal of interest from the outside world in favor of the self, and the latter by the patient's ability to invest real or imaginary objects, including the analyst, with libidinal and aggressive interest. Kohut's conceptualization of the "narcissistic transference" (1971), later designated the "selfobject transference" (1977), was intended to denote a mode of relatedness according to which patients with narcissistic neuroses, in Freud's sense, could develop a special kind of transference that rendered them treatable by psychoanalytic methods. In his earlier writings, Kohut (1971) stressed that in successful treatment, the narcissistic transference was followed by the engagement and working through of an "object-libidinal transference," so that narcissistic pathology ultimately gave way to the libidinal and aggressive conflicts associated with neurotic pathology, with the analyst serving now as a transference object proper.

Kohut's concept of selfobject transference requires the therapist, for at least a major portion of the treatment, to comply with the patient's childhood wishes by providing heretofore unmet needs: for mirroring, for affirmation, for an alter ego, and for a selfobject to idealize. Only through these empathic provisions can the patient's archaic narcissistic structures (e.g., the primitive grandiose self) evolve into mature narcissistic structures capable of sustaining a healthy, reality-tested sense of self-worth. Commensurate with this treatment orientation is the need to refrain from interpretations that might prematurely rupture the patient's narcissistic defenses. As noted by Bach (1994), "premature confrontations often lead to narcissistic rage reactions in the overinflated patients and a pseudoacquiescence in the depleted patients, but not to structural growth. Effective interpretation of libidinal and aggressive conflicts become possible only when the patient begins to really understand that *the same reality can be viewed in different ways by different people and that his point of view and the therapist's point of view can both have reality and legitimacy.* Before that time, such interpretations are often counterproductive and, indeed, may spring more from the therapist's countertransference than from the patient's needs" (p. 9, *emphasis added*).

As might be gathered, the narcissistic patient presents in many ways the greatest challenge for the psychodynamically oriented psychotherapist. Patients with severe anxiety, phobias, depression, or obsessive or compulsive systems readily acknowledge their suffering and need for treatment. The adverse impact of their symptoms on their functioning is clear both to themselves and to their therapists; these symptoms can readily be connected with both developmental history and current life stresses, and psychopharmacological agents are available that can reduce their severity and facilitate psychodynamic treatment. By contrast, narcissistic patients present with neither clear-cut symptoms nor clearly identifiable dysfunctional behavior. Some patients sense that there is something wrong with them but don't know what it is; often, these patients' family members and friends are largely unaware of their psychopathology. In other cases, however, these others are far more aware of the disturbed functioning and relationships than are the patients themselves. Although this state of affairs—in particular, the tendency to ego-syntonicity and the lack of clear-cut symptoms or dysfunction—is to some extent shared with other patients who fall into the broad diagnostic category of personality disorders, certain aspects of the pathology of narcissistic patients—in particular, the tendency to self-absorption and grandiosity—significantly impair their ability to engage in psychotherapy, thereby diminishing the possibility of a favorable outcome. It is generally agreed that psychopharmacological agents are of limited use in the treatment of such patients. Some authorities consider psychoanalysis the treatment of choice, because often these patients can benefit only from intensive, long-term treatment. However, because psychoanalysis is often not feasible and, in any event, is not offered by most psychotherapists in private practice, the treatment possibilities for narcissistic patients are, in point of fact, severely limited.

Case Example

History

Ms. V, the patient, was a well-groomed, brisk woman of 45. Married with no children, this aspiring actress had held several low-level clerical jobs, had had roles in a few amateur theatrical productions, and was currently engaged in an extramarital affair.

Brought up in a small southern town by her mother in the home of her maternal grandparents, Ms. V reported that she was never told anything about her father, although he and his family lived in the same town. She learned about him only when he died and a high-school friend advised her to attend the funeral. She believed her mother had intimated then that he had deserted them when the patient was 2 years old. Her mother had held a light manufacturing job throughout the patient's childhood and was an important source of income to the family. The patient recalled her as cold, distant, and suspicious, as well as being angry and contemptuous toward men. By contrast, Ms. V always had many friendships, several quite close and of long duration. She described herself as even-tempered; she never cried, and maintained a humorous, story-telling, wisecracking attitude with friends. She believed that they, like her husband, found her attractively tough.

Ms. V's narcissistic personality disorder met the DSM-III criteria. She had an exaggerated sense of self-importance, believing herself to be a great actress on the basis of a few roles in semi-amateur companies and expecting a career as a star when none of her performances had even been mentioned in reviews in the local newspapers. Her need for attention and the fragility of her self-esteem were apparent in her constant wisecracking and her catastrophic reaction to having to wait for her husband to pick her up. A lack of empathy was evident in her relationships with her husband and mother, as will be seen in the specimen session below. The vacillation between idealizing and devaluing objects was shown most clearly in her conviction that she was worthwhile only when her husband was around, which alternated with a conviction that he was worthless because he treated her so badly.

The psychotherapy sessions were all about Ms. V's husband; they were attempts to understand *him* in order to save her marriage. All of her concerns were interpersonal. She talked about her therapy sessions with friends, using their opinions to define her reality. She described having similarly used her friends to "check out" her mother's perceptions and explanations when she was growing up. She connected waiting for her husband when he was on a business trip or when he was late for a date with her with waiting for the father who never came when she was a child.

Themes of abandonment pervaded Ms. V's life narrative. Struggles emerged between a fear of being abandoned—repetition of the trauma—and attempts at reversal by abandoning others. At the end of a year of psychotherapy, she declared herself much better and began to talk of ending treatment within a few sessions. Interpretations of her need to repeat the abandonment were to no avail. She referred to the feared separation from her husband as "his going away, his leaving me" and, later, as "when he left." Ms. V left the therapist and then provoked her husband to leave her. She was away from treatment for 6 months. When finally she returned, it was for help in coping with the breakup of her marriage.

Her therapy had resulted in an impasse. Ms. V's persistent lack of insight convinced the therapist that she could not be helped by psychotherapy precisely because of the narcissistic disorder that had driven her to treatment. In these extreme circumstances, it seemed that if anything could work, it would be analysis. It was with the hope that her narcissism was analyzable that this recommendation was made. After a brief consultation, analysis was initiated on a four-times-per-week schedule, on the couch, which was maintained for 6 years. The legal process for a divorce was initiated several months after the analysis was begun.

Course of Analysis

Ms. V alternated transference attitudes from the very beginning of her analysis. Some weeks she would present herself as misunderstood, a helpless victim, beginning each session with a demand for help. In other sessions, her attitude and manner of speech were imperious in an infantile, omnipotent way. These distinct attitudes never overlapped in the same session and initially were extremely impenetrable, lasting from session to session and from week to week. Imperious, mirroring sessions would begin with such opening lines as "I *have* to tell my mother to go to Florida to live" or "I *know* why I don't get along with my husband. It is the birth order factor." Desperate, idealizing sessions would open with such lines as "I had a terrible dream" or "I had a traumatic phone call." A feature of the idealizing sessions was that she would call the analyst "my wizard." The quality of the session was predictable from the opening statement or question.

In the imperious mood, with the mirroring transference, Ms. V reported that when her husband came home from work an hour late, saying, "You be nice to me and I'll be nice to you," she screamed at him. She was surprised to hear that the analyst considered this response an expression of rage at her husband. In this mood, her manifest complaints dealt always with the other person, never with her own feelings. The way she dressed in the imperious mood was stylish but severe. Her posture, gestures, and tone of voice were definite, dramatic—and severe.

In her beseeching, idealizing mood Ms. V would speak of her fears. One session she began by saying that if her husband left her, her mother would move in and take over her life. She implored the analyst to protect her; she painted such a frightening picture of a cold, demanding mother that the listener could only tremble for her. One especially dramatic scene was reported after a weekend visit from her mother; the patient woke up in the middle of the night to see her mother standing at the foot of the bed, staring at her. Terrified, she sat bolt upright on the couch as she had on the bed. The analyst behind the couch became as powerful a figure as the mother at the foot of the bed. If the analyst helped her, she would be great; if not, she was nothing. When she manifested the idealizing attitude, the patient presented herself as an innocent requiring rescue from the intrusive, demanding mother. She dressed in printed silk little-girl dresses with bobby socks and running shoes over her stockings. Her posture was flaccid, her voice high-pitched.

Following is an example of a complete session from the first months of the analysis, in which Ms. V took an imperious, angry, isolated position, manifesting a mirroring transference.

> Ms. V began by saying, in a defiant tone, "I didn't call my mother on Mother's Day. And I didn't like her calling me and saying she was afraid I was sick." She then described her mother's conciliatory attitude, to which she had nonetheless responded with rejection. Although she complained that her mother was cold and indifferent, she herself was not at all that way. Refusing to talk to her mother made her feel better. She felt less left out, less isolated, when she didn't have to talk to her mother.
>
> Ms. V then spoke about her husband. He was being difficult, refusing to discuss the young woman who was his new assistant at work. She wanted him to explain himself, to tell her why he had to work late so many evenings, to promise her that he wasn't having an affair with this young woman. She wanted also to tell him that she was jealous of a client of his she had read about in a promotional piece he had done for the client. In this account, the client was a superwoman. Although Ms. V realized that it was necessary for her husband to present his client in the best possible light, she resented the fact that he'd done his job so well. She was sure that her husband admired this "perfect" woman more than he admired her.
>
> Ms. V complained that the analyst would misunderstand and think that she was just feeling in need of bolstering up because she felt guilty about the affair she was having, and that neither her mother nor her husband understood how much she needed to be admired. The analyst intervened—for the only time in the session—to connect the idea of guilt with the need to be admired for doing something she

> thought was wrong. Scornfully admitting that this was correct, Ms. V pointed out that she had provoked her mother by not calling her on Mother's Day and had also provoked her husband, by accusing him, with no evidence at all, of having an affair with his assistant. She ended the session by describing how nice she really was to her husband: she had allowed him to eat his lunch an hour late on Saturday when he was working at home, not interrupting him as she usually did.

In this session, the patient's defiant tone of voice was the first indication of her transference attitude, and her statement that she had not called her mother on Mother's Day clearly challenged a social norm she believed the analyst accepted. So she went on to describe her mother's conciliatory attitude. Her next statement, however, that her mother was the cold and indifferent one, contradicted her description of their roles in this incident. Clearly, she was challenging the analyst either to accept her self-contradictory view or to challenge her. She then repeated this self-contradictory narrative twice over, each time with a new set of characters: first her husband and his assistant, and then her husband and his superwoman client. Each time she gave evidence that she had wronged someone; each time she accused the victim of what she herself had done. This evoked in the analyst a mounting countertransferential wish to protest, to set her straight, to show her that she was contradicting herself. The patient's expectation that these contradictions would go unchallenged left the analyst feeling gulled and humiliated. That Ms. V wanted simply to be mirrored rather than responded to seemed evident; any response at all would have produced a confrontation that would be used to preclude her understanding the self-accusation she was defending herself against. Her aggressive stance seemed to afford her sufficient pleasure to keep her functioning well. When the patient projected the idea that she felt guilty about the love affair onto the analyst and then saw this as an accusation, the interpretation aimed to elucidate the defense. The scornful exhibitionism and challenging unreasonableness of her characterization of the events she narrated were revealed to the patient as a cover for her guilt, as an invitation to the analyst to punish her for it, and as a discharge of aggression. Interpretation of the transference attitude at this point would have been premature, affording the patient just the nugget of reality that would convince her that she had to fight this out not with her superego but with the analyst. Nonetheless, some interpretation connecting the exhibitionism or mirroring transference attitude with the guilt was necessary so that her need to maintain that attitude might be diminished.

This session began with a defiant account of her controlling and punitive behavior toward her mother. At the same time, she was controlling and punishing the analyst; her description of her mother as cold and rejecting was a warning to the analyst of how any intervention at that point would be received. The session's only intervention was indeed met with scorn. The attempt to connect her need for approval with her guilt was a beginning at revealing to her the superego aspects of the conflict that undermined her self-esteem. She finished the session with an anecdote in which she again described her angry control of a love object; this time, however, she was able to allow a small concession—a late lunch—which only served to accentuate the degree of control she had been exercising.

Thus, in this session she manifested coldness, superiority, and the tendency toward self-consciousness and shame that Kohut considered diagnostic indicators of the grandiose mirroring transference. Yet the analyst's interpretation of her defensive use of this posture, linking it to guilt over a sexual transgression, had the effect of softening her attitude. Extreme grandiosity thus appears to be an artifact of the treatment, as does its eventual toning down.

Another early session began with an account of a mortally ill woman who doesn't dare ask for help. The patient was low-key in her manner, evoking a countertransferential wish to help, even to rescue. She described herself as pitiable. Again, only one interpretation was made in the session—that she experienced the analyst as bound to her by pity. This time, the interpretation was received in a helpless way, not at all rejected and possibly even confirmed by the production of a relevant memory. Again, the session ended with a slight modification of her stance; instead of merely accepting, she was actively confirming. Just as she had been unaware of being angry at her husband even as she was delivering tirades against him, so she was only dimly aware of how much her helpless, needy feelings directed her behavior and how her behavior evoked specific responses from others.

Although this alternation of attitudes continued right up to the end of treatment, the attitudes themselves became less extremely divergent. In the first year of the analysis, this modulation first became apparent in a session she opened by announcing, "I'm glad I don't have tantrums any more." During that session, she explored her sexual jealousy of her husband and was able to grasp the unconscious meaning of her suspicion that he was having affairs: she was envious of his ability to have sex with a woman, envious indeed of his penis. She began to complain that he kept his closets too organized, that he scheduled his appointments too closely, and that he was excessively conscientious in attending to the administrative details of a fraternity to which he belonged. She noted, however, that as he became more organized, he advanced in his career. She was able to realize that she preferred her lover, who suffered from premature ejaculation, because he didn't make her feel as envious as did her virile and efficient husband.

By the next session, though, she had returned to the complaints, expressing them now with a penitent "I see what's wrong now." Her mood had shifted back to the infantile, dependent state. Now, instead of being the imperious, envious, and spiteful one, she was the victim. She listed all the complaints her husband might have about her. She described in detail how 1) her field was not as prestigious as that of her husband, 2) her position in her field was not as advanced as her husband's in his, 3) her salary could never compare with his professional fees, and 4) although he said he didn't want the encumbrances of a house or family, she was the one he could blame for their childless state as well as for their failure to invest in a house. Her despair over these complaints—which her husband had never actually made—was total. She could not believe that if she was this bad, she could have any redeeming features whatever. When these pronouncements were interpreted as fantasy, she bitterly accused the analyst of believing that her self-reproaches were only cover-ups for the reproach that she had not been faithful to her husband. She had the fantasy that her sexual transgressions would be repeated in the analysis, as analyst and husband were equated. This fantasy was then traced back to a fantasy that her father would accuse her of sexual activity with her mother. She recovered a memory of sleeping in the same bed with her mother until adolescence.

Later on, she began to challenge the analyst by missing appointments and by arranging her schedule and finances so that she couldn't help leaving treatment. She left a job that provided insurance that allowed her to pay a full fee for one providing no insurance at all. When the analyst agreed to accept a reduced fee so that she could accept a job with more responsibility but without health insurance, she became suspicious. She feared that she would have to reciprocate, as she would if a friend lent her money or invited her to stay with her. A decision about whether to leave the analysis engendered a transference crisis. A new phase of treatment was ushered in by her understanding of the offer as a seduction similar to her fantasied seduction by her mother. She was then in the third year of treatment, the second of analysis. As she became aware of her sexual yearnings toward the analyst, her fear of them, and her need for a man in her life to protect her from the fulfillment or even awareness of these wishes, her negative oedipal desires came into focus. The helpless stance or idealizing transference was a wish to be loved; the imperious or mirroring transference was the wish to be the active lover.

A session after the transference crisis, in which the idealizing, dependent stance was modified by her emerging capacity to see complex compromises between good and evil, power and weakness, in the analyst as well as in other people in her life, began this way:

> I want to talk about Bill—with him I can really see what you said last time. I *do* demand more and reject him for not giving me more than he really owes me!

A significant shift in her understanding of her interpersonal difficulties appeared later in the same session:

> Janet can't understand me—she has acquaintances, friends, and a best friend—me. She can't understand why I put people into only two categories—in and out. She thinks it's okay to see people every couple of weeks for a drink, enjoy it, and not want more from them. Not *all* her relationships are that way, but she can enjoy the ones that are!

Later yet, a modulated form of the mirroring transference appeared in a session that began this way:

> Funny how I think—can't really understand it. First I get so angry at things, then when I think about it, I'm not really angry at all.

She drew comparisons between her attitudes toward the analyst and her attitudes toward other people in her life:

> It's just like asking about my father. I knew it was so painful not to know—but I was afraid I'd learn something unbearable if I asked. I couldn't stand asking. But I'd have been so much better off! I really put myself through a lot of pain unnecessarily because I couldn't ask! Like asking you about my vacation sessions. I thought you'd hate me because I was going away at the wrong time. And tell me I was bad—and you didn't. I was so relieved! I should have done it before!

Later in the analysis, idealizing sessions began with such statements as "I have to tell you. I really believe *one* thing you said now," or her remark about Bill: "With him I can really see what you said last time." Such statements are restricted. No longer the all-knowing wizard, the analyst is now given credit for knowing *one* thing or saying something that applies to *one* of the patient's relationships. Thus, she began to see that her former way of characterizing the analyst as either all-good, all-giving, and all-knowing or as all-bad, depriving, and destructive was not the only way to relate to her. The same applied to other people. She could see that she had experienced her husband, and now her lover, as simply not there when she was angry because disappointed by them.

She persisted in characterizing her own affects by contrasting them with her mother's attitudes, but now by modulation rather than through simple reversal. She was able to see her splitting of affects as unusual; it was beginning to be dystonic to her that she could not tolerate the ambivalence of human relationships by maintaining an intermediate distance between herself and other people—neither being overly demanding nor shutting them out, neither idealizing nor scorning.

Ms. V's depressive affect was expressed mostly in complaints about her inability to work, a craving for drinks in the afternoon, and a conviction that her rival would get promoted before she would, thus forcing her to quit a job she enjoyed because of the humiliation of being passed over. This paranoid attitude was modified sufficiently for her to see that her rival was not omnipotent and to give up the conviction that she would be passed over for promotion because of what she considered the invincible self-esteem of the rival. Now she was able to bear the interpretation of her projection as well as the inference that she was in charge of the powers that would decide her fate. By the end of the analysis, she was neither imperious nor imploring. She was more indulgent toward her own feelings. She neither had to project so rigidly nor required the sharp division of her world into all good and all bad. She became capable of more empathic understanding of others as well as able to expect more from them. The latter capacity allowed her to ask for such things as vacations rather than taking as reality her fantasy that her requests would be denied.

Summary

Ms. V's analysis was conducted using a classic psychoanalytic technique. The 1-year psychotherapy that preceded the analysis was an analytic psychotherapy in that the patient was encouraged to explore her ideas and feelings. She never received any advice or special help. She was never the recipient of any special empathy. No educative attempts were made. Transference interpretations were balanced by interpretations that clarified affect, linked affect to the gratification of instinctual wishes, and explicated superego fears. It was the patient's gradual shifting and remodeling of her views of the world and her own experience in it that resulted in her change of behavior.

The transference developed from a set of rigid postures in which the analyst was either the all-powerful, idealized parent or the scorned, impotent one. While various figures of the patient's childhood were experienced in both guises, the attitudes themselves softened. At times the all-powerful, idealized figure represented the mother, at other times the grandfather, and at still other times the father. The most dramatic change resulting from treatment was a drastic revision of the patient's early history. Able to ask her mother about her early life in short conversations over a period lasting from the second through the fourth years of treatment, she discovered that her father had, in fact, been present; he had visited frequently in the home she and her mother shared with her grandparents. She eventually came to recall sitting on his lap while he read her the funnies. Indeed, her humor was traced to an identification with this powerful figure doing the reading.

The transference deepened and was enriched by the many threads of transferences from all the objects of the patient's early life. A major feature was the development of an ability to experience anger and disappointment toward the analyst despite the fear of losing that beloved figure, whom she might psychically kill off as she had her father. The reorganization of her inner life came about through a gradual removal and replacement of warped strands with new ones in the fabric of her understanding. Thus, this patient uncovered, disconnected, and reconnected her affects, wishes, and fears, and her memories and fantasies, to form a more viable mental tapestry.

For Further Study

Bursten B: Some narcissistic personality types. Int J Psychoanal 54:287–300, 1973

Freidman JA: The idea of narcissism in Freud's psychoanalysis. International Review of Psycho-Analysis 15:499–514, 1988

Glassman M: Kernberg and Kohut: a test of competing psychoanalytic models of narcissism. J Am Psychoanal Assoc 36:597–626, 1988

Meissner WW: A case of phallic narcissistic personality. J Am Psychoanal Assoc 33:437–469, 1985

Robbins M: Narcissistic personality: a symbiotic character disorder. Int J Psychoanal 63:457–473, 1982

Rothstein A: An exploration of the diagnostic term narcissistic personality disorder. J Am Psychoanal Assoc 27:893–912, 1979

Schwartz L: Narcissistic personality: a clinical discussion. J Am Psychoanal Assoc 22:292–306, 1974

Spruiell V: Theories of the treatment of narcissistic personality. J Am Psychoanal Assoc 22:268–278, 1974

References

American Psychiatric Association: Diagnostic and Statistical Manual: Mental Disorders. Washington, DC, American Psychiatric Association, 1952

American Psychiatric Association: Diagnostic and Statistical Manual of Mental Disorders, 2nd Edition. Washington, DC, American Psychiatric Association, 1968

American Psychiatric Association: Diagnostic and Statistical Manual of Mental Disorders, 3rd Edition. Washington, DC, American Psychiatric Association, 1980

American Psychiatric Association: Diagnostic and Statistical Manual of Mental Disorders, 3rd Edition, Revised. Washington, DC, American Psychiatric Association, 1987

American Psychiatric Association: Diagnostic and Statistical Manual of Mental Disorders, 4th Edition. Washington, DC, American Psychiatric Association, 1994

Bach S: The Language of Perversion and the Language of Love. Northvale, NJ, Jason Aronson, 1994

Fenichel O: The Psychoanalytic Theory of Neurosis. New York, WW Norton, 1945

Freud S: Three essays on the theory of sexuality, I: the sexual aberrations (1905), in Standard Edition of the Complete Psychological Works of Sigmund Freud, Vol 7. Translated and edited by Strachey J. London, Hogarth Press, 1953, pp 135–172

Freud S: Psycho-analytic notes on an autobiographical account of a case of paranoia *(dementia paranoides)* (1911), in The Standard Edition of the Complete Psychological Works of Sigmund Freud, Vol 12. Translated and edited by Strachey J. London, Hogarth Press, 1958, pp 3–96

Freud S: On narcissism: an introduction (1914), in The Standard Edition of the Complete Psychological Works of Sigmund Freud, Vol 14. Translated and edited by Strachey J. London, Hogarth Press, 1957, pp 67–102

Freud S: Neurosis and psychosis (1924), in The Standard Edition of the Complete Psychological Works of Sigmund Freud, Vol 19. Translated and edited by Strachey J. London, Hogarth Press, 1961, pp 148–153

Freud S: Libidinal types (1931), in The Standard Edition of the Complete Psychological Works of Sigmund Freud, Vol 21. Translated and edited by Strachey J. London, Hogarth Press, 1961, pp 215–220

Glassman M: Kernberg and Kohut: a test of competing psychoanalytic models of narcissism. J Am Psychoanal Assoc 36:597–626, 1988

Hartmann H: Comments on the psychoanalytic theory of the ego (1950), in Essays on Ego Psychology. New York, International Universities Press, 1964, pp 13–141

Kernberg OF: Borderline Conditions and Pathological Narcissism. New York, Jason Aronson, 1975

Kohut H: The Analysis of the Self. New York, International Universities Press, 1971

Kohut H: The Restoration of the Self. New York, International Universities Press, 1977

Moore B: Toward a clarification of the concept of narcissism. Psychoanal Study Child 30:243–278, 1975

Chapter 13

The Patient With a Neurosis

Gerald A. Melchiode, M.D.

Current Psychodynamic Perspectives

Where have all the patients with neuroses gone? I have difficulty locating them in our present nosology. They are like a lost tribe, dispersed and forced to wander through the nomenclature and forbidden to settle in one place. Anxiety, phobic, and obsessive-compulsive neuroses are found among the anxiety disorders. Hysterical neurosis–conversion type and hypochondriacal neuroses are under the somatoform disorders and the hysterical neuroses; hysterical neurosis–dissociative type is under the dissociative disorders. Descriptive classifications, albeit important for other reasons (e.g., research), distract us from a psychodynamic perspective, which is useful in understanding and treating individual patients.

Anxiety has always been the hallmark of the neuroses, and the various defense mechanisms employed to deal with the anxiety give each neurosis its unique form. Anxiety is a subjective sense of apprehension with a concomitant activation of the autonomic nervous system. Some authors make a distinction between fear and anxiety. Fear is the affect state caused by anticipation of an external danger, whereas anxiety is the affect state elicited by awareness of an internal danger. These internal dangers relate to the calamities of childhood and include 1) loss of a need-fulfilling person or object, 2) loss of love, 3) castration anxiety, and 4) superego anxiety (Brenner 1982).

Neuroses are unique to the human condition for two reasons. First, compared with other species, humans have a relatively long period of dependence on parents. In early development, the child must be able to master its instinctual needs with regard to its adult caregivers. This dependence sets up a situation in which a sense of helplessness is created when those needs come into conflict with the child's internal representation of the early caregivers.

The second reason for this uniqueness is the human capacity for language, meaning, and symbolism. Here the child, because of faulty cognitions and magical thinking, has the capacity to distort both drive derivatives and the mental representations that oppose those drives. The first basic anxiety of the child relates to the loss of the object. Around the age of 1–1½, the baby perceives at some level that it desperately needs the mothering person to relieve tension, and that without this person, it will be overwhelmed by its own needs. Around the age of 2–2½, a more sophisticated step is reached in which the child realizes that not only the parents' care is required, but also their love. Without that love, the child feels alone and forsaken. The toddler must learn to relinquish that which is pleasurable in order to win the parent's love. Toilet training is the prototype for this conflict. Thus, the second basic anxiety relates to *loss of love.*

Between the ages of 2½ and 6, the child is preoccupied with physical injury, especially to the genitals. During this stage, the child is masturbating and fantasizing about an exclusive intimate relationship with the parent of the opposite sex and has aggressive feelings for the parent of the same sex. Because of magical thinking, the child believes that the parent of the same sex knows what he or she is thinking and will retaliate. The anxiety during the oedipal stage is called *castration anxiety.*

During the ages of 5 and 7, an internalization of the conscience occurs with the resolution of the oedipal stage. Now the child fears punishment from his or her own internalized parental images. Anxiety relating to such fears is called *superego anxiety.*

Each of these traumatic states has in common an overwhelming sense of helplessness. Until about 7 years of age, the child does not have the requisite ego development (e.g., cognitive development) and independence to work out or even to consider other options for dealing with its helplessness.

The classic psychoanalytic view postulates that the neurotic core conflict occurs during the oedipal period with the consolidation of the superego as an internal agency. However, this core conflict is colored by the preoedipal stages that precede it: for example, individuals who have the most intense separation anxiety also have the greatest amount of castration anxiety. Psychoanalytic theory posits that this childhood neurosis is repressed, but not without extracting a heavy toll, because the neurotic needs and wishes continue to press for discharge. The person will tend to turn his or her reality into the image and likeness of his or her oedipal struggles. This is what Freud called the "repetition compulsion."

The person then goes through life until he or she encounters an external situation that reverberates intrapsychically with his or her past. When this occurs and the old infantile wishes and the archaic prohibitions are triggered, the ego signals with anxiety. The ego must then satisfy the wishes of the id and the prohibitions of the superego, yet temper the anxiety. This maneuver is called a "compromise formation." Defensive or adaptive mechanisms are used to effect such compromise formations. The type of defensive mechanism employed gives the neurosis its form. Repression alone can be used. Here the person still experiences the anxiety but unconsciously blocks out of his or her mind the ideational content of the wish. This is called an "anxiety neurosis." Repression is viewed as the primary defense mechanism in all of the neuroses; the other defenses constitute so-called second-line defense mechanisms. If repression is used and symbolic displacement is added, this results in a hysterical neurosis such as conversion disorder. In other words, the person blocks out the ideational content of the wish but the wish is deflected to a body part or function. The result is a paralysis of that body part or function, which may be understood also as a punishment for the wish. For example, when a person has unacceptable aggressive impulses that are only partially repressed, the mind tries to bind the anxiety by deflecting the aggressive wish onto a body part, and the hand may be curled into a fist. Yet the hand is involuntary rigid and paralyzed in that position (the punishment for the wish).

In *phobic neurosis*, repression is employed, but when it begins to fail, other defenses are added—namely, externalization, displacement, and avoidance. In other words, a current situation in the patient's life stimulates aggressive wishes that are unacceptable. The ego tries to repress these wishes but is only partially successful. The aggressive wishes are deflected outside of the person. For example, in Freud's case description of Hans (a boy with a fear of horses), Hans's aggressive wish was externalized to his father. That maneuver was unsuccessful because his father was often present, so Hans had to deflect the wish from father to horses, which were less a part of his immediate environment. Hans then used the defense of avoidance to distance himself further from horses, which now contained his original aggressive impulses (Freud 1909/1955).

Obsessive-compulsive neuroses are the most complex of the neuroses. Again, for the purpose of explanation, a current situation calls forth an unacceptable hostile wish. Repression is deployed, but again it is only partially successful. A host of secondary and tertiary defenses come into play: reaction formation, undoing, magical thinking, and intellectualization. A harried mother's child becomes sick, which stimulates certain unconscious death wishes toward her own younger siblings. Her ego attempts unsuccessfully to repress these wishes, but anxiety breaks through, and she automatically employs reaction formation and becomes overly solicitous toward her ill child as a way of warding off her hostile feelings. The mother then cannot sleep at night because she fears that she left the gas stove on. She goes to the kitchen and turns the gas on (an expression of her hostile wish) and then off again as a way of undoing her wish. She must do this 10 times as a way of binding her anxiety. It is as if this were a magical ritual to ensure her child's safety—a derivative of omnipotent magical thinking which she explains to herself (intellectualization) as behavior that demonstrates her concern for her child.

In each of these examples, aggressive wishes are used for simplicity, clarity, and consistency. Sexual wishes could also have been used, and clinical experience has shown that wishes are often a mixture of aggressive and sexual impulses.

In summary, this presents the structural theory of neurosis, which postulates that the functions of the mind are the result of component forces. In healthy functioning, the forces are not observable. In neuroses, however, the vectors of forces are drives, governing forces, and adaptive forces. In the structural theory, these are—respectively—the id, the superego, and the ego. The meaning that one attaches to external reality can also be included as a factor. A diagram of the structural theory would look like this:

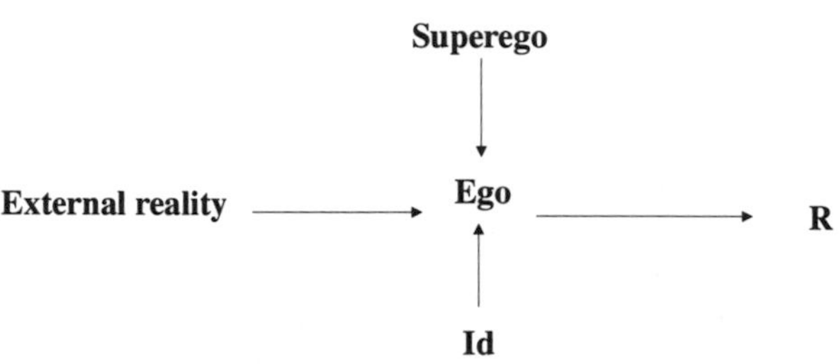

In this chapter, R = the neurosis; thus, the neurosis is a compromise—the result of the various forces. A diagram of an anxiety neurosis would look like this:

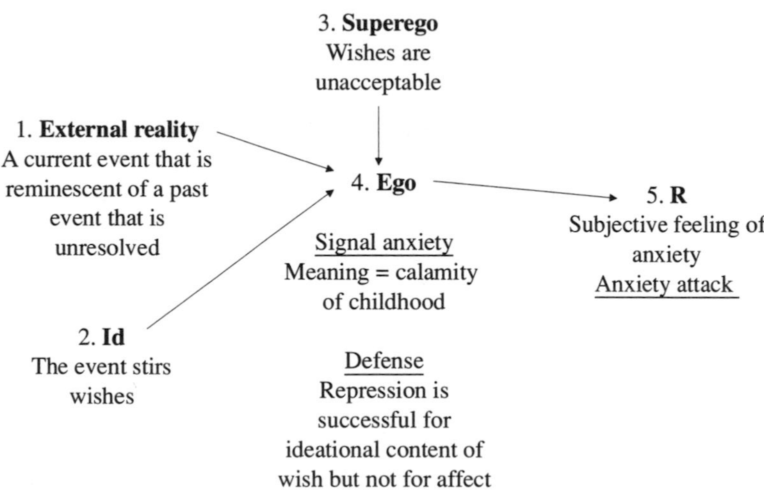

These agencies—id, superego, and ego—do not exist in a place in the brain. One should not attempt to reify these terms—they are abstractions that help categorize functions of the mind.

Historical Review

Residents during the middle and the end of the 19th century studied a psychiatry textbook by Griesinger (Kaplan and Sadock 1981), in which they learned that the mental disorders, such as the neuroses, are caused by the degeneration of nervous tissue, which in turn is caused by constitutional factors. Such problems are irreversible, and nothing can be done for patients but to diagnose and classify them. The great German diagnosticians, such as Kraepelin, came from this school of thought. Treatments were nonspecific (rest, hydrotherapy, and good nutrition). There was no reason to talk to a patient other than to make a diagnosis, since the patient's thinking was viewed as nothing more than the rambling of a lunatic whose neurons were degenerating.

Griesinger influenced Meynert, and Meynert taught Freud. After medical school, Freud underwent training in neurology and received a traveling fellowship to Charcot's clinic in France. Charcot was the leading neurologist of his time, and in his clinic, Freud witnessed something that must have been, for him, extremely remarkable. Charcot took patients with degenerative mental disorders, hypnotized them, and made the symptoms disappear. Therefore, Freud had to rethink his conception of mental illness.

Janet offered an alternate explanation. He postulated that there was a split in the mind—that certain aspects of the psyche operated unbeknownst to other aspects of the psyche. Janet believed that this property of mental functioning was constitutionally determined.

Around the same time in Vienna, Breuer was treating neurotic patients with hypnosis. Breuer told Freud about a patient, Anna O. (Bertha Pappenheim), whom he had treated with such a method, and the two began treating similar patients and writing up their cases. These cases appear in the first volume of the *Standard Edition* of Freud's work. Freud and Breuer devised a new theory of psychopathology—a "hydraulic" model in which the mind is conceived of as if it were a pressure cooker: A person encounters an upsetting event in his or her current life to which he or she is unable to react emotionally, and the memory of the event (with its concomitant feelings) is split off from consciousness. The unreleased energy, unable to be expressed, is bottled up within the person's system and emerges as a physical symptom. Freud hypnotized such patients, led them to remember the traumatic event in their current life, and then encouraged them to abreact to it. The symptom would subside. Freud found that it was not necessary to induce hypnosis because the same goal could be accomplished by having patients recline on a couch and say whatever came into their minds. Thus, he evolved a traumatogenic theory for neurosis: It was a reaction to an upsetting external event. Freud never gave up the notion of constitutional factors, but considered them to be predisposing rather than precipitating factors. For the first time, physicians had a medical reason to listen to their patients for more than a description of symptoms.

Freud was forced to revise his theory when his clinical experience led him to realize that actual traumatic events did not always precede the onset of neurosis. In fact, this clinical observation still holds today. There is a current misunderstanding of Freud's position on trauma. Some writers, such as Masson (1984) and Miller (1986), have accused Freud in particular and psychoanalysts in general of denying that real traumas are causative factors of illness. But one must remember that Freud was writing about neurosis, and now, just as then, some neurotic patients have endured trauma whereas others have not. Thus, external real trauma is not a universal factor of all neuroses.

Freud's second theory of neurosis was an intrapsychic one. In it he divided the mind into conscious, preconscious, and unconscious elements. The conscious part of the mind is that of which we are immediately aware; the preconscious contains those things that we are not aware of immediately, but that we can call to mind easily; and the dynamic unconscious is that part of the mind that is cut off from consciousness, but that continually presses for expression. The function that cuts off the unconscious from the system conscious–preconscious is called repression. When unconscious sexual impulses cross the repression barrier, they cause neurotic symptoms (as the conscious part of the mind tries to bind the unpleasure released by the impulses). This theory is known as the "topographic" model of the mind.

Using this model, Freud faced a problem that did not make sense clinically. His patients were not always conflicted by an unconscious wish on the one hand and by something conscious on the other; more often, *both* parts of the patient's conflict were unconscious. His attempt to resolve this dilemma led him to devise the structural theory of the mind described earlier—namely, dividing the mind into the id, ego, and superego functions (Sandler et al. 1973).

Differential Dynamic Diagnosis

Because many organic factors can give rise to anxiety, these must be ruled out in evaluating a patient. For guidance regarding such assessments, the reader is referred to standard texts in psychiatry, as this section deals mainly with a dynamic differential.

A useful approach is first to differentiate the symptom neuroses from the functional psychoses and the character neuroses or personality disorders, and then to differentiate the symptom neuroses from each other. To differentiate neuroses from functional psychoses and personality disorders, a number of aspects can be examined:

How do others view the patient? Vaillant once remarked that a patient with a neurosis is like someone who gets on an elevator with a pebble in his shoe—he is uncomfortable, but no one else on the elevator notices—whereas the patient with a personality disorder is like someone who enters an elevator smoking a smelly cigar—he is content, but everyone else on the elevator is uncomfortable. In other words, the person with a neurotic illness suffers in silence for the most part; it is as if the disorder is well encapsulated and hidden from the world, and the person may be seen as "normal" by others. In contrast, the patient with a personality disorder (or a functional psychoses) is disturbing and viewed by others as unusual.

How does the patient view his or her own symptoms? It is common for neurotic patients to be embarrassed by their symptoms and to view them as foreign. As a result, they often have difficulty volunteering information in the interview. A person who is embarrassed by his phobia to drive across bridges may tell the psychiatrist that he has not taken a driving vacation for years. Only later in the interview are the true symptoms revealed. This patient's attitude with regard to his symptoms is termed "ego-alien" or "ego-dystonic." Patients with a personality disorder, by contrast, are unaware of their psychopathology. It is actually lived out in relationship to others. It is as if the psychopathology were woven into the fabric of their personality. This attitude is called "ego syntonic." We can also apply that term to patients with functional psychoses. A psychotic patient who is delusional and believes that the DAR is plotting to kill her is unable to step back and view this belief as unusual—in fact, she may take measures to protect herself from the DAR. Thus, for a functionally psychotic patient, symptoms are ego-syntonic.

How accurate is the patient's perception of reality? For patients with a neurosis or a personality disorder, reality testing is intact. For patients with a functional psychosis, reality testing is impaired by delusions and/or hallucinations.

Does the patient exert appropriate control of impulses? Neurotic patients struggle with—and are conflicted over—their impulses and often appear inhibited. Impulse control may be impaired in the personality disorders (e.g., borderline and antisocial personality disorders). Impulse control can also be affected in the psychoses—for example, a psychotic patient with delusions of persecution may attack someone in order to protect him- or herself.

Does the patient have good object relations? Although patients with a neurosis are involved with others, they use the neurosis to manipulate others. For example, an agoraphobia patient might exploit her illness by insisting that her husband accompany her everywhere she goes. Personality disorder patients have disturbed object relations—it is as if the personality disorder were being acted out in their relations with others. On the other hand, psychotic patients have withdrawn from others and will isolate themselves, consumed with their delusions or hallucinations.

How are affects manifested? Depressive and anxious affects can be found in each disorder. In the neuroses, depressive and anxious affects can signal defense. Patients with a personality disorder can become depressed or anxious secondary to how others react to or disappoint them, whereas patients with a psychosis are overwhelmed with anxiety or depression and attempt to bind these affects with primitive defenses.

It is important not to base a diagnosis of a neurotic disorder solely on the presence of neurotic symptoms. A patient may have a psychosis and at the same time present with neurotic symptoms. Basing a psychodynamic diagnosis only on the presence of neurotic symptoms may cause the clinician to miss an underlying psychotic process entirely.

> Mr. W, an obese, withdrawn 23-year-old man, presented with obsessive-compulsive symptoms. He was preoccupied with a fear of dirt, bathed compulsively, and was unable to touch objects, such as door knobs, that were commonly touched by others. In fact, he carried tissues, which he wrapped around door knobs and door handles before using them. However, realizing that tissues were porous and did not provide a complete barrier from dirt, he usually would stand by a closed door, hoping someone else would open it first so that he could walk through it without touching anything.
>
> Mr. W's bathing rituals consisted of washing himself and then washing a path from the shower to his bedroom so that he would not contaminate himself in walking from his bathroom to his bedroom. He used so much water bathing that he was thrown out of a number of apartments and was reduced to swabbing himself with rubbing alcohol.
>
> Mr. W was unable to work as a musician because he could not put his instrument down during the breaks—he feared that the instrument would get dirty. His travel was restricted. He could not travel on public transportation during rush hour because he was afraid someone would bump into him and thus dirty him. He wore a heavy overcoat in public, even during the summer months, in order to protect himself from contamination. He was unable to sit on a chair in the analyst's office because he feared the chair might be dirty.
>
> Mr. W's symptoms had begun while he was taking care of his father, who was dying of rectal cancer. The patient was required to help his father with his surgical dressings. It was at this time that he began to worry about touching anything his father touched. What appeared initially in treatment as an obsessive-compulsive neurosis was really a well-organized delusional thought disorder that the patient later revealed. He believed that being contaminated by dirt would "lower his resistance." If his resistance were lowered, he could contract a virus, and he had read somewhere that viruses cause cancer. In other words, Mr. W believed that he would get cancer and die like his father.

If one follows the psychodynamic differential in this case, one finds that this patient meets the criteria of a functional psychosis rather than a symptom neurosis. For example, others viewed this man as very unusual. In addition, his symptoms were ego-syntonic: he neither found them embarrassing nor saw them as unusual. In fact, Mr. W viewed his symptoms as a completely reasonable way to avoid contamination. He had a break in reality testing—a delusion—and he had isolated himself from others.

It should be kept in mind that a patient can buy a ticket for a psychosis and at the same time buy a ticket for a neurotic symptom, but not the other way around—that is, a patient cannot buy a ticket for a neurotic disorder and at the same time buy a ticket for a psychosis.

What defense mechanism does the patient use? Vaillant's hierarchy of defenses is useful here. The patient with a neurosis uses one of the so-called neurotic defenses, such as repression, reaction formation, intellectualization, or undoing. In the personality disorders, the patient employs the so-called immature defenses, such as acting out. The psychotic patient uses the so-called narcissistic or psychotic defenses, such as denial and delusional projection (Vaillant 1977).

Within the class of neuroses, each neurotic illness can be differentiated primarily by the cluster of defenses used. In the anxiety neuroses, one sees the defense of repression, which is only partially successful. In the phobic neuroses, the cluster of defenses includes externalization, displacement, and avoidance. In hysterical neurosis–dissociative type, the defenses include repression and dissociation. In hysterical neurosis–conversion type, one sees repression, somatic displacement, and identification. The obsessive-compulsive neuroses contain the largest cluster of defenses: isolation of affect, magical thinking, undoing, reaction formation, and intellectualization. One should bear in mind that the source of the anxiety or depressive affect does not differentiate the various neuroses, since any one or combination of the calamities of childhood can trigger these affects, which in turn trigger the defenses.

How does the patient's superego function? In the neuroses, superego functions are rigid and harsh, and these patients experience great distress. In the personality disorders, the superego functions vary—they are lax in antisocial personality disorder, harsh in obsessive-compulsive disorder, and self-defeating in masochistic personality disorder. In psychotic patients, superego demands are projected and can account for delusions in which the patient believes that the police are watching him or her.

Can the patient develop a transference and an observing ego? Patients with neuroses are capable both of forming a transference in psychotherapy and of developing an observing ego to explore the transference in treatment. The ability of personality disorder patients to do so depends on the strength of their ego functions. For example, a person with a high-functioning histrionic personality disorder may be able to develop such structures, whereas a patient with a severe borderline personality disorder may quickly form a transference but initially lack the capacity to step back and examine it. Although Freud believed that psychotic patients were incapable of forming a transference, clinically this has not proven to be so. These patients can develop a very intense transference that is greatly distorted by primitive defenses; such a transference can quickly lose its "as if" quality. For example, a psychotic patient may develop a delusional transference and believe that the therapist has hypnotized him or her.

These differentiating factors mean that the choice of psychotherapy differs for each variety of the disorder. In the neuroses, insight-oriented psychotherapy is the treatment of choice. For the personality disorders, psychotherapy varies from insight-oriented to supportive, depending on the ego strength of the individual with the disorder. For the psychoses, the treatment of choice is supportive psychotherapy. Because the emphasis in this chapter is on psychodynamics, the issue of medications is not addressed here. However, the author firmly believes that medication should be used where indicated and should be combined and integrated with the psychotherapy.

Case Examples

In this section I use case material to demonstrate the psychodynamics in various neuroses. The patient material is drawn from the kinds of cases that residents and psychiatrists encounter in busy clinics or practices. These cases illustrate how an understanding of these dynamics is essential in one's approach to the patient, whether that approach is purely psychotherapeutic or combines psychotherapy and pharmacotherapy.

Anxiety Neurosis

While filling a guest staffing assignment on an inpatient unit, a resident presented the case of Ms. X, a somewhat shy 22-year-old woman who suffered from anxiety. The resident claimed that the patient's first anxiety attack erupted out of the blue. He could find nothing that precipitated it. When she experienced her first anxiety attack, she was just sitting at home.

Later in the conference, the interviewer asked the patient to reconstruct the events around her first anxiety attack. She replied that she was indeed alone at home, sitting and reading a book. He then asked her to tell him about the book. The patient said that it was a science fiction book about a giant meteor hurtling through space on a collision course with the Earth. The people on earth felt trapped and helpless to avoid destruction. When asked what was going on in her life around that time, she admitted that she had been disappointed in her marriage and was considering a separation. However, she found herself pregnant, believed herself to be unattractive, and was economically dependent on her husband. She recommitted to the marriage, but then discovered that her husband had been unfaithful, and he became abusive toward her. Could it be that the plight of the people in the novel struck a chord in her? Like them, she too felt trapped and helpless. Her own early history revealed that her father had abandoned the family when she was a youngster. She remained with her mother, who took out her own anger of being abandoned on her daughter, the patient. The patient's expressed feelings were very similar to those she was feeling at that time in her life.

The psychiatrist constructed the psychodynamics for this patient: The precipitating event was discovering the husband's extramarital affair. It is not completely clear what this event meant intrapsychically to her. One might speculate that the pregnancy and the subsequent change in her body image made her feel defective (perhaps a derivative of castration issues). At the same time she felt defective, she may have also felt unloved. The current situation is reminiscent of the earlier time in her life when she was abandoned by her father and—more importantly—stuck at home with her mother. The affect that she could repress only partially was helpless rage, which she could not direct toward her mother because she was so dependent—just as she is now dependent on her husband. The story line in the science fiction novel served as a perfect metaphor for her predicament. The content of the drive derivative was repressed, but not the unpleasure or anxiety that accompanied it.

Should medication be used in this case? Of course, if this patient requires it to reduce the extreme anxiety. But to stop at that measure would be to do a disservice to her, because it would leave her with the belief that something was wrong with her, that she was defective and unlovable, and also that she was helpless in her anger. Psychodynamic therapy can enable her to understand her predicament in terms of her past, to look at her childhood with her adult eyes, and to appreciate that her perception of herself is understandable in terms of her past experiences. She can then see that she is frozen developmentally in reacting to her husband as if he were her mother. In the transference, the patient can feel her dependency on the therapist and be unable to express angry feelings toward the therapist because she fears abandonment. The therapist uses the exploration of the transference as a tool for the patient to deal with these issues in the safe environment of treatment. Accomplishing this, she would then be able to make a decision about her marriage that was based on rational issues and not feel compelled to make choices because of her neurotic anxieties and faulty perceptions.

Hysterical Neurosis, Conversion Type

Most of the patients with this disorder are encountered in psychiatric consultations in general medical wards and clinics.

> Ms. Y, a thin, 20-year-old Filipino student nurse, was admitted to a hematology service for an anemia workup (which was negative). She fainted while walking on the medicine wards to work her shifts—a curious symptom because she does not faint at any other time nor in any other situation. Both she and her sister, also a student nurse in the same program, were admitted for graduate studies. Now that Ms. Y was ill, she could not pursue her studies, but instead would return to the Philippines and take care of here aging father, whom she adored. She seemed not in the least upset over her plight.

The psychiatrist constructed the dynamics: the drive derivative was the wish to be her father's favorite and to beat out her rival sister. This wish aroused an affect for anxiety, which was accompanied by the idea of punishment for her strivings. She employed the defense of repression because all of the thoughts and feelings were unconscious and displaced onto her body in the symptom of fainting. The symptom enabled her to express the forbidden wish (to return home and take care of her father) and at the same time to express the punishment for her competitive wishes (her fainting and inability to pursue her studies). She was unconcerned about her symptom because it was a perfect solution for her; it enabled her to have her father all to herself without fighting it out with her sister.

> Ms. Z, a 42-year-old woman who was seen on a neurosurgery ward, complained of sternal pain and numbness and tingling in the fingers of both hands. The neurosurgeon suspected a spinal mass but found nothing. It was determined that the tingling in her fingers was caused by hyperventilation. But what would account for the pain in her sternum? Ms. Z revealed an ambivalent relationship with a younger brother, who was born when she was 3 years old. Her brother had died recently, just prior to the onset of her symptoms. He had developed cancer, and much of his care had fallen to the patient. After his death, Ms. Z was afraid that she too would die, and the psychiatrist believed that this fear is what precipitated her anxiety attacks. When asked what death would be like, she replied that it would be a reunion with her dead brother. When asked to point to where she felt the pain, Ms. Z moved her hand up and down her sternum, in the midline from her throat to her abdomen. Her brother had died of cancer of the esophagus.

In this psychodynamic formulation, the precipitating event was the death of the patient's brother. The drive derivative connected to the event was the patient's own aggressive feelings, which must have been close to the surface. The affect was anxiety with an unconscious content of castration anxiety and superego punishment. The defenses were repression (since she was unaware of the content of her wishes), somatic displacement, and identification with the dead brother through her symptom.

Phobic Neurosis

> The department of surgery referred Ms. A, a frightened, 25-year-old medical student, because she was missing time from work with a number of excuses, none of which made much sense. A careful history revealed that she was phobic. Ms. A was made anxious by patients who were about to vomit. A patient in the process of vomiting did not bother her, but a patient, especially a female patient, who was about to retch—whose face was red, veins protruding, and eyes bulging—created the most intense anxiety for her. She dealt with her anxiety by avoiding such patients, but she was too embarrassed to tell anyone. Such behavior created the impression that Ms. A was irresponsible and lazy. Further history revealed that when the patient was 5 years old, her mother had become pregnant with her younger brother. The mother had suffered excessively from morning sickness, and the patient had vivid memories of her mother running to the bathroom about to vomit. These episodes filled the little girl with dread, because she believed that her mother was about to die. This belief corresponded with hostile, competitive oedipal wishes toward her mother. In her current life, the medical student was struggling with her own ambitions and wishes to enter surgery as a career.

The drive derivative here is the patient's competitive wishes, which are tantamount in her mind with something bad happening to her mother. The affect is anxiety, which was connected in her unconscious with castration fears. Her superego finds her competitive strivings unacceptable. She defends against the anxiety with displacement—that is, with the idea "It is not mother who will die, but these other women." The patient then employs the defense of avoidance to distance herself from the vomiting female patients.

The residents asked about the use of behavior therapy in cases of simple phobias, because there is a vast behavioral literature supporting the successes of such treatment in alleviating this type of symptom without apparent symptom substitution. The psychiatrist said that using behavioral treatment would have done this particular patient a disservice by staying at the level of her symptoms without exploring their deeper meanings. Doing so would also have left this patient with feelings about herself as being defective, with inhibitions around her competitive strivings, and with a specialty choice dictated more by irrational fears than by mature decision making.

Obsessive-Compulsive Neurosis

Ms. B, a very agitated woman in her mid-40s, presented with an unusual neurosis. She took sips of water in multiples of three; turned a light switch off and on in multiples of seven; and went down to the basement of her house and turned the basement light on and then off. All of this had to be accomplished before she left for work in the morning, and because it was a multiple progression, the rituals took so long that at the end of the week, she had to set her alarm an hour earlier on Friday morning. Ms. B was free of the compulsions on the weekend and reported no compulsive rituals at work.

(As an aside, there are currently biological theories for obsessive-compulsive disorder. One wonders what biological theory would explain the selectivity of this patient's weekday neurosis.)

To continue with Ms. B's story, at the time she was first seen, she lived with her aging mother, who was developing symptoms of congestive heart failure. The patient was the one chosen in her large Italian-American family to remain single and stay at home to take care of her parents. Ms. B did this without protest, but her association belied her superficially altruistic position: She spoke with some regret of missed opportunities to have a family of her own.

Also around this time, she began a clandestine affair with a married man in the stairwells of the office building in which she worked. Developmentally, Ms. B was always the good girl who did whatever she was told and never complained. Her siblings found her "goody-goody" attitude irritating at times. The patient developed hyperthyroidism at the beginning of adolescence, and she carried wet tissues with her that she would suck on in a ritualistic manner. Earlier, at the age of 6, she had two memories: one in which she awoke in her bed with her nightgown pulled up and discovered her father standing over her, and another in which she discovered her father having intercourse with her aunt. She divulged these two events to no one. Prior to these events, she was an energetic, mischievous child, but afterward she grew quiet, pensive, and restrained in her behavior.

Ms. B lived her life keeping these secrets from her mother and behaving in such a way as to not call any adverse attention to herself. Following her father's death when she was in her 20s, she devoted herself to her mother's care, much to the relief of her brother and sister, who pursued their own interests, married, and had children.

The psychiatrist constructed the following psychodynamics: The drive derivative was Ms. B's wish that her mother would die and free her to pursue a more personal relationship with the man at work. This wish caused her anxiety, especially now that her mother's heart had begun to fail. Her anxiety was associated with her fear of punishment for her sexual wishes toward her own father, which were stimulated by her father's sexual misconduct, and the childhood secrets kept these feelings very much alive in her own mind. Her death wishes toward her mother paralleled similar wishes she had had when she was 6. The real trauma at age 6 resulted in the dramatic personality change at that time from a "naughty" girl to a "too-good-to-be-true" girl.

She defended against her current anxiety with reaction formation—that is, by being overly solicitous toward her mother. The patient also used the compulsions as if they were magical rituals to protect her mother while the patient was away at work. The ritual contains an expression of the drive (i.e., to kill the mother by turning off the light, and the undoing of that wish by turning the light on). Her choice of numbers and the sips of water seemed to be a way of alleviating her anxiety that carried over from behavior used to deal with the anxiety associated with her adolescent hyperthyroidism.

Understanding the patient's rituals as protecting her mother helps one to appreciate why she did not need them on the weekend, since she could be with her mother then. Also, on the weekend the patient did not meet with her lover, a man associated in her mind with her father.

Her treatment took place years before the advent of the serotonergic agents that are being used now to treat obsessive-compulsive disorders. Could they have been used to treat this patient if they were available then? Yes—but not without integrating them with psychodynamic psychotherapy, because it was only with a psychodynamic understanding that this patient was able to unburden herself of the secrets that she had held for 40 years. Through her psychotherapy, she was able to understand how her "secrets" pervaded her life, changed her personality, and constricted her. Most importantly, her work in therapy gave her an understanding of the uncontrollable compulsive behavior that made her believe she was losing her mind.

Ms. B's therapy lasted about 4 years. Initially, she was reluctant to look for an intrapsychic cause for her illness, but the fact that her compulsions did not occur on the weekends piqued her curiosity. This observation prompted her to explore her deeply ambivalent relationship with her mother. As her (previously defended against) resentment emerged, she developed more conscious guilt. The psychiatrist then directed his efforts toward lessening the guilt by exploring its developmental roots.

(In a once-per-week psychotherapy, one does not work in such a focused way with the transference as in a psychoanalysis. Rather, much of the work is done by examining the displacement of the transference in the patient's external life.)

So it was for Ms. B. Although therapist and patient had many examples of guilt-ridden relationships with peers to work through, they also saw derivatives of these relationships in the transference. She was always prompt for her appointments and paid her bill a month in advance. As for Ms. B's relationship with her father, patient and therapist were able to work through and achieve an understanding of her relationship with the unavailable married man at work. However, she did develop a symptom in the therapy that enabled her to better appreciate her early relationship with her father. She lost control of her right hand and arm and began to flail as if fighting off an attacker. This symptom was a reexperiencing in the session of Ms. B's memory of trying to protect herself when she discovered her father standing over her bed.

Some years after treatment had successfully ended, Ms. B returned. Her mother had died and she was worried that she would become severely depressed. It did not happen. During a period of normal bereavement, the psychiatrist saw Ms. B in brief supportive therapy. Although the patient missed her mother, she was at peace with herself. She had new energy to devote to her many nieces and nephews. Ms. B's relationship with her family and peers was far less controlling, and her relationship with the man at work ended when it became clear that he was not willing to leave his wife to marry her. The obsessive-compulsive symptoms did not return.

Summary

In each of the case studies presented above, the patient's neurotic symptoms may be understood as consisting of 1) a drive derivative—a wish that derives from each patients' unique experience, 2) an unpleasurable affect connected to a calamity of childhood, 3) defenses, and 4) superego injunctions. The question of medication was raised in two of these cases, and I concluded that medication alone could not have freed these patients from their pasts. However, the opposite question is just as valid—that is, is it fair to understand a patient's dynamics yet prolong his or her suffering? Where indicated, combined approaches are the treatment of choice, and in other cases, psychotherapy alone is preferable.

For Further Study

Frosch J: The neuroses, in Psychodynamic Psychiatry: Theory and Practice. Madison, CT, International Universities Press, 1990, pp 293–359

Gabbard G: Anxiety disorders, in Psychodynamic Psychiatry in Clinical Practice. Washington DC, American Psychiatric Press, 1990, pp 199–226

References

Brenner C: The calamities of childhood, in The Mind in Conflict. New York, International Universities Press, 1982, pp 93–108

Freud S: Analysis of a phobia in a five year old boy (1909), in The Standard Edition of the Complete Psychological Works of Sigmund Freud, Vol 10. Translated and edited by Strachey J. London, Hogarth Press, 1955, pp 1–149

Kaplan HI, Sadock BJ: Historical and theoretical trends in psychiatry, in Modern Synopsis of the Comprehensive Textbook of Psychiatry, 3rd Edition. Edited by Kaplan HI, Sadock BJ. Baltimore, MD, Williams & Wilkins, 1981, pp 1–12

Masson JM: The Assault on Truth. New York, Farrar, Strauss & Giroux, 1984

Miller A: Thou Shalt Not Be Aware. New York, New American Library, 1986

Sandler J, Dare C, Holder A: The Patient and the Analyst: The Basis of the Psychoanalytic Process. New York, International Universities Press, 1973, pp 11–20

Vaillant G: Adaptive ego mechanisms: a hierarchy, in Adaptation to Life. Boston, MA, Little, Brown, 1977, pp 75–90

Chapter 14

The Depressed Patient

David S. Werman, M.D.

Current Psychodynamic Perspectives

The impressive efficacy of psychotropic medication in relieving the symptoms of depression has had the unfortunate effect of contributing to a trend in which the focus on symptom relief often leads to a neglect of the inner turmoil of the depressed patient. As a consequence, the importance of underlying factors that may have played a part in precipitating the depression may be overlooked. Furthermore, when psychiatrists do explore possible precipitants, these are often limited to such external events as the loss of a job or the death of a spouse, while critical symbolic or fantasied matters are ignored. Not only is the depressive illness itself often regarded as unrelated to the patient's psychological life, past as well as present, but the possibility that the patient may be suffering from intense conflicts, a devalued sense of self, destructive or unfulfilling relationships, and/or unrelenting misery may not be entertained. The current catchphrase "chemical imbalance" convinces both the patient and the psychiatrist that the patient is little more than a collection of depressive symptoms, and that the only interventions of therapeutic value are those that aim at correcting the "imbalance."

There is no longer any need to stress that when antidepressant medication is indicated, it should be prescribed. For many severely depressed patients, psychotherapy only becomes feasible when the symptoms are alleviated with medication. Indeed, there is no inherent conflict between the use of somatic treatments and psychotherapy. The indications for the former are relatively clear; in contrast, those for the latter are less so because they depend on a careful psychodynamic—and therapeutic—evaluation of the patient, a procedure that is difficult to carry out when the patient is in a state of psychomotor retardation or highly agitated. Out of necessity, such an assessment can only be done effectively when the patient has begun to improve. But during this early phase, before the patient's full cooperation can be enlisted, family members or others who are closely associated with the patient should be called upon to provide information relating to the patient's illness.

The immediate focus in the evaluation of the depressed patient is to establish a diagnosis according to DSM criteria so that if somatic treatment is to be instituted, it can be begun promptly and appropriately. The psychiatrist then progressively assesses the patient and begins to develop a psychodynamic formulation from such data as can be obtained. This assessment includes factors that may have had a precipitating role in the patient's illness as well as the patient's current life situation, significant past history, important recent and past losses, and the nature of the patient's relationships. At the same time, the psychiatrist attempts to evaluate whether the patient needs and can benefit from some form of psychotherapy. If it is indicated, a determination is made as to the direction of therapy: toward either the supportive or the insight-oriented end of the psychotherapeutic spectrum. (It should be understood, in this context, that the concepts of supportive and insight-oriented psychotherapy are not two totally distinct modalities of treatment; rather, they are on a continuum—they may blend, overlap, and change at any time, depending on the patient's total psychological status.)

If the patient is to be hospitalized, it is more than likely that the stay will be limited to a few weeks. During this time, the psychiatrist has the opportunity of establishing rapport with the patient, attempting to understand the onset of the patient's depression, learning something about the patient's life, and beginning to plan for the patient's discharge and subsequent outpatient treatment. If the patient has been seen initially as an outpatient, the psychiatrist may progressively embark on the modality of psychotherapy he or she has considered indicated.

Historical Review

Psychiatrists have long discussed the relative weights of heredity and experience in the etiology of depression. Although there are important scientific implications in these discussions, what is paramount for the clinician is that certain individuals seem to have a vulnerability to depression. Particularly striking is the frequency with which one discovers early life experiences that seem to propitiate the illness. Over the past 75 years, psychoanalysts have contributed a number of seminal concepts that serve to illuminate the long-range repercussions of previous—and usually, but not exclusively, early life—experiences on the onset of later depressive illness. These concepts provide the clinician with valuable guideposts in his or her attempts to work with depressed patients. A description of some of the most prominent of these contributions follows.

Freud (1917/1957), like Abraham (1911/1968) before him, was struck by the clinical similarities between depression ("melancholia") and mourning, with one critical difference: unlike the grief-stricken individual, the depressed patient experiences "a disturbance of self-regard" characterized by self-reproaches,-

self-devaluation, and an expectation of punishment. In contrast, mourning is typically a reaction to the death or loss of a loved one, but may also be due to the "loss of some abstraction which has taken the place of one, such as one's country, liberty, and ideal and so on" (p. 243). Although depression may follow the actual loss of a loved person, it is more likely to be a response to the loss of *the love* of a beloved person, even though the depressed subject may not be conscious of the loss. The subjective experience of bereaved individuals is of a world that has become "poor and empty"; by contrast, depressed individuals feel as if they themselves have become "poor and empty." Freud conceptualized the depressive process as originating from a significant disappointment with a loved person from whom one's love has been detached. At that point, rather than being displaced onto another person, the disappointment is brought into the individual's psyche, where it serves to set up an identification with the abandoning object. In this way, the experience of the loss of the object becomes a sense of "ego loss"—that is, of a loss of some part of oneself, leading to feelings of impoverishment and devaluation.

Freud believed that this process required two conditions: first, a strong emotional investment in the beloved object, and second, the fragility of that investment, in that the original love for the object is largely based on narcissistic, self-serving needs. Such circumstances would result in an intensely ambivalent love/hate relationship with the object. The identification with the lost object substitutes for the object's love. Freud also noted that depression characteristically extends beyond the loss of a loved one to include all those people and situations in which one has felt "slighted, neglected, or disappointed," leading to more generalized mixed feelings of love and hate. Although Freud understood the foregoing developments as the consequences of life experiences, he was careful not to dismiss the possible role of constitutional factors. In summary, Freud's concept of depression rests on three factors: 1) loss of an object or the object's love; 2) ambivalent feelings toward the object; and 3) displacement of feelings from the object onto oneself.

Abraham (1911/1968) observed that in contrast to the anticipation of something frightening, characteristic of anxiety states, depression relates to one's reaction to a feared event that has already occurred. In this state, the patient experiences him- or herself as incapable of being either loved or loving and despairs of both the present and the future. Abraham (1924/1968) noted that in all of his depressed patients, the depression proceeded from an attitude of hate that paralyzed the patient's ability to love. Empirically, he saw depression as precipitated by a disappointment in love, such as the loss, in one way or another, of the beloved. This particular mode of reacting, he observed, represents a "repetition of an original infantile traumatic experience" (p. 456). Additionally, Abraham hypothesized a constitutional factor that was less implicated in depressive illness as such than manifested in a disposition toward an accentuation of orality. This factor, in turn, tends toward the development of intense oral needs, with a fixation at the oral level of development, and more or less inevitable frustrations and disappointments in the infant's first love relationship. Depression occurring in later life would represent a repetition of the earlier disappointments, now precipitated by events whose resonance is similar to that of the earlier experiences.

Melanie Klein (1935/1948) postulated that very early in life, the infant introjects (takes in) both the good and the bad aspects of the mother—aspects which in fact represent the infant's own loving and aggressive impulses. At some point the infant becomes aware of its own aggressive impulses, and this awareness leads to a "depressive fear" that those impulses may lead to the loss of the mother.

The advent of ego psychology gave rise to several new hypotheses. Bibring (1953) conceptualized depression as an affective state that is operative in all forms of depressive illness. The fundamental issue was an individual's perception of him- or herself as falling significantly short of earlier established deals of being loving, lovable, and competent. This belief leads to an experience of helplessness and powerlessness.

Zetzel (1965/1970) echoed Bibring's views but distinguished 1) depression as a reactive symptom, 2) depression as a syndrome of depressive illness, and 3) depression as a "depressive character structure," a concept that is currently being advanced by some psychiatrists. Zetzel also described certain individuals who seem to be unable to "bear depression."

Bibring's conceptualization of depression was faulted by Jacobson (1971), who was critical of Bibring's neglect of aggression. Jacobson understood depression as "the outcome of an aggressive conflict, caused by a lack of understanding and acceptance by the mother that reduces the child's self-esteem" (p. 180). She argued for a multifactorial approach that would encompass a variety of constitutional, somatic, and psychological factors. Most recently, Brenner (1991) stressed the view that depression is an affect, not an illness per se. Loss of the love of the loved object, loss of the object, castration, and (after superego development) punishment are the four major "calamities" that may lead to depression. Depressive affect, Brenner noted, may accompany any psychic conflict; what varies is its role in the resulting "compromise formation."

From this brief review of some of the significant psychoanalytic contributions to the understanding of depression, some general conclusions can be drawn:

1. There are probably constitutional precursors to depressive illness.
2. Early, overwhelming experiences seem to become fixed and act as a nidus for later depressive illness.
3. These experiences typically entail some form of loss—for example, loss of a loved object; loss of the love of that object; a sense of bodily harm, mutilation, or castration; or loss of one's sense of competency or ability to love and be loved.
4. Depressive illness is probably precipitated by events—real, symbolic, or fantasied—that resonate with the initial overwhelming experiences.

Differential Dynamic Diagnosis

These broad concepts can provide the psychiatrist with a road map to assist in understanding the psychodynamics of any patient's depressive illness. However, they can serve only as guidelines to help in exploring the sources and meanings of the illness. Indeed, in the initial assessment of the depressed patient, it is frequently difficult, if not impossible, to reach an understanding of the psychogenesis or psychodynamics of the patient's illness; the patient's cooperation may be markedly impeded by severe depressive symptoms and can only be enlisted progressively as the symptoms begin to diminish following antidepressant medication or electroconvulsive therapy (ECT). But when the patient becomes able to participate in the interview, the psychiatrist may begin to learn something about what lies behind the depressive symptomatology, as well as the immediate antecedents to the depression. The evaluation can then move from a diagnostic assessment toward a "therapeutic" one.

It is through the therapeutic evaluation that the psychiatrist determines the modality of psychotherapy that will be most beneficial for a given patient. From a psychodynamic perspective, the treatment spectrum ranges from largely supportive therapy, through mixed and shifting forms of supportive and insight-oriented treatment, to largely insight-oriented therapy, and finally to psychoanalysis. (Implied in the foregoing is the concept that there is a continuum along which these modalities lie—a concept about which there is no unanimity.) It should be understood that these modalities typically do not exist in "pure culture," but often represent admixtures that may change over time; in addition, elements of one modality may briefly appear during a treatment with another.

Patients for whom insight-oriented psychotherapy is indicated tend to demonstrate most of the following characteristics, to at least a moderate extent:

1. A motivation to understand themselves, rather than a wish only to be relieved of their depressive symptoms.
2. An ability to be introspective, to be curious about their behavior, to recognize that the principal source of their psychological difficulties is within themselves, and, accordingly, to see that to a significant extent they are the stewards of their psychological existence and the agents of such psychological changes as they would like to have take place.
3. A minimal use of primitive and highly maladaptive defense measures, such as projection, splitting, and denial, and a more frequent use of several "higher" level defenses, such as repression, isolation, reaction formation, intellectualization, and rationalization.
4. The ability to restrain drive impulses for immediate gratification of sexual or aggressive desires, to delay such imperative demands, and to permit thought, considered as trial action—time to evaluate the behavior anticipated.
5. The ability to tolerate moderate levels of sadness, anxiety, frustration, and other painful emotions.

6. The capacity to maintain mental representations of others with some degree of equilibrium and constancy (i.e., good object relations).
7. The ability to differentiate reality from fantasy, and possession of a strong sense of reality.
8. A life history that supports the ability to sublimate drive impulses and intense affects through appropriate activities such as work and play.

The diagnostic and therapeutic evaluation, whether more or less completed during the first few interviews or occurring over the course of the patient's progressive recovery from his or her depressive illness, should enable the psychiatrist to determine 1) whether or not there are significant conflicts or other psychological disturbances that are ego-alien to the patient, and 2) whether or not these difficulties can be helped by psychotherapy. If the answers to these two questions are generally positive, the psychiatrist should then determine which modality of psychotherapy is indicated at that time: either a treatment that tends largely toward the supportive end of the spectrum or one that is mostly directed toward the insight-oriented end. Such decisions should be regarded as tentative because after an early phase of treatment, an initial decision may prove to have been incorrect or inexact. Additionally, over a period of time, a patient in insight-oriented psychotherapy may reveal that he or she is too fragile for such work; or, to the contrary, a patient in supportive treatment may reveal him- or herself as capable of doing some exploratory work.

The essential issue is that regardless of the severity of the depression, all depressed patients should be fully evaluated to determine whether their illness has an identifiable psychodynamic basis and whether they are disturbed by significant conflicts. Such an assessment may likewise reveal noteworthy developmental deficits for which supportive psychotherapy may also be indicated. Neglecting to explore these aspects of the depressed patient's mental life in effect deprives the patient of what could prove to be a meaningful therapeutic experience with wide-ranging effects on his or her future. Moreover, by not exploring these dynamic and developmental areas, the psychiatrist forgoes a potentially enriching and gratifying professional experience.

Case Examples

The following vignettes illustrate some of the more frequent clinical situations encountered in work with depressed patients:

Case 1

Mr. C, a 52-year-old married man who owned a small retail business, was referred to the hospital for evaluation for ECT. His chief complaint on admission was that he did not "feel that life is worth living." In his first interview, he was tearful and showed slight psychomotor retardation. He reported early morning awakening, decreased appetite with a weight loss of 5 pounds, and a reluctance to be with people. His sexual drive, he said, was unchanged.

Mr. C dated his present illness to a time, about 4 years before his admission, when he began to feel sad and was no longer able to enjoy his work and leisure activities—especially fly fishing, his cherished hobby. About 4 months before entering the hospital, these sad feelings became more intense and he began to have fantasies of killing himself by carbon monoxide poisoning in order to put his suffering to an end. Two months later, he actually headed toward his garage to carry out a suicidal plan; instead, he managed to call his doctor. During the 6 months before his hospital admission, he had been treated with various antidepressants; at the time he attempted to commit suicide, he had been feeling slightly less depressed, with more energy than previously.

The history obtained by the admitting resident noted that Mr. C's father had died 5 years earlier—that is, about 1 year before the beginning of Mr. C's present illness. Mr. C described his father as a caring but tightly controlling man whom the patient had found virtually impossible to please. In contrast, he described his mother as a "warm and fun-loving person," but she was often unavailable to him because of bouts of depression and heavy drinking.

Both Mr. C and his wife regarded their marriage as generally successful except that, like his mother, Mrs. C had for several years been a binge drinker. Mr. C also admitted that he was disappointed in their three grown children, and he was particularly in conflict with the youngest son, who had dropped out of school and seemed unable or unwilling to hold down a job. Their arguments had been bitter and painful, and had resulted in the son's going off to the West Coast and refusing to communicate with his parents.

Mr. C was evaluated for ECT, but in light of his recent improvement on medication, it was decided that he should continue on the same regimen but at a slightly higher dose. When the prospect of psychotherapy was introduced, he expressed some curiosity about it and was especially interested in the possibility that therapy might prevent a recurrence of depression. However, he was somewhat skeptical because his previous visits to his psychiatrist had consisted chiefly in the doctor's inquiring about the status of his depressive symptoms and the presence of side effects from the antidepressant medication.

During his hospital interviews, Mr. C showed some ability to examine his thoughts and feelings. His principal defenses were isolation and intellectualization, he had no history of significant impulsive behavior, and he described several pleasurable activities that suggested some well-developed sublimatory resources. When it was pointed out to him that after his father's death, he seemed to have begun to assume his father's controlling manner, Mr. C expressed surprised and said that he would like to talk some more about that.

With the agreement of his psychiatrist, it was decided that Mr. C would be referred to another psychiatrist for psychotherapy, but that he would continue to see his original psychiatrist to monitor his medication. It was agreed that Mr. C would benefit from a form of psychotherapy that would permit him, at the least, to develop a greater understanding of his behavior and his feelings.

Having one doctor manage medication and another conduct psychotherapy is generally regarded as an optimal arrangement, albeit one that is not often possible. The advantage in such an arrangement is that it permits the psychotherapist to maintain a more "neutral," less directive posture with a patient.

Furthermore, the giving of medication can in and of itself have a variety of psychological meanings; for example, it may be seen as nurturing and caring or as controlling and parental). Whenever a patient in psychotherapy receives medication, it can be useful to explore with the patient the meanings of the medication for him or her.

To his psychotherapist's surprise, Mr. C proved to be much more comfortable in insight-oriented psychotherapy than had been expected. The major resistance encountered early in treatment was his desire to please his doctor. This reaction formation apparently had developed in the patient's childhood and youth as a defense against his rage at his father's constant attempts to control his life. Later on, it served him well in his marriage and in his retail business, where he tried to please even his most demanding customers.

Underneath his usually affable and compliant manner lay a long-smoldering resentment toward his father, and also toward his mother for her drinking and her failure—or inability—to protect him from his father.

Equally hidden from awareness was Mr. C's sense that he had been cheated out of a joyous and normal childhood. When he found himself in conflict with his own children, he was aghast at the extent of his outrage against them, and in therapy began to recognize how he had identified with his father's behavior. This behavior was hateful to him and resulted in a conflict from which he was unable to extricate himself.

His father's death 5 years prior to the onset of his present illness had had a profound impact on him when he realized that the recognition he had yearned for from his father was now irrevocably unattainable. Mr. C slowly and painfully came to understand that his self-esteem had to come chiefly from himself, although he was aware of the significant validation he received from his wife. After 2 years of psychotherapy, Mr. C felt he had reached a plateau and decided to end treatment. The termination phase revealed that he had formed a deep attachment to his doctor, whom he had unconsciously experienced as the loving father of whom he had been deprived, and thus, his feeling in therapy of being accepted and found to be worthy seemed, to some useful extent, to have been internalized. His relationships with his children were only slightly improved, but Mr. C was hopeful that he would be able to develop greater rapport with them.

Case 2

Ms. D, a 34-year-old married woman with two children, was referred to a psychiatrist by her family doctor. She had been experiencing progressive weakness and loss of energy. A careful history and physical examination revealed no organic basis for her symptoms. Previously a meticulous housekeeper, she now slept late, neglected her children and household chores, and increasingly avoided her friends and outside activities. Her appetite was sufficiently poor that she had lost 25 pounds over the previous 4 months.

Additionally, there were other vegetative symptoms, such as early morning awakening, as well as a complete loss of interest in activities.

Her psychiatrist diagnosed a major depression and prescribed a tricyclic antidepressant. After 5 weeks, most of Ms. D's symptoms had disappeared, and she stated that she was feeling almost "back to [her] old self." Her doctor attempted to explore the possible precipitants of Ms. D's depression, but she was neither able to provide him with relevant information nor interested in pursuing the matter further now that she was feeling well. Her psychiatrist continued to see her weekly for brief visits, chiefly to monitor her medication. After 3 months, she called and said that since she "felt fine," she could see no reason to continue her regular visits, and that her family doctor would manage her medication. The psychiatrist encouraged Ms. D to return for at least one more visit, but she declined.

Ms. D showed both a lack of motivation to look beyond her immediate symptoms and an inability to be introspective. Her only goal was to free herself from the pain of her depressive symptoms, and she regarded exploratory psychotherapy as intrusive.

Case 3

Ms. E, a 35-year-old married woman, was referred for evaluation because of repeated episodes of depression over the previous 5 years. During that time, she had been hospitalized twice following attempts to commit suicide, and on both occasions she had received a full course of ECT. As an outpatient, she had been receiving antidepressant medication, and therapy on an irregular basis, which seems to have been in the nature of counseling.

Ms. E's first depression had followed her infatuation with a physician who, with his wife, were close friends of Ms. E and her husband; the two couples had become friendly some years earlier, when the physician had been Ms. E's obstetrician. When Ms. E first manifested serious symptoms of depression, she went to this doctor, who began to treat her with antidepressant medication. When the patient avowed her love for him, he revealed that he was in love with her, but that since they both were married, it was not possible for them to become lovers. When Ms. E pressed her suit, the doctor referred her to a psychiatrist. Feeling both abandoned and painfully guilty, Ms. E then made her first suicide attempt.

Growing up as an only child in an extremely religious home where sin and punishment were frequently spoken about, she felt guilty whenever she had any aggressive or sexual thoughts or fantasies. Ms. E described her father as a decent but reserved man with whom she had never managed to establish any closeness. Seeking to avoid being under his wife's thumb, he tried to stay out of the house as much as possible.

Ms. E had had her first sexual relationship shortly after beginning college, and felt that she had sinned. Discovering that she was pregnant, she and her boyfriend decided to get married. Although his parents were supportive of the young couple,

Ms. E's mother never lost an occasion to remind her daughter of the premarital pregnancy.

Ms. E was not hospitalized after her initial visit but was advised to continue taking the medication she had been prescribed, though at a somewhat higher dose. She expressed a strong wish to "finally get rid of" her depressive episodes, and having heard about psychoanalysis from a relative, she thought she should try it since she had tried everything else. Accordingly, she was evaluated for analytic treatment and found to be strongly motivated and reasonably self-reflective. Questions were raised about her two suicidal attempts, but these were the only impulsive acts of significance in her history. Although she showed only a moderate ability to tolerate psychological distress, she was a thoughtful and generally energetic person who was enterprising and creative when not depressed.

Her analysis, carried out four times a week for 4½ years, was regarded by both the patient and her analyst as successful. Early in treatment, her oedipal conflict, appearing in derivative forms, began to be recognized as a central issue in Ms. E's psychological life. Her strong libidinal desires gave rise to prominent guilt feelings that were assuaged by self-inflicted punishment. Her guilt feelings usually led to depressive moods, as she saw herself as a "sinner," equating her fantasies with actual behavior.

This view of herself as a bad and unworthy person extended into many areas of her life in which she felt inadequate and incompetent. Even banal pleasurable activities such as eating gave rise to guilty and depressive feelings.

Through a series of externalizations and displacements, Ms. E frequently found herself envious and resentful of other people whom she perceived as able to "have their cake and eat it too." These feelings were also displaced onto her analyst in an intense transference. Through an extended process of exploration of this reaction, Ms. E began to understand much of her neurotic behavior, and struggled to integrate this understanding into her daily life.

Ms. E returned for follow-up visits about once a year for the next 4 or 5 years, and reported that although she still experienced episodes of depression, they were much less frequent, less severe, and of shorter duration than before treatment. She also said that she was generally able to understand what had precipitated these episodes, and found that she was able to tolerate them and did not think of suicide at those times. She had also been able to engage in valuable community activities that provided her with an excellent form of sublimation. Despite her previous contacts with psychiatrists, apparently no one had ever attempted to establish a psychodynamic formulation of Ms. E's problems and conflicts—in particular, those relating to aggression and sexuality—but had focused only on her depressive illness.

Case 4

Ms. F, a 22-year-old single woman, was brought to the psychiatric outpatient clinic by her mother after she had, once again, made several superficial cuts on her wrists. Since puberty, Ms. F had had frequent brief depressive episodes, typically following the breakup of a relationship. During these episodes, which usually lasted 6–8 weeks, she cried, locked herself in her room, and refused to eat. When the depressive episode abated, she promptly attached herself to another man with whom yet another exploitative relationship developed.

Ms. F grew up in a chaotic home in which her alcoholic father was verbally and occasionally physically abusive of his wife and their three children. There was some suspicion that Ms. F had been sexually abused by her father, but she had no memory of anything like that having happened. When the patient was 9 years old, her father died and her mother proceeded to have a series of lovers. Ms. F herself had her first sexual relationship when she was 13. She was regarded as an indifferent, although fairly intelligent student, and dropped out of high school when she was 16. She then held, for 3 or 4 months at a time, a number of relatively unskilled jobs. From time to time, she took various street drugs, and about once a month she drank enough to pass out.

The initial assessment led to diagnoses of dysthymia and borderline personality disorder, for which Ms. F fulfilled most of the DSM-III-R (American Psychiatric Association 1987) criteria. Especially prominent was her use of such primitive defenses as denial, splitting, projection, and externalization. She possessed little insight into her behavior and disavowed any responsibility for the difficulties in which she found herself. Nevertheless, she was experiencing considerable pain, and the resident following her believed that supportive psychotherapy was indicated to shore up her need for soothing, to bring home to her a keener sense of reality in regard to her self-destructive relationships, to assist her in controlling the dangerous behavior she engaged in, and to help her deal with everyday problems. Supportive work with patients such as Ms. F sometimes evolves to a point where they become able to engage in a somewhat more exploratory therapeutic process, and useful insight work may then be carried out. Ms. F's tendency to deal with stress by acting out in some way or another unfortunately became the mode with which she dealt with the potential stress of psychotherapy, and so was unable to avail herself of it; after several months, she stopped coming.

About 8 months later, Ms. F returned to the clinic of her own accord and asked to see the resident who had treated her previously. When told that she was no longer working in the clinic, having finished her residency, she refused to see anyone else and walked out.

Case 5

Mr. G, a 42-year-old computer programmer, was admitted to an inpatient psychiatric unit with the diagnosis of major depression. His wife had brought him to their family doctor because of Mr. G's repeated statements that he intended to take his life. A voluntary commitment was effected, despite some initial protests by the patient.

On admission, Mr. G was moderately agitated, was uncooperative in the early interviews, and expressed paranoid views about the staff. Therefore, all the information was at first provided by Mrs. G. She said that she had no idea as to what might have precipitated Mr. G's depression, the first such episode she had observed since their marriage some 15 years earlier. She stated that their marriage was reasonably satisfactory, that their sexual relationship was mutually gratifying, that Mr. G enjoyed his work and felt he was fairly paid, and that the couple's relationship with their two teenage daughters was excellent. The information Mrs. G supplied on her husband's family background was limited to a few facts: Mr. G had a brother, 1 year younger than himself, with whom he had always gotten along well, aside from the usual brotherly rivalry. Mr. G's parents had been dead for 7 and 10 years and his contacts with his brother, who lived in the Southwest, were limited to annual visits by both families and occasional phone calls on holidays and birthdays.

After an appropriate evaluation, Mr. G was begun on a course of ECT, to which he responded well. He underwent 12 treatments and was discharged from the hospital virtually free of depressive symptoms. During his hospitalization, Mr. G began to recover and became more responsive and articulate. The resident who had been seeing him twice a week had primarily focused on the status of Mr. G's symptomatology, assessing its progressive abatement. Toward the end of Mr. G's hospital stay, he asked the resident if he could discuss some "personal" things with him. When encouraged to do so, he revealed that he had been having a love affair with a woman who worked alongside him in his office. From the outset of the relationship, he had felt intensely guilty but had not been able to discuss it with anyone. About 4 months before his admission to the hospital, his lover began to urge Mr. G to divorce his wife and marry her. He felt trapped, unable either to abandon his wife or to give up his lover. He was unable to stand the anger of the latter and dreaded a confrontation with the former, which he knew would cause both of them considerable distress. He was also unable to tolerate the idea that his wife might throw him out of the house.

He related a lifelong history of anger—bordering on hatred—toward his brother and his parents. His brother had been a sickly child and, accordingly, had received considerable attention from their parents. Moreover, they had spent a great deal of money on medical and rehabilitation services for this boy, which had had significant material and psychological repercussions for Mr. G. For example, he had had to attend a state university rather than the Ivy League school to which he had been admitted. Growing up, he had kept his anger and resentment to himself, and had sought his parents' favor by being compliant and, as he said, by being a "straight arrow."

Mr. G's current love affair was the first time in his life that he had done anything that was "really wrong," and it reverberated with the guilt feelings he had harbored because of the hostile fantasies he had earlier entertained about his parents and brother.

Mr. G said that he felt a great need to understand why and how he had gotten himself into such a "mess." He worried about how, if ever, he could extricate himself from it, and was troubled at the thought that his depression might recur, because his problems were still unresolved. Although not suicidal, he was afraid that the earlier urge to take his life might recur. He felt that he had to get his life in order so that he could develop a better relationship with his children.

At the time of his discharge, Mr. G was referred to a psychiatrist to begin psychotherapy. The hospital stay and the ECT had been successful in treating his symptoms, but all of his conflicts, character difficulties, and current life problems remained. The course of ECT had enabled him to emerge from his depression and permitted him to undertake psychotherapy, which held out at least the possibility of steps toward increased maturity and relative freedom from his disabling neurotic conflicts.

Summary

The foregoing clinical vignettes suggest the range of situations that the clinician may encounter in working with depressed patients. As the case of Ms. F illustrates, depression can accompany any psychiatric diagnosis; similarly, the underlying psychodynamic configurations relating to depression are widely varied. Consequently, optimal management of the depressed patient requires a thorough diagnostic and psychodynamic evaluation. The patient, as a complex human being, can too easily be lost behind his or her depressive symptomatology and emerge from a somatic treatment relatively free from symptoms but still mired down in the very psychological conflicts that may have been influential in the occurrence of the depression.

Not all depressed patients can benefit from psychotherapy, and not all who may be helped by such treatment are prepared to undertake it. But it is the psychiatrist's obligation to explore these issues; to do less is to deprive the patient of the optimal help psychiatry can offer.

For Further Study

Jackson SW: Melancholia and Depression: From Hippocratic Times to Modern Times. New Haven, CT, Yale University Press, 1900

Jacobson E: Transference problems in depressives, in Depression: Studies of Normal, Neurotic and Psychotic Conditions. Edited by Jacobson E. New York, International Universities Press, 1971, pp 284–301

Klein M: Mourning and its relation to manic-depressive states (1940), in Love, Guilt and Reparation and Other Works, 1921–1925. New York, Free Press, 1975, pp 344–369

Leff MJ, Roatch JF, Bunney WE: Environmental factors preceding the onset of severe depressions. Psychiatry 33:293–311, 1970

Maltsberger JT, Buie DH: Countertransference hate in the treatment of suicidal patients. Arch Gen Psychiatry 30:625–633, 1974

Perry SW: Combining antidepressants and psychotherapy: rationale and strategies. J Clin Psychiatry 51 (no. 1, suppl):16–20, 1990

Schwartz L: Case report: normalization of dexamethasone suppression test associated with social support system improvement. Psychiatr J Univ Ottawa 9:45–46, 1984

Stone L: Psychoanalytic observations on the pathology of depressive illness: selected spheres of ambiguity or disagreement. J Am Psychoanal Assoc 34:329–362, 1986

Wolpert EA: On the nature of manic-depressive illness, in The Course of Life: Psychoanalytic Contributions Toward Understanding Personality Development, Vol 3: Adulthood and the Aging Process. Edited by Greenspan SI, Pollock GH. Adelphi, MD, National Institute of Mental Health (DHHS Publ No ADM-81-1000), 1981, pp 443–451

References

Abraham K: Notes on the psycho-analytical investigation and treatment of manic depressive insanity and allied conditions (1911), in Selected Papers. London, Hogarth Press, 1968, pp 137–156

Abraham K: A short history of the development of the libido, viewed in the light of mental disorders (1924), in Selected Papers. London, Hogarth Press, 1968, pp 418–501

American Psychiatric Association: Diagnostic and Statistical Manual of Mental Disorders, 3rd Edition, Revised. Washington, DC, American Psychiatric Association, 1987

Bibring E: The mechanism of depression, in Affective Disorders. Edited by Greenacre P. New York, International Universities Press, 1953, pp 13–47

Brenner C: A psychoanalytic perspective on depression. J Am Psychoanal Assoc 39:25–43, 1991

Freud S: Mourning and melancholia (1917), in The Standard Edition of the Complete Psychological Works of Sigmund Freud, Vol 17. Translated and edited by Strachey J. London, Hogarth Press, 1957, pp 239–258

Jacobson E (ed): Depression: Studies of Normal, Neurotic and Psychotic Conditions. New York, International Universities Press, 1971

Klein M: Contribution to the psycho-genesis of the manic-depressive states (1935), in Contributions to Psycho-Analysis 1921–1945. London, Hogarth Press, 1948, pp 282–310

Zetzel ER: On the incapacity to bear depression (1965), in The Capacity for Emotional Growth. New York, International Universities Press, 1970, pp 82–114

Chapter 15

The Substance-Abusing Patient

Leon Wurmser, M.D.

Current Psychodynamic Perspectives

Definitions

Before we can deal with the psychoanalytic study of the problem of substance abuse, we must define the scope of the concepts used.

Substance abuse is a social, legal, and political term with strong derogatory and judgmental explicitness, not just connotations. Some authors define substance abuse as any use of a substance that affects the mind for reasons that are not medically accepted and that go against prevailing social and legal standards (e.g., Jaffe 1965). In contrast to this definition based on conformity to certain external standards and rules of behavior, it is more consistent with medical tradition, logically and practically, to define substance abuse proper as *the use of any mind-altering substance for the purpose of inner change if such use leads to any transient or long-range interference with social, cognitive, or motor functioning or with physical health, regardless of the legal and social standing of the substance* (Wurmser 1978). This definition places the focus on the person and the act instead of on arbitrary societal standards: the criterion here is one of the impairment of functioning and health, and hence of the definition of psychological normality and illness, transcending the act's conformity with and adaptation to external rules.

We first must briefly review the vast range of activities and behaviors subsumed under this omnibus term of "substance abuse" and then narrow our scope for the purposes of this chapter. The clinically most useful classification is that used in the Second Report of the National Commission on Marijuana and Drug

Abuse (Shafer et al. 1972–1973, pp. 95–97). This definition distinguishes five groups of substance use:

1. **Experimental use** refers to a self-limited trial of drugs (mind-altering, potentially interfering substances, including alcohol and nicotine), primarily motivated by curiosity or the desire to experience new feeling or mood states.
2. **Social or recreational use** occurs in social settings among friends or acquaintances who desire to share an experience perceived as both acceptable and pleasurable. Such use usually occurs on a more frequent basis than experimental use.
3. **Circumstantial-situational use** is task-specific and is motivated by the wish to cope with a specific, sometimes recurrent, situation or condition of a personal or vocational nature.
4. **Intensified use** is defined as the regular, long-term, patterned drug use, at a minimum level of once daily, that is still compatible with social and economic integration and apparent compensation.
5. **Compulsive use** refers to a pattern of high-frequency drug use, at high-intensity levels of relatively long duration, that produces physiological or psychological dependence such that the individual cannot at will discontinue such use without experiencing physiological discomfort or psychological disruption. Compulsive substance use is characterized primarily by significantly reduced individual and social functioning.

Using these five classifications, we can state that for practical purposes, the first of the two groups (experimental and social users) appear not to be particularly associated with serious preexisting psychopathology, whereas the latter two most definitely are, and very many of the third group (situational) are as well. Thus, we are dealing with a continuum—a curve of compulsiveness steeply inclining between groups 2 and 4.

It is evident that many of the current views on substance abuse are in urgent need of revision. There is no such thing as "alcoholism as a disease," in the sense of a unitary entity with a clear and singular cause, course, and treatment (Fingarette 1988). There is no such thing as an addictive personality with clear and common dynamics and one preferable treatment approach for all. There is no linear relation between one set of causal factors and the symptoms of addictive behavior. There is no sharp line between specific addictions and addictive behavior in general, except for the contingencies of the physical effects induced by specific drugs; but there is also no sharp line between addictive behavior and the neurotic process. Treatment experiences with the more severe forms of neurosis—those that now are often singled out as either "narcissistic" or "borderline" disorders (Abend et al. 1983)—are not *principally* different from those with the milder forms, and the problems associated with the treatment of drug- and alcohol-dependent patients represent, for the most part, simply a special form of these severe neuroses (Wurmser 1987a, 1987b, 1988).

Deficit Versus Conflict

Turning now to the current psychodynamic perspectives on "compulsive" or "addictive" drug use, we can divide these perspectives into two classes: 1) those that emphasize the *defect* or *deficit* nature of the underlying disturbance, and 2) those that stress the *conflict* nature of this compulsiveness. Proponents of both views would generally agree with what Krystal and Raskin (1970) succinctly expressed: "We are dealing with sick people and the drug is not the problem, but is an attempt at self-help that fails" (p. 11). In the former view, the drug use is an artificial means of coping with the underlying deficit, one that acts as a kind of prosthesis, and the therapeutic approaches are seen as attempts to remedy such defects—to make up for them, in socially and personally more useful ways. In the latter view, the drug use is seen simultaneously as fulfilling some unconscious wishes (id), as protecting against the anxiety elicited by those wishes and serving as a defense against them (ego), and as satisfying the demands of punishment and expiation for such wishes (superego); the therapeutic approaches focus on elucidating the underlying conflicts and the compromise character of their attempted solution in the form of symptoms and attitudes.

The deficit viewpoint was summarized by Kohut (1971) as follows: "The drug serves not as a substitute for loved or loving objects, or for a relationship with them, but as a replacement for a defect in the psychological structure" (p. 46). Correspondingly and more specifically, Khantzian (in press) emphasized the role of *the defect in self-care and self-regulation:* "The act of using such drugs is less the function of a motivated behavior to actively harm [the] self, [and] more an indication of developmental failures and deficits that leave such individuals ill equipped to take care of themselves . . . substance abusers' self-protective, survival deficiencies are the consequence of deficits in the capacity for self-care" (see also Khantzian 1974, 1977, 1978).

Krystal (1977) mentioned also the deficit in the "self-helping" function, but his major contribution lies in the study of affect pathology: "I have found that as a result of massive childhood psychic trauma, these individuals experienced arrest in affect development and an impairment of affect tolerance. These produce, in effect, a fear of feelings, and [the] need to block them" (p. 95). He described the phenomenon of "affect regression" and differentiated three categories of this entity: *resomatization, dedifferentiation, and deverbalization* (Krystal 1974, 1975, 1988, in press). In resomatization, "the reaction is somatic, with little reflective awareness of it, as if this self-perceptive function of the ego were inactivated" (Krystal, in press). In dedifferentiation, "as in the infant, there is little or no differentiation between depression and anxiety. Instead, one sees a generalized 'unpleasure' response, primarily on a lower than adult level of integration" (Krystal, in press). In deverbalization, the third category of affect regression, the affect fails to serve signal functions; in the sense of "alexithymia," the feelings cannot be linked to words and symbolic expression.

Because my presentation in this chapter is mostly founded on the conflict model of explanation, I can be brief in this introductory part. Wieder and Kaplan (1969, 1974) stressed this view of drug use as conflict solution: "When an individual finds an agent that chemically facilitates his preexisting, preferential mode of conflict solution, it becomes his drug of choice" (Kaplan and Wieder 1974, p. 29). In their explanatory scheme, these authors attempt to balance defensive and wish-fulfilling aspects and to correlate the regressive states attained with drugs with developmental stages as conceptualized by Margaret Mahler. In the recent literature, substance abuse studies that use the conflict model have been quite sparse in comparison with those using the deficit model.

Historical Review

Throughout the older psychological literature and even today in the popular literature, the emphasis has been and is on the wish-fulfilling nature of drug abuse—drug use as an "expensive search for cheap pleasure" (Wurmser 1978). In analytic terms, the focus merely shifted from conscious to unconscious wishes.

Freud very early called masturbation the "primal addiction" (S. Freud 1898/1962, p. 276) but also mentioned the use of a drug as a love object (S. Freud 1912/1957, p. 188), attributing such use to constitutionally heightened orality (S. Freud 1905a/1953, p. 182). Through a basic change in mood and the ensuing removal of inhibitions and undoing of sublimation, alcohol allows regressive wish fulfillment in general (S. Freud 1905b/1960, p. 127).

Rado (1926) stressed the "orgiastic effect of intoxicants": "In comparison with the abrupt curve of genital orgasm, the course followed by pharmacotoxic or pharmacogenic orgasm is generally a long drawn-out one" (p. 401). The crucial orgiastic gratification lies not in the oral zone but rather in a "hidden and mysterious pleasure" brought about by sucking—the "alimentary orgasm." In a later paper (1933), however, he gave more weight to the defensive aspect—that is, to how the pharmacogenic pleasure effect lifts the patient suddenly and magically out of a chronic state of painful, "tense depression": "The ego is, after all, the omnipotent giant it had always fundamentally thought it was. In the pharmacogenic elation the ego regains its original narcissistic stature" (Rado 1933, pp. 7–8).

Simmel (1929) and Glover (1932/1970) were the first to stress the importance of aggression. According to Glover, drugs represent in concrete form "repressed aggressive or sadistic interest[s] . . . this would suggest that in the choice of a noxious habit the element of sadism is decisive" (Glover 1932/1970, p. 206).

A particularly valuable older study of the dynamics of drug addiction—specifically, addiction to heroin—is found in the monumental work of Chein and colleagues (1964), *The Road to H.* These authors stressed that "all addicts suffer from deep-rooted, major personality disorders" (p. 14). They summarized the causation of drug taking as "the challenge of the risk; the attractiveness of the forbidden; the glamour of defying authority; the power of self-destructive needs given a socially validated channel of expression; the drawing power of illicit subsociety to lonely individuals alienated from the mainstream and the lure of its ability to confer a sense of belonging, interdependence of fate, and common purpose to individuals who would otherwise feel themselves to be standing alone in a hostile world" (pp. 6–7). The adaptive or functional use of narcotics lies in their suppression of anxiety: the drug use represents "an enjoyment of negatives" due to "the opiate's capacity to inhibit or blunt the perception of inner anxiety and outer strain. In this sense, the drug itself is a diffuse pharmacological defense" (pp. 229–233).

Differential Dynamic Diagnosis

Core Phenomena of the Neurotic Process

When we examine severely ill patients who show what we would call "addictive behavior," we notice that this behavior is really synonymous with severe *compulsiveness* insofar as it refers to outside factors and entails severely self-destructive consequences (Wurmser 1987b).

Compulsiveness itself belongs, however, to the very essence of the neurotic process. As Kubie (1954) stressed, the stamp of the neurotic process is *its compulsiveness—its insatiability, automaticity, and endless repetitiveness.* To this one might add that the second criterion for the neurotic process consists in *the polarization of opposites*—the dichotomizing of the judgments of good and bad, of pure and impure, of sacred and demonic, of God and Devil, the extreme quality of love and hate, of trust and distrust. Closely connected with that criterion is a third: the *absoluteness and globality* of most experiences—the claim of totality for affective or cognitive comprehension of self and world. Wishes and affects have a particularly overwhelming, global, and all-encompassing nature; they cannot be contained. Put differently, there is an *overvaluation,* an overestimation of self or others; such global experiencing constitutes a transgressing of the limits—a dissolution of the boundaries—in value, truth, and action.

These three, then—compulsiveness, polarization of opposites, and global overvaluation—are criteria for *describing* the neurotic process, as it becomes conspicuously evident in severely regressive patients—typically, those with problems of compulsive substance abuse.

Principal Phenomena of Compulsive Drug Use

If we go beyond the observable *core phenomena,* which are characteristic of the neurotic process in general, and turn to what is on this phenomenological level specific for patients with drug abuse, we find as the lowest level of specificity the following primary, easily visible dynamic features (Wurmser 1982):

1. Drugs generally are used as an artificial *affect defense*—that is, they are compulsively taken to bring about relief from overwhelming feelings. Drug use is ultimately only a pharmacologically reinforced denial and blocking of affect. This presupposes not only a specific proneness for these particular defenses but also an inclination to massive affect regression, with some specificity between the prominent affect and the drug preferred (Wurmser 1974, 1978).
2. In most persons with an addiction, a *phobic core* can be seen as infantile neurosis underlying the later pathology—typically, the fears around being closed in, captured, and entrapped by structures, limitations, commitments, physical and emotional closeness, and bonds. The compulsive *search* of individuals with an addiction is like a mirror image of the compulsive *avoidance* of persons with a phobia. Whereas the latter condense all their dangers into one object or one situation and arrange their lives around that object's or situation's avoidance, those with an addiction do exactly the reverse: their lives' entire content and pursuit—that which they seek and depend on above everything else—becomes condensed into one object or one situation (Wurmser 1980; Wurmser and Zients 1982).
3. Where there are phobias, there are *protective fantasies*—either of personal protective figures or of impersonal protective systems—specifically counterpoised to those threats. This search for a protector against the phobic object or the anxiety-provoking situation almost inevitably leads to a compelling dependency once such a factor has been found—be it a love partner, a fetish, a drug, a system of actions, or the analyst. Most typically, drug addiction enacts the protective fantasy that most potently defends the phobic core. Given the extent of the dependency placed on them, such protectors must be highly *overvalued*—that is, they are "narcissistic objects," selfobjects, and are experienced in extremes: all-powerful, all-giving, and all-forgiving or all-destructive, all-condemning, and all-depriving.
4. The helplessness of being uncontrollably overwhelmed and/or traumatized is defended against by a thick crust of *narcissism*—of grandiosity and entitlement, resentment and coldness, or idealization and submission. Often this narcissism is papered over with the superficial amiability, friendly compliance, and flirtatious charm of the "sociopath."
5. Torn between fear of the condemning and humiliating powers on the outside and of the defensive, narcissistic needs from within, the personality assumes a strikingly unstable and unreliable quality. Periods of high integrity and honesty suddenly give way to episodes of ruthless coldness and criminality. The discrepancy may be so extreme as to constitute a *split or multiple personality*. There is correspondingly a remarkable discontinuity of the sense of self, a global lability without mediation and perspective. This quality is manifested in an unreliability that infuriates others and that humiliates and

depresses the individuals themselves. These "ego splits" or "ego discontinuities" constitute not a defense but a functional disparity and contradictoriness derived from denial above all.

6. *Acute narcissistic crises*—feared or real disappointments in others and in oneself—usually trigger these overwhelming affects and thereby launch the individual into compulsive drug use.

Major Defenses

The next level of specificity is of a higher level of abstraction: the nature of the predominantly used defenses. Three of these defenses are particularly prominent:

1. *Drug use is a pharmacologically reinforced denial and blocking of affect*—an attempt to get rid of feelings and thus of undesirable inner and outer reality.
2. The mechanism of *turning passive into active* is a cardinal defense in severe psychopathology in general, especially against traumatic reality and aggression from within, much as repression represents the primary defense in the less-severe forms of neurosis, mostly against libido.
3. With *externalization,* "the whole internal battle ground is changed into an external one" (A. Freud 1965, p. 223); externalization is the defensive effort *to resort to external action in order to support the denial of inner conflict.*

Central Conflicts

It has proven pragmatically most accurate to group the pathogenic conflicts—as those most relevant for this group of patients—under the following broad headings:

1. There is the preeminence of the problems of—and therewith the conflicts about—*affect regulation.* We notice throughout a problem with *intolerance* toward affects, especially those of the nature of unpleasure. I often have the impression that such affects are a kind of psychoanalytic bedrock, transcending the power of verbal mastery and both preceding and overwhelming the ability of symbolization. Although they certainly often seem to result from issues of later provenience (e.g., anal or oedipal problems), I still presume that they antedate these.

   Conflicts about global affects lead to mental phenomena that are typically viewed and descriptively encompassed as "oral" and "narcissistic." Conflict exists *between clashing, overwhelming affects that cannot be contained*—typically, rage versus anxiety or guilt, love versus humiliation, pain and shame versus excitement. Moreover, there is the conflict between the often irresistible tendency to spiral down into *overwhelming affect* and the desperate efforts at controlling such affects, which, if these efforts fail, results in shame about losing one's *inner control.* Finally, there is the problem of being overrun—"infected"—by the affects and the moods of the immediate environment; this represents the collapse of the defense against affect transmission from the outside. This is a very archaic—in fact, the most archaic—group of conflicts.

Intrinsic to this massiveness and intolerability of affects and, especially, of moods is the particular severity of conflicts, originally of outer conflicts (with the immediate environment) but then more and more of inner conflicts. The more severe the dysregulation, the more extreme—archaic—the ensuing conflicts, and the more radical the affective judgments of good/bad, safe/terrifying, pleasurable/unpleasurable, admirable/contemptible, shamefully weak/guiltfully strong, and so on—that is, some of the phenomena explained by many today as "splitting." I shall come back shortly to this topic.

2. One important culmination point of such conflicts and of the opposite forms of danger involved is the period in which there is a clear opposition between *the need to belong and the need to be oneself*—that is, the so-called separation and individuation period, with its convergence of early castration concerns, anal-sadistic investments, probably some early oedipal strivings, the revolutionary acquisition of symbolization, and the emergence of shame and other early superego manifestations. It appears that during this period some of the massive and archaic identifications occur that will later shape the entire character. These identifications are typically global and will subsequently necessitate large-scale forms of denial and the mask of the "false self." Such identifications represent one prominent way of coming to terms with these *conflicts about union and separateness.*

   One consequence of these conflicts is the prevalence of two antithetical equations. According to the first, separateness—being an individual with his or her own will—is absolutely evil: *success = separating oneself = injuring and killing the other = dying = immense guilt* (Modell 1984). Every self-affirmation is eo ipso defiance and therefore something very bad. The second equation, by contrast, states that *submitting = passivity = dependency and weakness = loss of control, of identity, of one's self = shame and humiliation.* Such feelings of shame are the price one pays in order to be loved.

3. In clinical observation, the main dynamic aspect can be found in episodes during which feelings of a vague tension or of an unaccountable anxiety—of a generalized depression or dysphoria, of a kind of unhappiness, mostly with one's own performance—become overwhelming. Among the broad groupings of anxious and depressive affects are two that stand out because of their recurrent and prominent appearance: 1) feelings of severe inferiority and devaluation in comparison with an ideal, hence of a fear or sense of exposure as well as of humiliation, either impending or already inflicted—*shame* (Wurmser 1981); and 2) feelings of being no good, of being unable to perform what ought to be done, or of doing things injurious to others—*guilt.*

More typically, those anxious and depressive versions of shame and guilt refer only to screen events that conceal dynamically more important ones. Their real causes are hidden—are unconscious. During such episodes, an overbearing inner authority and the ideals carried by that authority seem to have become intolerable, the anxiety about that pressure overwhelming, and the sense of guilt or of shame about having miserably failed such peremptory demands particularly harsh. During what can be described as an impulsive action sequence, there is a kind of defiance against—a temporary *overthrow* of—one part of such a particularly burdensome and chafing inner authority figure in the hope of thereby reaching some fantasy identity that is free of the inner tyrant. This period of respite may last as long as the drugs help with the denial—the not-perceiving—of those features of reality that contradict such a fantasy identity. As soon as the power of suppression and denial wanes with the fading of the drug's effect, however, the original pressures resurge with added fury. The "inner judge" has now even more reason to condemn the patient's self (Wurmser 1984).

This bursting out from a confining stricture is the other side of the coin of what we know as *claustrophobia:* one important symbol for the superego is limitation—an enclosure, a confining structure, the *claustrum.* Not only are forms of claustrophobia found in most drug users, but it is also significant that the sensation of dread is usually displaced further to metaphorical enclosures. Many such individuals feel stifled, smothered, and uncomfortably hemmed in by any human warmth and by any physical and emotional closeness. When another person gets too close (including in intensive psychotherapy), they must beat a frightened or angry retreat or burst out. Any gesture of closeness may be experienced as a suddenly concrete threat of being engulfed and swallowed up by the other.

Dynamically important is the equation of such a "devouring claustrum" with the superego and all its representations and representatives. It appears that this equation forms part of a central fantasy of great specificity: the superego is limitation par excellence, hence the main referent for a claustrum. The battle against *"claustrum = limits = superego = confining external world"* is thus an indispensable psychodynamic factor. Behind this symbolic equation there is a deeper equation of *"claustrum = overstimulation = anxiety"* (Wurmser 1980).

Relief from this claustrophobic anxiety could only come from protection, yet such protection would again be sought in external structures, in outside controls and limitations. In this search, individuals retain the hope that someone else will take over, constrain them, and thus shield them against that dark and overwhelming inner demon. The tragic paradox is, of course, that all such protection is bound to become once more a new claustrum and therefore again a source of terror.

Behind the defensive efforts against the superego, we often find deep *conflicts within conscience, especially in the forms of the opposition of severe feelings of shame and guilt* and of massive *loyalty conflicts.*

Case Example

> For so long I have thought it was impossible to let anybody know what my fantasies were because they were so different from what reality is and what the laws would allow. I was afraid I would be called down, so I concealed them. I hid them but enacted them at the same time.

So spoke Mr. H, whom I started seeing in analysis when he was around 27 years old; his addiction to a whole panoply of drugs had lasted about 15 years. The treatment ended after 3½ years in terrible failure. Every advance on the part of the patient was followed by a yet worse setback, even more provocative and dangerous actions, still more alarming entanglements in serious criminality, and loss of all the money advanced to him by parents and friends. Eventually, he broke off the analysis and, for another 3 years, led a very stormy and marginal life in which he underwent a number of other treatment efforts, all of them unsuccessful; these, in turn, were followed by unremitting failures and several near-fatal overdoses. Finally, Mr. H entered an inpatient facility on the West Coast and was put on a narcotics antagonist and an antidepressant. On his own, he decided to return from the West Coast and to resume therapy with me, but with the adjuncts of drug treatment and Alcoholics Anonymous (AA). He resumed his profession, although now in a much more subordinate capacity than before his breakdown.

For 1 year Mr. H did very well. The insights he had gained in the previous analysis combined with the other treatment approaches and the more supportive therapy now to make him feel more stable, in control, and healthy than ever before. He remarried and his wife soon became pregnant. She, herself a former drug addict and a quite disturbed woman, put a lot of pressure on him, and he had another brief episode (lasting about 2 weeks) of narcotics use and gambling. Although he recovered from this and again seemed to be doing well (he became the father of a girl and moved into his own house), his marriage gradually fell apart, escalating into increasingly more horrible fights involving the police and courts. Mr. H went back on methadone and stopped therapy.

The critical trauma of Mr. H's life was the divorce of his parents; his mother had sent his father—a kind, rather passive man—away when the patient was 5 years old. The child (he was the only one from that marriage and remained, in fact, his mother's only child) was inconsolable and, in a number of destructive actions, took highly effective revenge on his mother. When she remarried, he paid her and his stepfather back by his sullen and wrathful withdrawal.

The humiliation brought about by his testing and his provocations was a small price to pay for his success in reuniting the original family. In fact, every recurrence of drug taking and every financial and legal calamity had that effect: to bring his two parents back together again.

Mr. H's castration anxiety was throughout his life massive and remained conscious. I presume that his invitation of humiliation and other forms of punishment—through the drug abuse and other law violations—served partly as a screen for this massive castration anxiety:

> Don't mutilate me. See, I offer myself already as the victim. I humiliate and harm myself in all other regards. I am a weak, helpless child who has relinquished all controls and must fail.

This dynamic must be viewed against the foil of Mr. H's double oedipal victory—first by successfully getting rid of his mother and sleeping with his father, and then by having his mother all to himself. Yet both victories not only were transient and in themselves spurious, they were also fraught with a sense of guilt for which he had to atone.

What was the source of this crescendo of guilt that drove him again and again into dangerous actions? After sustaining another severe setback about 8 years after the first attempt had begun, Mr. H decided to resume analysis. One of his first important insights consisted of the following:

> Why this need to destroy every success? Because I don't deserve it. Yet why? I felt guilty because I was being treated differently from the other children. The grandparents on both sides spoiled me, slipped secret presents and sums of money to me; my grandfather got me every day in school and took me out for a separate and special lunch. It was hard for me to find my way with that. I felt different from the other children, as an outsider, and as that I felt ashamed. And at the same time I was favored and put into a special position, and for that I felt guilty.

He was placed in a chronic conflict of conscience—opposite expectations, opposite self-images, opposite forms of self-condemnation.

Yet that conflict of conscience went farther and deeper: Mr. H took, unconsciously, the guilt for the breakup of his parents' marriage upon himself—and at the same time felt overwhelmed by rage and despair when his mother continued to go out every night, oblivious to his screaming out the window, hour after hour. Connected with that conflict of conscience was a most powerful fantasy, the uncovering of which went a long way to further his understanding of his severe castration anxiety and his near-inability to have sexual relations once he became committed to a woman:

> Here my rage is fulfilled—she has a bloody hole; she is injured. I don't want to be responsible, yet my wishes of revenge against my mother have been carried out.

Since the age of 8, Mr. H had had a recurrent nightmare of a pulsating thing haunting him, growing and diminishing and growing again, a terror reemerging during the withdrawal states. On the other hand, he thought that his mother actually did have a penis or even several of them, and he maintained that belief until late in his childhood. Thus aggression, guilty fear, and reparation through denial formed a central and deeply character-forming fantasy.

Later, Mr. H saw himself as caught in unending loyalty conflicts between the new families his father and mother had each formed, yet unwelcome and the outsider on both sides.

Even now, years later, his mother knows how to play the wounded, suffering, and self-sacrificing mother and to manipulate him in all her unending schemes:

> Do this for me! Please, do me the favor! Don't tell my husband, don't tell anybody, and I'll send you the money.

By appearing hurt if he hesitates, she keeps appealing to his loyalty toward her—she, who has been a paragon of disloyalty toward three husbands and toward her child. In the 1½ years of his marriage, Mr. H himself succeeded in weaving a similar web of power and guilt, of demands for love and forgiveness, of resentment and rage between himself and his wife. In Mr. H's words, "almost every close relationship is tinged with guilt," and even today the *loyalty conflicts,* the contradictory emotional commitments, are too numerous to count.

When Mr. H's sense of guilt growing out of those four deep roots—the guilt about his mother's leaving and his parents' divorce; the guilt about his rage and vindictiveness against the untrustworthy mother, which ostensibly had been transformed into reality by her "bloody injury"—the "castration"; the guilt about his claims for preferential treatment that were fulfilled by his grandparents; and the guilt about his parents' incessant yet irreconcilable claims for his allegiance and loyalty—overwhelms him with its irresistible tide, he tries to turn it around in the form of destructive fury, of catastrophic defiance, and of making those close to him feel absolutely powerless and utterly betrayed.

All of these conflicts of conscience are played out behind a facade of narcissistic entitlement, but this "selfishness" is in reality little more than a screen concealing storms of conflict. Thus, it is not astonishing that Mr. H feels continually trapped and enclosed—caught by a web that he tries in vain to tear asunder with desperate rage—and that an intense anxiety, like an evil shadow, persistently haunts him.

The sequence in Mr. H's case is similar to that observed in many other cases of substance abuse—a state of overwhelming anxiety, acts of flouting and overthrowing outer and inner authority, culminating in provoked massive punishment and the eventual attainment of forgiveness and acceptance. Although this sequence/explanation is not necessarily true for *all* cases of compulsive drug use, it has proven to be an extremely useful structure ordering many observations in the patients I have seen.

Treatment Strategies

The insights presented in this chapter permit treatment strategies that combine solid analytic knowledge with other, radically different approaches, many of which are viewed as antithetical to analysis. Although analysis addresses the conflicts, auxiliary measures may need to be employed to help with the regulation of the overwhelming affects. Outer structures as well as chemical substances are needed as such auxiliary regulators. It is as if the *vertical* approach of analysis needs to be supplemented with a *horizontal* approach—especially one using behavioral methods including antidepressants, family involvement, behavioral therapy, AA, and antagonists such as disulfiram (Antabuse) or naltrexone (Trexan). Our function as therapists is to incorporate both of these dimensions in our treatment strategy in ways and forms that allow us to help patients resolve their neurotic conflicts in a space tolerably protected against terror and despair.

Special care must be taken not to assume too much of a *real* superego role, and especially not to be maneuvered into the dilemma between permissiveness and punitiveness, between collusion and prohibition. Rather, insofar as is possible, therapists should analyze the externalized or projected superego functions as they are manifested in the transference—that is, instead of *using the superego transference,* they should analyze it. Aggression is not treated primarily by confrontation or by direct drive interpretations, but by defense and superego analysis. The focus is on the many layers of conflicts and on the specific range of affects they lead to. There is no assumption of a superego defect—a superego lacuna—nor is there an *a priori* assumption of visible, deep ego defects, except for the intolerance toward certain specific affects; only at the end of thorough conflict analysis is it possible to pinpoint possible ego defects. Deficit psychology and conflict psychology represent two different visions of the individual; they are complementary to each other rather than mutually exclusive, but they set very different goals and dictate quite different approaches. Much importance is given to a rational alliance and hence to a therapeutic atmosphere of kindness and tact, which facilitates such an alliance. With regard to programs such as AA or Narcotics Anonymous (NA), we should realize that their success rates are only between 14% and 18%, if all patients who get involved with them are counted. This does not detract from their value, only from their claim to be a panacea.

Summary

Finally, I attempt to condense the main thoughts presented in this chapter in the following points:

The main point I want to make is that of the depth of *anxiety* and other affects of unpleasure lurking behind the facade of criminality, sociopathy, and defect. In case after case, I have been struck by the importance of phobic symptoms and phobic character. In many instances, it is possible to draw some conclusions about the origin of this *phobic core structure.*

Then there is the importance of conflicts *within* conscience and between different ideals in the triggering of severely destructive, impulsive action sequences, especially those involving compulsive drug use. The presence of superego conflicts necessarily entails a different approach to understanding and treating patients than is usually taken.

Added to these points are the revolutionizing insights into the early development of infants, which allow conceptualizations and approaches that are empirically much better founded than many of the hitherto cherished retrospective speculations. Especially this applies to the value of an affect theory independent from any drive theory and a new view of what is the specific psychoanalytic concept of causality—*conflict causality.* According to this concept:

- The more severe the trauma, the more overwhelming the affects.
- The more radical and overwhelming the affects, the more intense the conflicts.
- The more intense and extreme the conflicts, the more encompassing (global) the defenses and the more totalitarian the demands of "the inner judge," that sadistic version of conscience we encountered in our patients. Thus, the trauma lives on in the severity and pitiless character of the conscience.
- The more extreme the aggression of the superego, the more prominent the core phenomena described in this chapter and the broader the problems of "narcissism," of "splitting of identity," and of resentment.

In the face of clinical reality, all the simple answers to such a difficult problem as addictive behavior, both in its broad sense and in its underlying dynamics, wither away:

> What is simple and unified is not true, can hardly be that. Only what is composite can perhaps be assumed to be that. (Pär Lagerkvist, *Pilgrimen* [1966])

For Further Study

Chein I, Gerard DL, Lee RS, et al: The Road to H. New York, Basic Books, 1964

Fingarette H: Heavy Drinking: The Myth of Alcoholism as a Disease. Berkeley, University of California Press, 1988

Kaplan EH, Wieder H: Drugs Don't Take People, People Take Drugs. Secaucus, NJ, Lyle Stuart, 1974

Khantzian EJ, Mack JE: Self-preservation and the care of the self: ego instincts reconsidered. Psychoanal Study Child 38:209–232, 1983

Krystal H: The genetic development of affects and affect regression, I. The Annual of Psychoanalysis 2:98–126, 1974

Krystal H: The genetic development of affects and affect regression, II. The Annual of Psychoanalysis 3:179–219, 1975

Krystal H, Raskin HA: Drug Dependence: Aspects of Ego Functions. Detroit, MI, Wayne State University Press, 1970

Wieder H, Kaplan EH: Drug use in adolescents: psychodynamic meaning and pharmacogenic effect. Psychoanal Study Child 24:399–431, 1969

Wurmser L: Psychoanalytic considerations of the etiology of compulsive drug use. J Am Psychoanal Assoc 22:820–843, 1974

Wurmser L: The Hidden Dimension: Psychodynamics in Compulsive Drug Use. New York, Jason Aronson, 1978

References

Abend SM, Porder MS, Willick MS: Borderline Patients: Psychoanalytic Perspectives. New York, International Universities Press, 1983

Chein I, Gerard DL, Lee RS, et al: The Road to H. New York, Basic Books, 1964

Fingarette H: Heavy Drinking: The Myth of Alcoholism as a Disease. Berkeley, University of California Press, 1988

Freud A: Normality and pathology in childhood: assessments of development, in The Writings of Anna Freud, Vol 6. New York, International Universities Press, 1965

Freud S: Sexuality in the aetiology of the neuroses (1898), in The Standard Edition of the Complete Psychological Works of Sigmund Freud, Vol 3. Translated and edited by Strachey J. London, Hogarth Press, 1962, pp 259–285

Freud S: Three essays on sexuality (1905a), in The Standard Edition of the Complete Psychological Works of Sigmund Freud, Vol 7. Translated and edited by Strachey J. London, Hogarth Press, 1953, pp 123–243

Freud S: Jokes and their relation to the unconscious (1905b), in The Standard Edition of the Complete Psychological Works of Sigmund Freud, Vol 8. Translated and edited by Strachey J. London, Hogarth Press, 1960, pp 9–249

Freud S: The tendency to debasement in love (1912), in The Standard Edition of the Complete Psychological Works of Sigmund Freud, Vol 11. Translated and edited by Strachey J. London, Hogarth Press, 1953, pp 179–190

Freud S: Neurosis and psychosis (1924), in The Standard Edition of the Complete Psychological Works of Sigmund Freud, Vol 19. Translated and edited by Strachey J. London, Hogarth Press, 1961, pp 149–156

Glover E: On the etiology of drug addiction (1932), in On the Early Development of Mind. New York, International Universities Press, 1970, pp 187–215

Jaffe JH: Narcotic analgesics, in A Pharmacological Basis of Therapeutics, 3rd Edition. Edited by Goodman LS, Gilman A. New York, Macmillan, 1965, pp 247–311

Kaplan EH, Wieder H: Drugs Don't Take People, People Take Drugs. Secaucus, NJ, Lyle Stuart, 1974

Khantzian EJ: Opiate addiction: a critique of theory and some implications for treatment. Am J Psychother 28:59–70, 1974

Khantzian EJ: The ego, the self, and opiate addiction: theoretical and treatment considerations, in Psychodynamics of Drug Dependence (NIDA Research Monograph 12). Washington, DC, U.S. Government Printing Office, 1977, pp 101–117

Khantzian EJ: The ego, the self and opiate addiction: theoretical and treatment considerations. International Review of Psycho-Analysis 5:189–198, 1978

Khantzian EJ: Self-regulation vulnerabilities in substance abusers: treatment implications. In press (to be published in monograph by American Psychoanalytic Association, The Psychology of Addictive Behavior (ed. S. Dowling)

Kohut H: The Analysis of the Self. New York, International Universities Press, 1971

Krystal H: The genetic development of affects and affect regression, I. The Annual of Psychoanalysis 2:98–126, 1974

Krystal H: The genetic development of affects and affect regression, II. The Annual of Psychoanalysis 3:179–219, 1975

Krystal H: Self- and object-representation in alcoholism and other drug dependence: implications for therapy, in Psychodynamics of Drug Dependence (NIDA Research Monograph 12). Washington, DC, Government Printing Office, 1977, pp 88–100

Krystal H: Adolescence and the tendencies to develop substance dependence. Psychoanalytic Inquiry 2:581–617, 1982

Krystal H: Integration and Self-Healing: Affect, Trauma, Alexithymia. Hillsdale, NJ, Analytic Press, 1988

Krystal H: Disorders of emotional development and addictive behavior. In press (to be published in monograph by American Psychoanalytic Association, The Psychology of Addictive Behavior [ed. S. Dowling])

Krystal H, Raskin HA: Drug Dependence: Aspects of Ego Functions. Detroit, MI, Wayne State University Press, 1970

Kubie LS: The fundamental nature of the distinction between normality and neurosis. Psychoanal Q 23:167–204, 1954

Modell AH: Psychoanalysis in a New Context. New York, International Universities Press, 1984

Rado S: The psychic effects of intoxicants: an attempt to evolve a psycho-analytical theory of morbid cravings. Int J Psychoanal 7:396–413, 1926

Rado S: The psychoanalysis of pharmacothymia (drug addiction). Psychoanal Q 2:1–23, 1933

Shafer RP (chairman), Farnsworth DL, Brill H, et al: Marijuana: A Signal of Misunderstanding; Drug Use in America: Problem in Perspective (First and Second Reports of the National Commission on Marijuana and Drug Abuse). Washington, DC, U.S. Government Printing Office, 1972–1973

Simmel E: Psychoanalytic treatment in a sanatorium. Int J Psychoanal 10:70–89, 1929

Wieder H, Kaplan EH: Drug use in adolescents: psychodynamic meaning and pharmacogenic effect. Psychoanal Study Child 24:399–431, 1969

Wurmser L: Psychoanalytic considerations of the etiology of compulsive drug use. J Am Psychoanal Assoc 22:820–843, 1974

Wurmser L: The Hidden Dimension: Psychodynamics in Compulsive Drug Use. New York, Jason Aronson, 1978

Wurmser L: Phobic core in the addictions and the addictive process. International Journal of Psychoanalytic Psychotherapy 8:311–337, 1980

Wurmser L: The Mask of Shame. Baltimore, MD, Johns Hopkins University Press, 1981

Wurmser L: The question of specific psychopathology in compulsive drug use. Ann N Y Acad Sci 398:33–43, 1982

Wurmser L: The role of superego conflicts in substance abuse and their treatment. International Journal of Psychoanalytic Psychotherapy 10:227–258, 1984

Wurmser L: Flight from conscience: experiences with the psychoanalytic treatment of compulsive drug abusers. J Subst Abuse Treat 4:157–179, 1987a

Wurmser L: Flucht vor dem Gewissen. Heidelberg, Springer, 1987b

Wurmser L: "The sleeping giant": a dissenting comment about "borderline pathology." Psychoanalytic Inquiry 8:373–397, 1988

Wurmser L, Zients A: The return of the denied superego: a psychoanalytic study of adolescent substance abuse. Psychoanalytic Inquiry 2:539–580, 1982

Chapter 16

The Panic Patient

Fredric N. Busch, M.D.,
and Theodore Shapiro, M.D.

Current Psychodynamic Perspectives

The differentiation of panic disorder from other anxiety syndromes in DSM-III, DSM-III-R, and DSM-IV (American Psychiatric Association 1980, 1987, 1994) represents part of an attempt to more systematically define psychiatric disorders on a descriptive basis. Panic disorder consists of recurrent panic attacks (discrete periods of intense fear or discomfort) accompanied by at least four characteristic associated symptoms. Panic disorder is often accompanied by agoraphobia, the fear of entering situations or places from which escape may be difficult and in which the individual fears developing an embarrassing symptom. As a result, the individual restricts his or her travel or activities. Although psychoanalysts have been aware of panic attacks and agoraphobia, they have not always clearly differentiated them from other forms of more chronic anxiety, such as generalized anxiety disorder. In part because these syndromes have not been clearly defined, little effort has been made by psychoanalysts to develop new dynamic theories for panic disorder and agoraphobia beyond the original formulations of Freud described below. In contrast, this area has been a focus of efforts for general psychiatrists and there has been a wealth of important new data. For this reason, the Cornell Panic–Anxiety Study group has been making a renewed effort to study psychodynamic perspectives in relation to the various forms of anxiety, particularly panic disorder (Busch et al. 1991; Shear et al. 1993). In this chapter, we develop a psychodynamic formulation consistent with recent findings on panic disorder and present a case study that demonstrates the value of a psychodynamic approach in understanding and treating this illness.

Historical Review

Freud's (1895b/1962) description of anxiety neurosis shares many similarities with the current DSM-IV definition of panic disorder, a fact that attests to the descriptive continuity of the disorder's presentation regardless of our formulation about its origin. Freud reported that patients feared "extinction of life, or of a stroke, or of a threat of madness" (pp. 93–94) and that these fears were accompanied by palpitations, shortness of breath, diaphoresis, shivering, vertigo, and paresthesias. He viewed anxiety neurosis, along with neurasthenia, as "actual neuroses": primary somatic disruptions related to sexual practices requiring nonpsychological treatments (a change in sexual behavior). Actual neuroses were contrasted with *psychoneuroses* (phobia, obsessive-compulsive disorder, hysteria) in which the anxiety generated by dammed-up libido (drive energy) was bound by psychic conflict. Thus, the psychoneuroses could first be approached with psychological treatments, and the underlying actual neuroses could then be treated by modifying behavior.

In "Inhibitions, Symptoms and Anxiety" (1926/1959), Freud developed a new theory of anxiety in which he viewed it as an intrapsychic mechanism for alerting the patient to the presence of psychologically meaningful dangers. He posited anxiety signals that prompted the ego to mobilize defenses against the danger of emergent forbidden wishes. In the new theory, anxiety was seen as a response to a series of significant dangers that were associated with various developmental stages: helplessness, separation, castration, and superego anxiety. The latter is an intrapsychic conflict that occurs only after resolution of the Oedipus complex in the tripartite mature mind. Although Freud continued to believe that under certain conditions, such as acute trauma, automatic anxiety could break through and be expressed as panic, many psychoanalysts, using the new theory, came to view any form of anxiety as secondary to the emergence of forbidden unconscious wishes, and thus as requiring a psychoanalytic therapeutic approach.

Freud also suggested several etiologies for agoraphobia, which often accompanies panic disorder. He theorized that agoraphobia may sometimes be secondary to acute anxiety (panic attacks), also a currently popular view: "In the case of agoraphobia, etc., we often find the recollection of an anxiety attack; and what the patient actually fears is the occurrence of such an attack under the special conditions in which he believes he cannot escape it" (Freud 1895a/1962, p. 81). He speculated that the avoidance of going out may be secondary to a fear of intensification of sexual impulses (Freud 1926/1959); thus, the fear of the marketplace is a displaced fear of sexual temptation and enactment in public. Additionally, Freud postulated that the defenses of projection and displacement were often involved in phobia formation. For example, Hans's anger at his father was projected from his inner conflicts and displaced from his father to horses (Freud 1909/1955, 1926/1959). Freud noted that one advantage of this substitution was that the anxiety was now conditional on the presence of horses, which through restriction of activity, were easier to avoid than the father.

In recent years, the development of neurophysiological and cognitive-behavioral treatments and formulations of panic disorder and agoraphobia has overshadowed the interest in psychoanalytic models and treatments. Psychopharmacologists view panic disorder as different from other anxieties; that is, as having a somatic basis—reminiscent of Freud's actual neurosis—that is responsive to psychotropic medications. Cognitive-behavioral theorists view panic as having a psychological etiology but see it as originating from catastrophic misinterpretation of somatic sensations rather than from intrapsychic conflict. Pharmacological and cognitive-behavioral treatments have been demonstrated to provide rapid and effective relief of panic symptoms in many patients in a series of treatment studies (Ballenger et al. 1988; Beck et al. 1992; Lydiard et al. 1988; Margraf et al. 1993), whereas little systematic empirical research has been conducted on psychoanalytic treatments of panic.

The psychoanalytic theory and approach, however, provides a way of understanding the meaning of the symptoms from a dynamic viewpoint that highlights conflicts, defenses, and idiosyncratic interpretations of life events that may lead to panic in a given individual or may, in general, add to panic vulnerability. In fact, psychoanalytic models are complementary to contributions from both neurophysiological and cognitive-behavioral approaches. Data collected from this approach could help resolve important questions and treatment problems unexplained by neurophysiological and cognitive-behavioral approaches—for example, the timing of the onset of the disorder, the importance of personality disturbances that appear to precede panic onset, and possibly the substantial post-treatment relapse rates. Additionally, there is evidence of high rates of related psychosocial difficulties in panic disorder patients (Markowitz et al. 1989), and treatments that focus on panic symptoms alone do not address these other impairments. It is possible that in the excitement of developing effective treatment for panic attacks, other problems of patients have been minimized or ignored.

Indeed, there are a number of case reports of successful treatment of symptoms consistent with the DSM-III description of panic disorder through psychoanalysis or psychodynamic psychotherapy (Abend 1989; Malan 1979; Mann and Goldman 1982; Milrod and Shear 1991b; Sandler 1988; Sifneos 1972; Silber 1989). Milrod and Shear (1991a) have recently reviewed the psychoanalytic literature and have noted several additional reports of effective psychoanalytic treatments. These reports indicate that psychodynamic psychotherapy can be an effective treatment for panic disorder and suggest that dynamic mechanisms may be important, both etiologically and clinically, in this disorder.

Differential Dynamic Diagnosis

One problem in evaluating current research on panic disorder is that it has tended to focus on variables that can be easily described and measured via structured diagnostic interviews and checklists. However, because such methods allow little room for the kind of psychodynamic exploration typically done by psychoanalysts, certain kinds of data relevant to panic disorder are not pursued. Nevertheless, over the past several years, clinical observation and some systematic research have been done in areas that hold promise for developing a complementary psychodynamic model for panic disorder and agoraphobia. Data pursued in this research include life events, premorbid personality traits, patients' perceptions of their parents, and studies of children of panic patients.

Several studies report that stressful occurrences in patients' lives typically precede the onset of panic disorder (Faravelli 1985; Last et al. 1984; Roy-Byrne et al. 1986; Solyom et al. 1974). Referred to as *life events,* these stressors often involve separations (a loss or rejection, a change in job or location) or a demand for more independent behavior (a job promotion). Life events may have a greater impact on individuals who are particularly sensitive to changes. In fact, clinical observers from various theoretical perspectives have suggested that panic patients may be unassertive or dependent well before the onset of their panic attacks. This theory can be contrasted with a popular current view that these traits are the *result* of the panic attacks. In England, Marks (1970), for example, reported that the majority of agoraphobia patients had a premorbid personality "variously characterized as 'soft,' passive, anxious, shy and dependent" (p. 541). In the United States, even Klein (1964) found that half of his patients retrospectively reported that they were "fearful and dependent children, with marked separation anxiety, and difficulty in adjusting to school" (p. 405). He noted that this group "seems to have suffered from a chronically high separation anxiety level throughout life and to have developed panic attacks under conditions where they were peculiarly vulnerable" (Klein 1964, pp. 405–406). These patients may also have difficulty tolerating anger and other intense affects. During the 1920s, the psychoanalyst Deutsch (1929) suggested that anger plays a central role in phobias and that the presence of a phobic companion unconsciously reassures the patient that his or her aggressive impulses have not harmed that person.

Premorbidly perceived unstable attachments to parents could lead to a vulnerability to intense anxiety states. Clinical observers have found that panic patients typically describe their parents as variously overprotective, restricting, controlling, critical, frightening, and rejecting. For example, Tucker (1956), described reports of a "lack of parental affection, overprotection and overcriticism by parents" (p. 827) in 77 of 100 phobic patients. More recently, questionnaires have been developed to more systematically assess patients' perceptions of their parents. When compared with control subjects, panic patients have been found to perceive their parents as having been more overprotective and less caring (Arrindell et al. 1983; Parker 1979; Silove 1986). In addition, children with school-avoidant anxiety were found to have mothers who were also anxious (Last et al. 1987). These data point to early identifications.

Prospective developmental studies by Kagan and colleagues (Biederman et al. 1990; Kagan et al. 1990; Rosenbaum et al. 1988) have shown that children whose parents have panic disorder and agoraphobia demonstrate a high rate of behavioral inhibition and autonomic arousal in unfamiliar situations very early in life. These characteristics are similar to those seen in a separate group of "inhibited" infants and children who "manifested long latencies to interact when exposed to novelty, retreated from the unfamiliar, and ceased play and vocalizations while clinging to their mothers" (Biederman et al. 1990, p. 21). Kagan and colleagues reported that this behavioral inhibition is typically maintained through infancy, toddlerhood, and elementary-school age. These studies also indicated that compared with control subjects, children exhibiting behavioral inhibition had a higher level of psychopathology, including an increased risk of multiple anxiety, overanxious, and phobic disorders.

The Cornell Panic-Anxiety Study group conducted a pilot study at Payne Whitney Clinic to further evaluate the importance of psychological factors and meaningful life events in panic disorder. Nine patients who met criteria for panic disorder were interviewed by trained analysts on videotape. These tapes were then analyzed with a focus on life events preceding panic, conflicts over sexuality and aggression, internal representations of parents, and difficulties in social and occupational functioning. Confirmatory evidence was found for the importance of life stressors in panic onset: significant life events were found to precede panic onset in all of the patients. In addition, such events were considered to be especially meaningful to patients because they represented threats to attachment that echoed the patients' early childhood experiences. These life events were similar to those reported in other studies, and involved separation from a significant other who had a caregiving or companion role or an increase in demands for more independent behavior. For example, one patient's panic attacks began while she was away from her husband on a business trip. The work was very intense and her supervisor was critical and demanding. She found the supervisor's behavior to be highly reminiscent of her mother's behavior when she was a child. Seven of the nine patients experienced concern about their angry feelings—worrying either that these feelings were not well controlled or that their expression would lead to rejection by others. Sexual conflicts were not found to be significant in panic onset and, when present, appeared to play a secondary role to anxiety about insecure attachment and angry feelings. The patients typically described their parents as temperamental, controlling, and frightening. Often, parents were noted to have been highly anxious themselves. The patients described significant problems in their relationships with others that appeared to be patterned after their conflicts with their parents, and these problems usually affected their occupational functioning.

Using a psychodynamic interview and the information described above, the Cornell group postulated both a neurophysiological and a psychological vulnerability to panic stemming from a particular constitutional predisposition and/or a specific set of early life experiences (Busch et al. 1991). The group suggested that a feeling of fearful dependency—an anxious state in which the parent was felt to be both necessary for protection and yet unpredictable in terms of availability—would place children at increased risk for panic disorder. The fearful dependency on the parent could develop either from an inborn excessive fearfulness of unfamiliar situations, as noted in Kagan's studies, or from the actual controlling, rejecting, or unpredictable behavior of parents (Bowlby 1973). In life, the source of the anxiety is not dichotomized in the manner outlined. The experience of the fearful dependency is blamed on the parent in order to avoid the narcissistic humiliation of the child's incapacity for handling the unfamiliar. Therefore, in both cases (the interaction of a fearful constitutional predisposition with ordinary failures of parental care or the interaction of an unremarkable predisposition with a particular group of traumatic developmental experiences), the child will internalize a representation of the parent as unstable, rejecting, and controlling.

Given this early psychophysiological configuration, the group suggested that individuals with such vulnerabilities would have particular difficulty tolerating angry affects. The perceived or actual rejecting, controlling, or frightening parental behavior engenders intense, angry feelings in the child—feelings that create guilt and anxiety because the child fears that their expression would further damage an already insecure bond with the parent. Defenses such as denial, displacement, reaction formation, and projection will typically keep the anger and its attendant anxiety under control. However, under certain circumstances, an escalating cycle of anxiety—narcissistic humiliation—anger—guilt—anxiety—fearful dependency can occur. Enacted separation anxiety escaping its signal function represents one attempt to control these feelings, as the child clings to the ambivalently held object. In adulthood, a life event that represents a threat to a fantasied attachment can trigger a state of regressive fearful dependency, leading to the arousal of the dormant dynamic postulated above. Here again, both anxiety about the actual or perceived loss and angry reactions toward the loss will occur. The escalating cycle described above will follow, leading to panic levels of anxiety. The panic attack itself is a compromise formation, as it represents both a plea for help and a denial of destructive rage as well as an expression of anger through intense demandingness. It also serves to deny angry feelings on the conscious level.

A conflict between anger and dependency is a dynamic well known to psychoanalysts. Individuals prone to panic appear to have an intense version of this conflict, as well as a particular set of object representations (i.e., the perception of others as controlling and rejecting) and a neurophysiological predisposition to panic. Although the study group considers that this formulation best fits the data of observation, other psychodynamic formulations may also be useful in understanding panic attacks. Sexual fantasies or other affects of sexual arousal that are perceived as intensely frightening because they are viewed as unacceptable may precipitate panic attacks. Self psychological concepts of annihilation anxiety and fear of self-fragmentation also have been suggested as possible theoretical explanations for panic attacks.

Case Example

Ms. J, a separated, 38-year-old woman, reported panic symptoms that had been occurring for the past 2 weeks. Although she had had intermittent panic attacks since she was 19 years old, it had been 2 years since she had last experienced an attack.

Ms. J was the second of two daughters (her sister was 19 years older) born to an Italian working-class family. She was always "Daddy's little girl." She described her father as temperamental, with recurrent angry outbursts and sulking; he had been very threatened when she attempted to leave home. Her mother was highly anxious and critical. As a child, Ms. J had experienced school phobia when she first started school but this had subsided and did not reappear. She met her future husband when she was 15 years old and married him secretly 4 years later, just before he went into the service, because she was afraid to tell her father. Her father became enraged when he found out, and 1 or 2 weeks later, he suffered a myocardial infarction.

She separated from her husband after about 6 years of marriage, stating that his family was not warm or close and that he did not want children. Although she had been separated for almost 6 years at the time she presented for treatment, she had not obtained a divorce and was still friends with her husband. Her boyfriend of 5 years was married with three children. Two years before she sought treatment, she had had an argument with her father about her boyfriend and as a result they stopped speaking to one another, even though she continued to live with her parents. She and her father had begun talking again about 2 months before her panic symptoms had reappeared. She had been discussing moving out of her home to live with her boyfriend, but was feeling increasingly guilty about leaving her parents.

Ms. J entered treatment with one of the authors (F.N.B.) 6 months after presentation, during which time she had been successfully treated with imipramine and tapered off. She showed some capacity for insight and there were ongoing interpersonal difficulties with her boyfriend and family that were thought likely to benefit from psychoanalytically oriented psychotherapy. Ms. J initially attended sessions irregularly. This resistance was interpreted as stemming from her disappointment with the switch in therapists: she saw her first therapist as more giving and the new one as more depriving. In fact, the first therapist did take a much more active stance in the use of medication. Her new therapist explained the difference between this active treatment and long-term exploratory treatment.

Early in the treatment, Ms. J became pregnant and then miscarried. During the next several months, she frequently spoke of her feeling that others were not responsive enough to her. She felt isolated but tended to recoil from discussing this, noting that she wanted to avoid these feelings because they were painful. Ms. J related how her mother responded to her neediness in a critical and attacking manner. There were also indications early on that Ms. J was quite conflicted about angry and guilty feelings close to the surface. For example, she was fearful that she would cause her boyfriend to have a myocardial infarction, just as she felt she had caused her father's. Ms. J reported that she always became nervous when people fought. She expressed anger indirectly at the therapist by coming late or missing sessions. If she were to express her anger directly, she felt, her therapist would withdraw like her father, who would go to his room and sulk for hours when Ms. J became angry with him.

After about 6 months, Ms. J's resistance diminished significantly and the therapist increased the meetings to two times per week, to which she came regularly. The central theme shifted from feelings of being isolated and unwanted to a focus on being deprived by others and angry about the deprivation. In the setting of the therapist's vacation 8 months into the treatment, she began focusing on her anger at her boyfriend and parents. She felt that this anger made her a "terrible person." At this time, she again became pregnant. She spoke of wanting to reduce the sessions to once per week, expressed a fear that hearing about the pregnancy would kill her father, and talked of quitting her job because she was angry about an incident that had occurred there. The therapist offered the interpretation that she needed to cut back her therapy in order to avoid damaging the therapist with her anger now that the relationship had intensified. Although she agreed that this might be the case, she insisted on reducing the frequency of visits.

One year into treatment, as the therapist's vacation approached, Ms. J missed three of four sessions. When she arrived at the session preceding the vacation, her anger at the therapist for going away was discussed. Two days after the therapist's departure for 2 weeks, her panic attacks recurred. She saw a covering therapist twice during this period. A decision was made to treat the attacks with psychotherapy alone because of her pregnancy. Ms. J's feelings of having been abandoned by the therapist and her attendant rage were openly discussed. She reported anger that, in her view, therapists encouraged dependence and then were uncaring when patients felt abandoned. As exploration of her anger continued with her regular therapist, her symptoms steadily decreased. Ms. J noted that her angry feelings at others were often followed by feelings of suffocation. Her primary panic symptom of fearing choking while drinking became more clear, as she recalled early intense, angry struggles at the dinner table over her not eating enough.

Ms. J's panic symptoms increased temporarily when her father was hospitalized for a brief period. She feared that she would harm him further at the same time she was angry at him for being ill. At this point, Ms. J had a dream in which she was walking with her boyfriend on the beach and a man was thrown from a wave onto the beach. She wondered if he would be harmed. The therapist's interpretation was that Ms. J might be anxious about harming her baby. She began to talk about her fears that she would harm the baby because of its demandingness and would be unable to care for it. Ms. J was asked whether her mother had had any problems with her delivery. Although she initially denied this suggestion, a few weeks later, out of curiosity, she asked her mother about it. She discovered that, in fact, her mother had rejected her initially when she was born.

With the interpretation of her fear of being angry toward and incompetent with the baby, the current panic episodes resolved. The time of her approaching delivery coincided with the therapist's graduation from residency. When this was announced, the patient stated that she would discontinue treatment after her delivery. Attempts to interpret this departure were unsuccessful and she missed three successive sessions. Two weeks after terminating, she called the therapist to report a recurrence of the panic symptoms 2 days after delivery. A decision was made to restart medications (diazepam [Valium] and imipramine [Tofranil]) to provide rapid amelioration of her panic symptoms while continuing with psychodynamic exploration. Work was done with her intense difficulties with anger at her baby's demandingness and the relation of this current anger to her anger at her father's demands. Although this dynamism had been discussed prior to the baby's birth, the new discussion appeared to be particularly helpful to her in the context of her actual experience with the baby. She also described her sense that the members of her family were abandoning her in her time of need. This fear was connected with her intense feelings of anger and rejection associated with the change in therapists. Her symptoms rapidly resolved and her acting out diminished, allowing her to continue with the new therapist.

After a brief period, Ms. J decided that she wanted to spend more time with her baby, and the new therapist converted her to monthly medication clinic visits. She was successfully tapered off medication after 1 year and was asymptomatic 5 months later, at which time she discontinued treatment. Although Ms. J was treated with two modalities, one panic episode was treated with psychotherapy alone. The timing of the resolution of this episode was clearly associated with interpretation and her recognition of her repressed fantasies and denied anger. Although she was shifted out of insight-oriented psychotherapy, there was evidence that her understanding of her emotional states had increased greatly, and she was more comfortable both with her relationships with her parents and her boyfriend and with caring for her new baby.

In terms of the formulation presented earlier, we can suggest that this patient suffered from an intense conflict between angry thoughts and feelings and fears of abandonment. Ms. J felt highly dependent on her parents and almost incapable of surviving without them, although she was in fact able to work and support herself. She feared isolation and loneliness and had to do much to avoid or deny these feelings. At the same time, she was enraged at her parents for their lack of empathy and their critical and demanding behavior. The rage at them was extremely threatening to her because she experienced it as potentially damaging and murderous to her parents and significant others. At times of perceived abandonment, she was caught between her intense need for others and her intense rage at them. This dilemma led to the vicious circle described previously, of fearful dependency, anxiety, narcissistic humiliation (at her inability to manage on her own), anger, guilt, anxiety, and fearful dependency, escalating to the level of a panic attack. The attack both represented anxiety about the intensity of her rage and served a defensive function, as she no longer experienced her rage consciously. It also represented an urgent call for help that kept her from the danger of intense isolation and met her dependency needs.

In reviewing this case, the tripartite structural model of Freud is valuable in understanding the course of treatment and its impact. We suggest that the patient had fantasies of harming others that were rendered unconscious because of the danger they represented to the ego. At certain points, the anxiety signal and the defenses were adequate; however, under conditions of perceived abandonment, the patient's rage intensified and its fantasied potential danger led to failure of the defenses and the onset of panic levels of anxiety. Mobilization of defenses, such as denial or repression of angry feelings, was inadequate to deal with this threat.

In the setting of the intensification of the analytic relationship, the patient developed a transference in which the therapist was seen to be as depriving and unhelpful as the patient perceived other figures in her life to be. Rageful fantasies triggered by the therapist's leaving on vacation led to the onset of symptoms. With the therapist's neutral stance, the patient could gradually learn that revealing her angry fantasies would not lead to abandonment. Given this increasing sense of safety in the therapeutic setting, the patient was able to hear interpretations about her unconscious angry fantasies toward the analyst and others. The discovery of her mother's rejection of her as a baby, prompted by her new curiosity and her own feared rejection of her baby, were also valuable to Ms. J. Once these events were revealed, the patient could see that the fantasies were not in fact a danger to the therapeutic relationship and also were not as dangerous to her other relationships as she had imagined. This realization led to a reduction in her panic attacks. In the subsequent episode of panic, the use of drugs as an adjunct to the psychoanalytically oriented psychotherapy provided immediate amelioration of the panic and also permitted further exploration in a setting of trust that her feelings of helplessness were not to be ignored.

It should be apparent that cognitive therapies would emphasize the miscognition and overvaluation of the estimate of danger, whereas interpersonal therapies would emphasize the helping benignity of the therapist, who would not attend to the transference rage. In this manner, other therapies address central aspects of the panic propensity but also protect the patient from further self-knowledge. The therapist's interest and benign, nonthreatening ministrations help the patient to feel protected regardless of what therapeutic modality is being used.

Summary

Given the formulation described here, addressing the patient's conflicts with anger and feelings of unstable attachment by using psychodynamic psychotherapy or psychoanalysis may well lead to a diminution in panic attacks. Depending on the level of the panic symptoms, the therapist may choose to proceed with medication or cognitive-behavioral treatments while continuing the psychodynamic assessment. To the extent that dependency and unassertiveness are longer-term problems that preceded the patient's panic attacks, psychodynamic exploration of conflicts may be more effective than medication or cognitive-behavioral treatments in addressing these traits over time. Indeed, the general psychiatrist, armed with appropriate tools to make a dynamic formulation derived from an adequate evaluation, can proceed with preliminary treatment goals by using dynamic exploratory procedures to provide further relief after the demanding imperatives of the distressing symptoms are understood.

These disparate effective approaches to panic/anxiety recommend that psychoanalytic researchers should proceed with more systematic investigation of the effectiveness of a psychodynamic psychotherapy in treating panic disorder. Such investigations would benefit from the use of a treatment manual. The hypotheses described above suggest certain themes that may be useful as a focus of interpretation. Additional studies are required to assess the presence of personality disturbances accompanying panic, the degree to which the various treatments affect these character issues, and the impact of intrapsychic conflicts and personality disorders on relapse rates. Such studies will help to elucidate where psychodynamic treatments can play a role in panic treatment, even in a setting where other treatments are available to alleviate initial symptoms.

For Further Study

Busch NF, Cooper AM, Klerman GL, et al: Neurophysiological, Cognitive-Behavioral, and Psychoanalytic Approaches to Panic Disorder: Toward an Integration. Hillsdale, NJ, Analytic Press, 1991

Bowlby J: Attachment and Loss, Vol 2: Separation, Anxiety, and Anger. New York, Basic Books, 1973

Compton A: A study of the psychoanalytic theory of anxiety, I: the development of Freud's theory of anxiety. J Am Psychoanal Assoc 20:3–44, 1972

Compton A: A study of the psychoanalytic theory of anxiety, II: developments in the theory of anxiety since 1926. J Am Psychoanal Assoc 20:341–394, 1972

Craske MG: Cognitive-behavioral treatment of panic, in American Psychiatric Press Review of Psychiatry, Vol 7. Edited by Francis AJ, Hales RB. Washington, DC, American Psychiatric Press, 1988, pp 121–137

Gorman JM, Liebowitz MR, Fyer AJ, et al: A neuroanatomical hypothesis for panic disorder. Am J Psychiatry 146:148–161, 1989

References

Abend SM: Psychoanalytic psychotherapy, in Handbook of Phobia Therapy. Edited by Lindeman C. Northvale, NJ, Jason Aronson, 1989, pp 393–403

American Psychiatric Association: Diagnostic and Statistical Manual of Mental Disorders, 3rd Edition. Washington, DC, American Psychiatric Association, 1980

American Psychiatric Association: Diagnostic and Statistical Manual of Mental Disorders, 3rd Edition, Revised. Washington, DC, American Psychiatric Association, 1987

American Psychiatric Association: Diagnostic and Statistical Manual of Mental Disorders, 4th Edition. Washington, DC, American Psychiatric Association, 1994

Arrindell W, Emmelkamp PMG, Monsma A, et al: The role of perceived parental rearing practices in the etiology of phobic disorders: a controlled study. Br J Psychiatry 143:193–187, 1983

Ballenger JC, Burrow GD, Dupont RL Jr, et al: Alprazolam in panic disorder and agoraphobia: results from a multicenter trial, I: efficacy in short-term treatment. Arch Gen Psychiatry 45:413–422, 1988

Beck AT, Sokol L, Clark DA, et al: A crossover study of focused cognitive therapy of panic disorder. Am J Psychiatry 149:778–783, 1992

Biederman J, Rosenbaum JF, Hirschfeld DR, et al: Psychiatric correlates of behavioral inhibition in young children of parents with and without psychiatric disorders. Arch Gen Psychiatry 47:21–26, 1990

Bowlby J: Attachment and Loss, Vol 2: Separation, Anxiety, and Anger. New York, Basic Books, 1973

Busch FN, Cooper AM, Klerman GL, et al: Neurophysiological, cognitive-behavioral, and psychoanalytic approaches to panic disorder: toward an integration. Psychoanalytic Inquiry 11:316–332, 1991

Deutsch H: The genesis of agoraphobia. Int J Psychoanal 10:51–69, 1929

Faravelli C: Life events preceding the onset of panic disorder. J Affective Disord 9:103–105, 1985

Freud S: Obsessions and phobias: their psychical mechanism and their etiology (1895a), in The Standard Edition of the Complete Psychological Works of Sigmund Freud, Vol 3. Translated and edited by Strachey J. London, Hogarth Press, 1962, pp 71–84

Freud S: On the grounds for detaching a particular syndrome from neurasthenia under the description "anxiety neurosis" (1895b), in The Standard Edition of the Complete Psychological Works of Sigmund Freud, Vol 3. Translated and edited by Strachey J. London, Hogarth Press, 1962, pp 85–117

Freud S: Analysis of a phobia in a five year old boy (1909), in The Standard Edition of the Complete Psychological Works of Sigmund Freud, Vol 10. Translated and edited by Strachey J. London, Hogarth Press, 1955, pp 1–149

Freud S: Inhibitions, symptoms and anxiety (1926), in The Standard Edition of the Complete Psychological Works of Sigmund Freud, Vol 20. Translated and edited by Strachey J. London, Hogarth Press, 1959, pp 75–175

Kagan J, Reznick JS, Snidman N, et al: Origins of panic disorder, in Neurobiology of Panic Disorder. Edited by Ballenger J. New York, Wiley, 1990, pp 71–87

Klein DF: Delineation of two drug-responsive anxiety syndromes. Psychopharmacologia 5:397–408, 1964

Last CG, Barlow DH, O'Brien GT: Precipitants of agoraphobia: role of stressful life events. Psychol Rep 54:567–570, 1984

Last CG, Hersen M, Kazdin AE, et al: Psychiatric illness in mothers of anxious children. Am J Psychiatry 144:1580–1583, 1987

Lydiard RB, Roy-Byrne PP, Ballenger JC: Recent psychopharmacological treatment of anxiety disorders. Hosp Community Psychiatry 38:1157–1165, 1988

Malan DH: Individual Psychotherapy and the Science of Psychodynamics. London, Butterworth, 1979

Mann J, Goldman R: A Casebook in Time-Limited Psychotherapy. New York, McGraw-Hill, 1982

Margraf J, Barlow DH, Clark DM, et al: Psychological treatment of panic: work in progress on outcome, active ingredients, and follow-up. Behav Res Ther 31:1–8, 1993

Markowitz JS, Weissman MH, Ouellette R, et al: Quality of life in panic disorder. Arch Gen Psychiatry 46:984–992, 1989

Marks IM: Agoraphobic syndrome (phobic anxiety state). Arch Gen Psychiatry 23:538–553, 1970

Milrod B, Shear MK: Dynamic treatment of panic disorder: a review. J Nerv Ment Dis 179:741–743, 1991a

Milrod B, Shear MK: Psychodynamic treatment of panic: three case histories. Hosp Community Psychiatry 42:311–312, 1991b

Parker G: Reported parental characteristics of agoraphobics and social phobics. Br J Psychiatry 135:555–560, 1979

Rosenbaum JF, Biederman J, Gersten M, et al: Behavioral inhibition in children of parents with panic disorder and agoraphobia. Arch Gen Psychiatry 45:463–470, 1988

Roy-Byrne PP, Geraci M, Uhde TW: Life events and the onset of panic disorder. Am J Psychiatry 143:1424–1427, 1986

Sandler AM: Aspects of the analysis of a neurotic patient. Int J Psychoanal 69:317–326, 1988

Shear MK, Cooper AM, Klerman GL, et al: A psychodynamic model of panic disorder. Am J Psychiatry 150:859–866, 1993

Sifneos PE: Short-Term Psychotherapy and Emotional Crisis. Cambridge, MA, Harvard University Press, 1972

Silber A: Panic attacks facilitating recall and mastery: implications for psychoanalytic techniques. J Am Psychoanal Assoc 37:337–364, 1989

Silove D: Perceived parental characteristics and reports of early parental deprivation in agoraphobic patients. Aust NZ J Psychiatry 20:365–369, 1986

Solyom L, Beck P, Solyom C, et al: Some etiological factors in phobic neurosis. Canadian Psychiatric Association Journal 19:69–78, 1974

Tucker WI: Diagnosis and treatment of the phobic reaction. Am J Psychiatry 825–830, 1956

Chapter 17

The Posttraumatic Patient

Jacob D. Lindy, M.D.,
Fred Moss, M.D.,
and Louis Spitz, M.D.

In recent years, posttraumatic stress disorder (PTSD) has skyrocketed from a low to a high priority for psychiatric educators and students. Massive, unmet posttraumatic needs of Vietnam veterans, crime victims, rape victims, incest survivors, and survivors of natural and man-made disasters continue to bring to the consciousness of contemporary psychiatrists the need to understand, diagnose, and treat responses to such overwhelming traumatic experiences.

In this chapter we describe the major features of PTSD and discuss the usefulness of dynamic concepts in understanding and treating the disorder. We also highlight several general principles of psychodynamics relevant to many disorders but perhaps best illustrated through work with posttraumatic patients.

Historical Review

The work of many psychoanalysts who have studied and written about trauma is evident in the phenomenology of the disorder.

Freud's (1920/1973) description of how trauma pierces the "stimulus barrier," overwhelming the ego, and his insistence on the primacy of the repetition compulsion in the formation of enduring symptoms are essential to the disorder. Janet (1889) carefully described dissociative phenomena following trauma, and placed these phenomena centrally in the origin of traumatic conditions. His distinction between automatic and narrative memory created a bridge to the biology of memory. Horowitz (1976) postulated a fluctuation between the intrusion and the denial phases of PTSD, and offered a cognitive processing model for the disorder's resolution that also contributed to the descriptions in DSM-III (American Psychiatric Association 1980; see below). Other psychoanalysts have contributed detailed descriptions of their individual work with trauma survivors, clarifying many of the ways in which dissociative phenomena express themselves in the treatment situation (DeWind 1969; Hoppe 1968; Klein 1968; Niederland 1968).

Differential Dynamic Diagnosis

Organized psychiatry began in 1980 a concerted effort to address an unmet need in research and treatment with a designation of the posttraumatic stress disorder diagnostic entity in DSM-III. Further refinements of the diagnostic criteria for this condition (i.e., in DSM-III-R and DSM-IV [American Psychiatric Association 1987, 1994]) continue to call for a stressor event that is sufficiently unique as to be outside the expectable range of human experience and sufficiently intense as to cause at least temporary psychological disturbance in most people so affected. The diagnosis of PTSD requires three types of symptom expression:

1. Intrusive repetitions of the event itself, returning in unbidden forms, interrupting sleep (as in nightmares) and/or distracting attention in wakefulness (as in flashbacks or reenactments).
2. Numbing or avoidance phenomena in which the survivor consciously or unconsciously acts so as to avoid reminders of the traumatic experience and/or becomes alienated from phase-appropriate tasks and relationships.
3. Autonomic hyperarousal in response to stimuli that constitute potential reminders of the trauma itself.

The very structure of the defining characteristics of PTSD is unique in the *Diagnostic and Statistical Manual* in that the precipitating event is causally connected with the essential features of the syndrome. Exploring the relationship between event and symptoms as it is enacted via reminders of the trauma in the present becomes one of the first areas of concern for the dynamic clinician. Discovering the specific relationship can be useful both in terms of improving the patient's cognitive grasp of the symptoms and in terms of improving the clinician's grasp of dynamic principles. Some precipitants are straightforward. For example, many survivors of a Memorial Day supper club fire outside Cincinnati, Ohio (in which 165 people were killed and more than 2,000 survivors exited with the pungent smell of burning flesh clearly imprinted in their memories) responded with anxiety months and years later when they smelled barbecued meat at spring picnics (Lindy and Titchener 1983). Similarly, some Vietnam veterans, in hot, sultry weather or while walking single file in wooded areas, reported anxiety as these reminders brought back moments of terror in the bush in Vietnam (Lindy et al. 1988).

When therapists point out the near-universality of such symptoms and their "plausibility" in light of past trauma, they provide structure and confidence for their patients, whose unsuccessful efforts to disavow the trauma have led to the appearance of their symptoms. Such interventions also assure the survivor that the therapist is reasonably well versed in the specific trauma constellation that he or she has suffered, and promote a beginning working relationship.

Some complex configurations that link current symptoms and their triggers with traumatic events are even more enlightening to survivors.

> For example, one survivor of the supper club fire mentioned above arrived at his appointment agitated and guilty that he had seen but not stopped the fighting of two teenagers on the sidewalk. When the therapist suggested a connection back to the fire, the patient explained that terrible fighting and pushing was going on as he exited the club. Further, he had made no effort to provide order or to stop the fighting. Many of those whom he saw fighting and pushing soon died in their unsuccessful attempts to escape. The distress he was feeling now after seeing the teenagers captured his agitation and guilt about making it out of the club while insufficiently acting to help the orderly escape of others.

The first symptom criterion of the diagnosis for PTSD is in the realm of intrusive phenomena. Here, aspects of the trauma are repeated in unbidden forms such as traumatic nightmares, uninvited thoughts, or intrusive images such as flashbacks, or in unconscious motor behaviors that repeat the event itself in reenactments. Dynamic understanding of the content and process of these intrusive phenomena is often crucial to the understanding of a given patient and to resolving the internal conflicts that these phenomena continue to stir in the patient's current life.

> A Vietnam veteran awakens in terror from a nightmare in which the face of a dying 12-year-old Vietnamese boy is coming toward him. In the traumatic dream, he was reliving a terrifying scene in which his own helplessness, rage, and guilt over having shot and killed a small boy during a perimeter action in Vietnam returns to haunt him. Additional history indicates that this survivor with PTSD is currently stressed by his difficulties in setting appropriate disciplinary limits with his own 12-year-old son. Hence, an unresolved aspect of the war trauma—namely, guilt over his aggression toward a boy in wartime (the killing of a presumably innocent child)—is activated in the context of current conflicts regarding discipline with his own son.

The second symptom criterion of PTSD, numbing or avoidant symptoms, may be thought of as repetitions of once-adaptive ego mechanisms designed to protect the psyche from the overwhelming impact of the event itself. A wide variety of symptoms come into play; these represent unconscious efforts of the ego to keep a safe distance from the traumatizing experience or reminders of it. There may be simple phobias related to the trauma. There may be the splitting off or blunting of intolerable affects in an effort to protect the ego from affect overload; similarly, there may be a disavowal of the meaning of trauma-related objects and aims. There may be amnesia. There is often a dissociation of images, affects, and thoughts connected with the trauma in an effort to maintain a psychoeconomic equilibrium. This state recapitulates the dissociation that occurred at the time the memory was first laid down.

Two important clinical facets of PTSD that to date have received less attention than they deserve in the PTSD literature may be thought of broadly within the numbing category. The first of these is *suicidal thinking,* often dynamically connected with a wish to join a comrade or even an enemy in death rather than face the difficulties of life in the present. A second facet concerns *somatic symptoms* among patients with PTSD, some of which actually bind anxiety by incorporating in their content particular aspects of the trauma itself.

> For example, a young woman developed severe, "steel-like" jaw pain after being raped and robbed. For her, the most traumatic part of the experience had been being forced to perform fellatio while the rapist held a knife at her face. She complained of her jaw symptoms long before she was able to put this aspect of her trauma into words.

The discovery of meaning in the various symptoms of PTSD is an enlightening experience for the patient and often brings hope where previously there had been only despair. In addition, such understandings provide the therapist with concrete examples of psychodynamics that can be brought home in terms of real-life clinical situations.

Illustrated in nearly every case of PTSD are two core psychoanalytic principles:

1. **The repetition compulsion,** as described by Freud (1920/1977)—the relentless drive of the patient to repeat unworked-through aspects of the traumatic event in the form of current symptoms (e.g., intrusive images, reenactments, nightmares). This phenomenon is a hallmark of the disorder.
2. **Defenses**—the ego's efforts to manage the strain of such repetitive intrusiveness. In other words, in the adaptive functioning of the ego, efforts are made to modulate and to keep under control the prospectively damaging influence of intrusive traumatic material. Horowitz (1976) describes these efforts as the movement from intrusive to denial phases.

Current Psychodynamic Perspectives

Recent empirical research has permitted us to describe in more detail the variety of ego responses to traumatic stimuli, with special emphasis on dissociative phenomena, splitting, disavowal, and the like. This new research has contributed to our knowledge of how the ego functions when satisfactorily resolving traumatic events and their impacts—namely, through increased emotional expression and the capacity to cognitively restructure those facets of the trauma that have been disturbing (Green et al. 1988). We have additionally become aware of the importance of social supports both during the period of acute trauma and its immediate aftermath and in the long term by virtue of the role of the recovery environment and the expressed attitudes of empathy or estrangement toward the survivor (Lindy and Grace 1985; Solomon 1988).

Childhood trauma has received special recognition. An increasing number of surveys are reporting a higher incidence of childhood trauma and more lasting effects from such trauma than were previously supposed (McNally 1992). Childhood trauma has been implicated in the development of borderline syndrome (Herman et al. 1989) and multiple personality disorder (Kluft 1985), as well as in PTSD. Research has also shed light on the relative role of preexisting childhood trauma in the development of PTSD in adulthood (Helzer et al. 1987), yielding some evidence that the vulnerable individual is more likely to experience the syndrome and less likely to recover promptly from it.

Empirical research highlights the crucial role played by guilt in the sustaining of PTSD symptoms (Pynoos et al. 1987; Terr 1985). Finally, contemporary understandings of PTSD place trauma in the context of an individual's altered assumptive world view (Lindy et al. 1988), fragmented self-structure (Ulman and Brothers 1988), and discontinuous character organization (Lindy et al. 1988). We shall return to some of these issues in the discussion of the case material below.

In recent years, investigators contributing to the psychodynamic understanding of PTSD with case-study data have reported some interesting findings. There is often a specific, dynamic configuration of some aspect of the traumatic event that functions as a core conflictual relationship theme (Luborsky 1984) and is contained within the traumatic experience itself as well as within the individual's affective response to repetitions (Lindy et al. 1988). In Vietnam veterans with PTSD, for example, such configurations may focus on betrayal of individuals in authority and inhibitions to intimacy. Another dynamic feature in other populations' often persistent symptoms of PTSD relate not only to the trauma's conflictual theme but also to earlier conflicts growing out of childhood. The pathogenesis of trauma-related pathology is not a static affair; rather, there is an interaction between affects associated with the trauma (e.g., helplessness and hopelessness) and restorative fantasies (e.g., vengeance, omnipotence, and omniscience) (Ulman and Brothers 1988). Trauma, restorative fantasy, and maladaptation become a dynamic sequence shifting with time (Pynoos and Nader 1988) and circumstance but sometimes become ingrained (Titchener and Kapp 1976). Adults who experience sufficient trauma—even those with previously well-functioning intrapsychic structures—nonetheless can sustain limited damage to those structures. For example, there may be damage in reality testing regarding perception, as in reminders of the traumatic experience; there may be an inability to process strong affects of a type aroused in the traumatic experience; and there may be shattering of one's assumptive world view.

A subject of special interest in the psychotherapy of PTSD is helping survivors to understand the multiple meanings of trauma-based guilt. Initially, a traumatized and bereaved survivor may lament, "If only I had . . . then the [trauma/death] would not have occurred." Later, the survivor may reflect that he is the weaker, less-deserving individual, yet he is alive while the more worthy one is dead. The patient may reflect that this brush with death has altered his life forever. A third possibility that may come to light is that some anger had been surfacing toward the dead friend prior to the accident, and that the survivor may have become so angry that he wished his friend dead. And finally, the survivor patient may reveal that, in fact, he made an important error that played into the traumatic circumstances.

The clinician must separately identify and empathize with each of these types of guilt: *narcissistic guilt* (the unconscious wish to control the uncontrollable), *existential guilt* (the irony of fate, the immediacy of near-death, and the death imprint), *neurotic guilt* (unresolved anger/competition/envy toward the deceased), and the *real guilt* all too often overlooked by the therapist's wish to be prematurely reassuring and accepting.

Psychotherapy with patients with PTSD becomes an intense "laboratory" in which the therapist becomes aware of the crucial roles of dosage and psychoeconomics in his or her interpretive work and learns how patients, through transference and countertransference, unconsciously test the therapist, forcing him or her, as it were, to take on a role in the trauma scene or to become a judge of the survivor's behavior in it (Wilson and Lindy 1994).

Case Example

In the following case illustration, one of the authors (F.M.), a resident in his third year of psychiatric training, narrates his experience working with a trauma survivor with PTSD. He describes how the diagnosis, although not immediately apparent, became clear; how the central role of numbing through somatization unfolded; and how survivor guilt, together with both real and neurotic anger, played central roles in the trauma and the transference. Of the remaining two authors, one (J.L.) supervised the psychotherapy and the other (L.S.) extracted from the case some general principles of dynamic psychiatry, which he presents in the case discussion and summary.

> As a third-year psychiatry resident working in an urban-based university clinic, I had the opportunity to work with a young man who presented with a symptom complex that I came to see as posttraumatically induced.
>
> Mr. K, a 24-year-old fundamentalist Protestant respiratory therapist, was currently disabled. Approximately 30 months before our initial encounter, while living in a West Coast city, he had received an electrical shock during a defibrillation procedure while working with a "code" team on a 42-year-old female patient who was in cardiac distress. He had had both of his hands on the patient's head (the left one on the breathing mask) and did not hear the "clear" signal. He felt nearly im-

mediate pain and then numbness in his left hand and forearm after the incident. He also experienced a headache, recurrent explosive vomiting (shortly after the accident), and intense anger at the doctor manipulating the paddles. The patient died at the scene.

Mr. K reported that these symptoms had worsened over the last 2½ years. On the day of the "code" death, he was seen in the emergency room and subsequently by the neurology, gastroenterology, family practice, and psychology departments. He had finally been given the diagnosis of a conversion disorder after extensive workup revealed no tangible organic factors that could explain the extent of his deficits. Although the mildly positive neurological findings noted shortly after the accident had cleared, he now continued to complain of complete inability to use his left arm effectively for any purpose. He reported that he was unable to hold down solid foods. His pulsating headache would at times force him to become bedridden for days, and did not respond to analgesics.

Psychiatric symptoms included decreased self-esteem, depressed mood, poor sleep and appetite, and anhedonia. He had become isolative and was not interested in friends or in having sexual relations. He had become increasingly dependent on his male roommate of 10 years to do the menial chores around the apartment and to drive him from place to place. He also required help from his roommate to get dressed and bathe each day. Mr. K felt hopelessness to the point of suicidal ideation.

In our initial visit, I was struck by Mr. K's detachment from his feelings. He remained superficial in his affect while he recounted the accident and its sequelae as he saw them. He stated that his previous optimistic outlook on life had been completely transformed to pessimism, but added that he worked very hard to keep this attitude hidden from others, "because so many people depend on me to be happy." He spoke of his fear of "losing my mind," his anger at being given a diagnosis that implied he was "faking," and his humiliation at having to depend on others to get his basic needs met, all with a numb affect. He did become slightly tearful when he mentioned that the worst part of the accident was that the woman died: "I can't get it out of my system, that I had something to do with somebody's death." His thoughts then naturally flowed into his somatic symptoms, which I have disclosed above.

Given the psychic numbing, and the intense feelings of guilt that seemed central to Mr. K's symptoms, I began at that time to consider a diagnosis of PTSD.

J.L., my supervisor, suggested that organizing a formulation around the trauma might help provide the focus for a brief psychotherapy. I then questioned Mr. K and learned of his ongoing, intrusive, repetitive nightmares with themes related to the accident and his tremendous fear of returning to the workplace because of overwhelming anxiety. I agreed that PTSD would be an appropriate working formulation.

When gathering historical data in the initial phase of our work, I learned of Mr. K's adoption in infancy and his overidealization of his adoptive parents. He had come to the conclusion that he had "the best parents anyone could ever ask for," and expressed no outward concern for his biological family. But Mr. K described how his mother could not talk to him at all since the accident because "she had nothing

> to be proud of . . . because I can't do my job anymore." Mr. K also expressed a fear that his mother might "disown" him. A failure/abandonment theme was clear, yet split off. Was failure and loss of his mother's attention related to intolerable feelings regarding the original parent and/or to feelings of failure and loss regarding the coded patient? Was Mr. K's reported reluctance and skepticism to get involved with me representative of this fear of loss?
>
> I also learned of an incident that had occurred 2 years previously, in which Mr. K's father was brought to the hospital with a cardiac arrest and required defibrillation for his resuscitation. Mr. K had never before thought of the possible connection between the related traumatic events.
>
> The likelihood that this defibrillation accident reminded Mr. K in some very important ways of the incident with his father needed to be considered and explored. How does the effect of a "successful" outcome of a trauma (his father lives) interface with an unsuccessful outcome (the coded woman dies).
>
> Through the first several sessions, my primary objective was to respond empathically to Mr. K's dilemma of loss and guilt over the death and shame over his subsequent dependency. In response, Mr. K reported feeling "like the world came off of my shoulders." He also reported a decrease in his depression and in the intensity of his headaches. However, he responded to my 2-week vacation with a return of symptoms even worse than in our first visit.
>
> My importance to Mr. K was intimidating for me. I also began to feel myself struggling with the "credibility" of his physical deficits and feeling increased frustration with his continued focus in the somatic realm and his stubborn reluctance to explore associated psychological factors. I arrived late to two consecutive sessions (inadvertently?).

In the supervisory group, the supervising clinician addressed the resident's frustration in two ways: 1) he suggested that rather than being off target, the somatic symptoms might contain some reference to the patient's private theory as to how the death occurred (i.e., that these symptoms represented a somatic enactment of the trauma), and 2) he pointed out that unexpressed anger, although part of the therapist's experience, might also be central to the patient's dissociated experience both with regard to the accident and at present.

> In session 4, I offered Mr. K a contract for a closed-ended, 15-session brief psychotherapy. This frame provided us with a built-in "loss" within the treatment and the opportunity to work on that issue as we later approached termination.
>
> I explored Mr. K's theory of how the death had occurred. His ideas appeared to be intimately related to the emergence of his somatic symptoms. He thought that by having his hand on the patient's neck and face, he had "stolen the arc from the chest, causing her brain stem to fry." His repetitive, flashback-type nightmare involved his "head exploding" as an outcome of the accident. Perhaps Mr. K was taking on within his own soma the imagined discharge path of the distorted electrical arc.
>
> In my view, Mr. K's headaches were multiply determined. My empathy helped relieve them and my inattention (lateness) made them worse. The headaches' ap-

parent response to tricyclic antidepressant therapy was atypical in its rapidity of onset. Further, I began to see the headaches as representatives of the intolerable feelings (i.e., guilt and shame) that Mr. K was unable to get "out of [his] head" as well as a manifestation of Mr. K's fear of "losing [his] mind."

As Mr. K became more comfortable with me, he also became increasingly capable of expressing his anger at the physician responsible for the shock, whom he firmly believed had never given the "clear" signal. His affect broadened considerably, and in approximately the sixth session, his anger at feeling generally not understood shifted toward the perceived perpetrator of the event, the doctor holding the paddles. I worked hard to encourage and validate the overwhelming feelings that were seemingly being exposed by Mr. K for the first time, and he again responded with symptom relief: "My headaches are tolerable and I'm sleeping better than I have for two and a half years."

Mr. K then told me of his ex-fiance, who had been killed 5 years previously by a drunk driver, and his vigilance since that time to ensure that his friends do not drive after drinking: "That has to be literal hell, knowing that you are the *cause* of someone's death. I don't want to have to live with the guilt of killing somebody."

I pointed out that he *was* indeed living with this kind of guilt.

In the next session, Mr. K expressed a great deal of anger toward me for "making me think about this guilt . . . feeling miserable about what I'd done," and told me that he had cried each night since our last session. He told me of a dream in which "a man's hand come out of a Coke machine, trying to kill me . . . He had a knife and was trying to kill me." (I often drank a Diet Coke during my session with Mr. K.) He expressed a wish for "the doctor to know the pain that I am in." I acknowledged his anger toward me.

Mr. K was then able to recall events of the day of the incident with remarkable clarity and affect. He remembered specific occurrences, nearly to the minute. He expressed anger at the doctor for failing to call "clear" and about the "negative workup" he had received in the other hospital departments. (Perhaps he had been experiencing a "positive" workup within our therapy.)

There was a notable shift in our next session, the tenth. He complained of worsening headaches. Mr. K was afraid that I knew him "more than my best friend," and referred back to his mother who had taught him to be "strong willed . . . not to tell anybody if she wasn't feeling well."

Retrospectively, I see this return of symptoms as a response to his realization that the termination phase of our work was upon us. I had now become very important to him, and my "loss" was imminent. Again, I suspect internal resonance with other important, heartfelt losses in his past, including those of his biological mother, his fiancee, the coded patient, his adoptive mother's attention, and his great fear of being "disowned."

In this session, Mr. K expressed an understanding of the "battle going on within [him]," which I soundly affirmed. He cried, telling me how much it bothered him "to depend on others." A reemergence of the original symptoms took place, including a significant detachment of appropriate affect, and an attempt was made by Mr. K to underestimate the importance of terminating our relationship.

The next three sessions were spread over 5 weeks. In session 12, he reexpressed his fear of being doomed to eternal damnation because of his role in the patient's death.

"What if God feels I am responsible? Will I go to hell?" he asked. "You mean, what if God misinterprets the facts?" I responded. Mr. K continued, "If I could see in an autopsy that her brain stem was not fried, maybe I wouldn't feel so guilty." I said, "So it's possible that your role is not central?" He replied, "You know, I sometimes wish that that doctor would have died instead of the woman."

In our next-to-last session, Mr. K acknowledged that his depression, headache, and weight loss had been considerably improved and that he now felt "near normal." He exhibited a much greater understanding of how somatic symptoms may indeed have important associated psychological factors. He was able to talk directly about his ambivalence regarding our termination, and to accept the termination as fact while being better able to tolerate the feelings of loss.

Mr. K then missed a scheduled session because of the death of an "ex-best friend." He was able to use our last session to acknowledge his newly found ability to manage his grief for his friend and to experience "feelings I've never felt before" at the funeral. He attributed this progress to the work done in our therapy.

Discussion and Summary

In the case study presented above, F.M., the therapist, describes a supervised focal therapy in which the number of sessions was eventually set at 15. His patient, Mr. K, had presented with a number of symptoms, including 1) an inability to use his left arm, 2) an inability to hold down solid food, 3) pulsating headaches that sent him to bed for days, 4) depressed mood with disturbed sleep and appetite, 5) low self-esteem, and 6) increased dependency on others for care. A diagnosis of conversion hysteria had been made by the previous physician.

Mr. K's symptoms plus his report of psychic numbness and his feeling that he had something to do with the woman's death in the particular episode he described led the therapist to consider an unresolved trauma (PTSD). The supervisor suggested that the patient's current state of mind and symptoms might be connected with the traumatic event. Clarifying for the patient the connection between his current symptoms and the traumatic event becomes a helpful organizing principle for sorting out the pieces, and can lead to further information. It is most instructive that the patient revealed upsetting, repetitive nightmares and the intense fear of returning to the workplace where he had been traumatized. The combination of clarifying the event and its associated feelings and of being listened to in a nonjudgmental, accepting manner not only helped the patient feel better immediately ("the world came off my shoulders") but also contributed to the development and solidification of the working alliance so crucial to progress in psychotherapy.

The therapist's departure on vacation led to a disruption of the developing alliance and a return of the symptoms. The patient felt even worse than he had when he started because of the anger mobilized toward the therapist, who had proved unreliable by going off on vacation.

Further supervision helped the resident with his frustration with the patient's continued focus "in the somatic realm and his stubbornness to explore psychological factors." The supervisor's comments gave the resident the cognitive understanding of another meaning that the patient's somatic symptoms might have—that is, that they might contain references to the patient's private theory of what had specifically happened during the traumatic event that led to the woman's death. The resident had felt that the patient's focus on his somatic symptoms represented a nonspecific resistance to exploring psychological factors. In addition, the supervisor pointed out that the resident's anger, while part of his own experience in conducting the therapy, might also reflect the patient's unexpressed anger regarding both the trauma and the current therapy.

Both of these suggestions pointed the resident to the specific nuances of the traumatizing event and the patient's attempt to fathom it. Undischarged anger was most important in that, of the many issues that fix the syndrome of chronic PTSD in place, the traumatic event and the period immediately following it are the most crucial. The individual is unable to appropriately or adequately discharge his or her feelings at the time of the trauma or directly thereafter, as was the case with this patient. Thus, by focusing the patient on the trauma and its aftermath, the therapist in essence forced the patient to reexperience the moments of the trauma—thereby affording the patient an opportunity to discharge his angry feelings and to gain insight into why the episode was indeed traumatic. In the treatment of posttraumatic disorders, the therapist and the patient may have to return to the trauma many times and often from different vantage points. In brief therapy, the therapist's opportunity for such extensive exploration is limited.

As pointed out in the description of this case, exploration of the patient's theory of how the woman died led him to the explanation of the arc that traveled to the patient's brain, causing it to "fry." This explanation helped both patient and therapist to make sense of the patient's repetitive nightmare of his head exploding.

In addition, the resident's understanding of what his own anger might reflect led the patient to express anger toward the physician who conducted the defibrillation procedure. The patient thus became able to express anger directly at the physician, with a resultant improvement in symptoms (i.e., the headaches became more tolerable and he reported sleeping better than he had in the last 2 years).

A key to understanding and treating patients with PTSD in the posttrauma period is the realization that it is not only that the patient was overwhelmed by a specific event or events, but also that a number of forces beyond those operating at the time of the trauma act to fix the syndrome in place. Thus most, if not all, of these contributing motivating or reinforcing forces must be unearthed for the symptoms to abate and for the patient to develop a new perspective about why the traumatic event affected him or her as it did.

During or shortly after a traumatic event, there is occasionally an *excessive* discharge of feeling in action, which represents an attempt to manage the experience of being overwhelmed. These excessive discharges that take place in actions have consequences of their own and often need to be uncovered and dealt with before the trauma itself can be revisited. For instance, Vietnam combat veterans (Lindy et al. 1988) occasionally handled the overwhelming terror they experienced during specific traumas by committing atrocious acts for which they later felt shame or remorse. These conflicts were reinforced by the societal reactions to which the veterans were exposed when they returned to the States.

It is common, after a major piece of psychotherapeutic work has been completed, for an important, related earlier experience—often one of traumatizing proportions—to surface. Reluctance to talk about this earlier event has to be dealt with so that various aspects of that experience can see "the light of day" and the link be made to the precipitating trauma. In this case, the patient, after communicating his theory of how the death occurred and expressing his anger at the physician, revealed another trauma—the accident in which his fiance was killed by a drunk driver. The two traumatic events were connected, and we would have to speculate as to how the deaths of the two women were linked in the patient's mind. There was the suggestion that the patient felt responsible for his fiance's death, in that he worried about his friends drinking while driving for fear that "they might end up feeling responsible for someone's death."

Another event of significance also figures into why the precipitating episode was so traumatic: the defibrillation of the patient's father. The patient responded to the surfacing of his concerns about feeling responsible for killing the woman with intense anger toward the therapist for compelling him to think about the episode and to feel miserable about what he had done. As is typical in these cases, after the two traumas were connected, the patient returned to the precipitating event and recalled the events of that day and of the incident with both remarkable clarity and intense feeling.

An important contributing factor in these cases is the individual's disillusionment and rage with whomever he or she holds responsible for the occurrence of the overwhelming event. These feelings must be worked through. In this particular case, Mr. K held the physician involved during the code responsible. This case material beautifully demonstrates that the patient felt better after expressing anger at the doctor he held responsible. Often, a developmental link can be established to the disillusionment and rage experienced after a trauma. This link is to the early experience of disillusionment with caregivers who did not protect the child from trauma. None of us pass through development without experiencing some of this disillusionment and anger, in that none of us can be completely protected from traumatizing events. In Vietnam veterans, the disillusionment and rage centered on the military and, later on, the government (Lindy et al. 1988). Further aspects of the working through of such disillusionment and rage have to do with understanding how the caregivers in the early environment helped a child after the traumas occurred. Poor handling of childhood trauma predisposes the individual to failure in mastering future traumas—that is, the individual has not internalized those techniques that would help him or her through a future posttraumatic period.

Another complication in working with such patients has to do with whether or not the patient was indeed responsible for the traumatic event that occurred (which was not so in Mr. K's case). If the patient was responsible, he or she must contend with a reality issue. Toward the end of this brief therapy, the therapist helped the patient to deal with these issues. Ultimately, Mr. K was able to see that his role in what happened with the woman who died was not central. This intervention came up after the patient wondered whether God was holding him responsible and whether he would go to hell.

By using formulations regarding PTSD that were developed with the supervisor's assistance, and by intervening empathically within the mode of brief insight-oriented psychotherapy, the resident was able to help the patient to make relevant gains and to experience significant symptom relief. The patient's progress and the overall learning experience with the patient were thus rewarding to student and educator alike.

For Further Study

Grinker RR, Spiegel JP: Men Under Stress, Philadelphia, PA, Blakiston, 1945
Haley S: When the patient reports atrocities: specific treatment considerations of the Vietnam veteran. Arch Gen Psychiatry 30:191–196, 1974
Herman J: Trauma and Recovery. New York, Basic Books, 1992
Kardiner A, Spiegel H: War Stress and Neurotic Illness. New York, Hoeber, 1947
Lifton RJ: Death in Life: Survivors of Hiroshima. New York, Random House, 1967
Lindy J (in collaboration with Green B, Grace M, MacLeod J, Spitz L): Vietnam: A Casebook. New York, Brunner/Mazel, 1988
McCann L, Pearlman LA: Psychological Trauma and the Adult Survivor. New York, Brunner/Mazel, 1990
Pynoos RS, Nader K: Children who witness the sexual assaults of their mothers. J Am Acad Child Adolesc Psychiatry 27:567–572, 1988
Terr LC: Too Scared to Cry. New York: Harper & Row, 1990
Titchener J, Kapp F: Family and character change at Buffalo Creek. Am J Psychiatry 133:295–299, 1976
Ulman R, Brothers D: The Shattered Self. Hillsdale, NJ, Analytic Press, 1988
van der Kolk B (ed): Psychological Trauma. Washington, DC, American Psychiatric Press, 1987

References

American Psychiatric Association: Diagnostic and Statistical Manual of Mental Disorders, 3rd Edition. Washington, DC, American Psychiatric Association, 1980

American Psychiatric Association: Diagnostic and Statistical Manual of Mental Disorders, 3rd Edition, Revised. Washington, DC, American Psychiatric Association, 1987

American Psychiatric Association: Diagnostic and Statistical Manual of Mental Disorders, 4th Edition. Washington, DC, American Psychiatric Association, 1994

DeWind E: The confrontation with death. Int J Psychoanal 49:302–306, 1969

Eitinger L: Organic and psychosomatic after effects of concentration camp imprisonment, in Psychic Traumatization. Edited by Krystal H, Niederland WG. Boston, MA, Little, Brown, 1971, pp 205–215

Freud S: Introduction to psychoanalysis and the war neuroses (1919), in The Standard Edition of the Complete Psychological Works of Sigmund Freud, Vol 17. Translated and edited by Strachey J. London, Hogarth Press, 1959, pp 205–216

Freud S: Beyond the pleasure principle (1920), in The Standard Edition of the Complete Psychological Works of Sigmund Freud, Vol 18. Translated and edited by Strachey J. London, Hogarth Press, 1973, pp 1–64

Green B, Lindy JD, Grace M: Long-term coping with combat stress. Journal of Traumatic Stress 1:399–412, 1988

Haley S: When the patient reports atrocities: specific treatment considerations of the Vietnam veteran. Arch Gen Psychiatry 30:191–196, 1974

Helzer J, Robins L, McEvoy L: PTSD in the general population. N Engl J Med 317:1630–1634, 1987

Herman JL, Perry C, van der Kolk B: Childhood trauma in borderline personality disorder. Am J Psychiatry 146:490–495, 1989

Hoppe K: Psychotherapy with survivors of Nazi persecution. Int J Psychoanal 49:324–329, 1968

Horowitz MJ: Stress Response Syndromes. New York, Jason Aronson, 1976

Janet P: L'automatisme Psychologique. Paris, Balliere, 1889

Krystal H, Niederland WG: Psychic Traumatization. Boston, MA, Little, Brown, 1971

Kluft RP: The natural history of multiple personality disorder, in Childhood Antecedents of Multiple Personality. Edited by Kluft RP. Washington, DC, American Psychiatric Press, 1985, pp 197–238

Klein H: Problems in the psychotherapeutic treatment of Israeli survivors of the holocaust, in Massive Psychic Trauma. Edited by Krystal H. International Universities Press, New York, 1968, pp 98–117

Lindy JD: The trauma membrane and other clinical concepts derived from psychotherapeutic work with survivors of natural disasters. Psychiatric Annals 15:153–159, 1985

Lindy JD, Grace M: The recovery environment: continuing stressor versus healing psychosocial space, in Disasters and Mental Health (DHHS Publ No ADM-85-1421). Edited by Sowder B. Washington, DC, U.S. Government Printing Office, 1985, pp 137–149

Lindy JD, Titchener JL: Acts of God and man: long-term character change in survivors of disaster and the law. Behavioral Sciences and the Law 1:85–96, 1983

Lindy JD (in collaboration with Green B, Grace M, MacLeod J, Spitz L): Vietnam: A Casebook. New York, Brunner/Mazel, 1988

Luborsky L: Principles of Psychoanalytic Psychotherapy: A Manual for Supportive-Expressive Treatment. New York, Basic Books, 1984

McNally RJ: Stressors that produce posttraumatic stress disorder in children, in Posttraumatic Stress Disorder in Review. Edited by Davidson J. Washington, DC, American Psychiatric Press, 1992, pp 57–74

Niederland WG: Clinical observations on the survivor syndrome. Int J Psychoanal 49:313–317, 1968

Pynoos RS, Nader K: Children who witness the sexual assaults of their mothers. J Am Acad Child Adolesc Psychiatry 27:567–572, 1988

Pynoos RS, Frederick C, Nader K: Life threat and post traumatic stress disorder in school-age children. Arch Gen Psychiatry 44:1037–1063, 1987

Schwartz HJ: Psychotherapy of the Combat Veteran. New York, SP Medical & Scientific, 1984

Solomon Z: Coping locus of control, social support and combat-related PTSD. J Pers Soc Psychol 55:279–285, 1988

Terr LC: Psychic trauma in children and adolescents. Psychiatr Clin North Am 8:815–835, 1985

Titchener J, Kapp F: Family and character change at Buffalo Creek. Am J Psychiatry 133:295–299, 1976

Ulman R, Brothers D: The Shattered Self. Hillsdale, NJ, Analytic Press, 1988

Wilson JP, Lindy JD (eds): Countertransference and PTSD. New York, Guilford, 1994

Chapter 18

The Depressed Male Homosexual Patient

Abraham Freedman, M.D.

Homosexual patients, like everyone else, seek treatment because they are experiencing depression, neurotic symptoms, or unhappiness in their life situation. Developmental and constitutional factors are usually enmeshed with these symptoms, as they are with all patients.

One of the major reasons that a person seeks treatment at a particular time is because of a disturbance in the equilibrium established over the course of that person's psychosexual development. For example, an early preoedipal attachment and a lack of healthy individuation render the individual especially sensitive to separation and object loss. Homosexual individuals who are narcissistic frequently see their lovers not only as a representative of themselves but also as that part of themselves that is identified with the early mother figure. These individuals are therefore exquisitely sensitive to the pain of separation and are prone to depression with despair over object loss. Oedipal conflicts may be successfully repressed by the development of a homosexual character structure and can generate neurotic illness when homosexual defenses are interfered with.

Current Psychodynamic Perspectives

Robert Stoller (1968, 1975), who followed children with gender identity problems and their families and supplemented these observations with social and anthropological studies, differentiated psychological gender identity from biological, chromosomal sexual determination. Gender identity might be established at birth when the doctor says to the parents "It's a boy" or "It's a girl." The family and society then treat the growing infant in accordance with its designated sex. Other elements of the family constellation continue to influence the development of the psychosexual orientation of the child. Stoller also studied a variety of variations in gender, including pseudohermaphrodites, whose conscious gender identity does not agree with their anatomic and endocrinological sex. His studies of transsexuals reveal a particular family constellation—that of a narcissistic mother whose male child represents her self-image as a beautiful, phallic female, and an absent or indifferent father. Both constitutional and developmental factors were influential in all of the subjects studied. Stoller's work was not based on the psychoanalysis of individual patients, although some of his subjects were followed in a longitudinal observational study for many years.

Charles Socarides (1978, 1988, 1991) developed his theories from the psychoanalysis of more than 50 homosexuals and over 350 subjects seen in consultation. Like Stoller, he postulated that the developmental problem in homosexuals is tied to a narcissistic mother who does not permit normal separation and individuation in the preoedipal period. Socarides described the heterogeneity of homosexual individuals and divided them into categories according to the quantitative differences between preoedipal and oedipal developmental psychopathology. Both Stoller and Socarides obtained their information from populations seeking treatment.

Differential Dynamic Diagnosis

Both the type of homosexuality and the choice of neurosis are determined by constitutional factors and psychosexual development. Boys with pathological attachment to a narcissistic mother are more likely to have a strong maternal identification and a more feminine personality structure. They will become the preoedipal type of homosexual. In later life, these individuals are more vulnerable to separation and are prone to succumb to depression. Developmental advance to an Oedipus complex, even though later repressed, results in the oedipal type of homosexual with strong phallic narcissism. In later life, individuals with this type of homosexuality are prone to neuroses stemming from castration anxiety and anxiety states. They are more conflicted about homosexuality and might change their sexual orientation under psychodynamic therapy.

Historical Review

The psychoanalytic theory of sexuality began with "Three Essays on the Theory of Sexuality" (S. Freud 1905/1953). The differences between sexual drive, aim, and object are essential to an understanding of psychological development. In infancy, everyone can be said to have been polymorphous perverse, because an infant shows pleasure from stimulation of any erogenous zone by anybody. Gender confusion can be related to an early developmental phase prior to differentiation of sexual aim and object. Freud believed in the universal bisexuality of human nature and that quantitative constitutional and experiential factors determined adult sexual disposition. In the study of a phobia in a 5-year-old boy, Hans (S. Freud 1909/1955), the variants of bisexuality accompanying the positive oedipal complex are clearly demonstrated. The relationship of hysterical fantasies to bisexuality is described in a 1908 paper, and Freud further elaborated on the infantile genital organization in 1923.

Anna Freud discussed the developmental basis of homosexuality in clinical papers written between 1949 and 1952 (A. Freud 1949, 1952, 1949–1950/1952). A general knowledge of various theories that attempt to explain homosexuality cannot be obtained by only reading psychoanalytic papers. A recent survey that can be helpful is Ruse's book, *Homosexuality: A Philosophical Inquiry* (1988), which explores the constitutional, endocrinological, experiential, and sociological origins of homosexuality. A knowledge of psychosexual development is necessary for the treatment of patients with gender confusion or homosexuality. Many excellent papers on the subject have been published in *The Psychoanalytic Study of the Child*—for example, see Greenacre's 1968 paper on the genetic and dynamic background of sexual functioning as well as her 1952 paper on pregenital patterning.

Case Examples

The mode of treatment selected is determined by the character strengths and pathology of the individual patient. Treatment can vary from supportive psychotherapy to full psychoanalysis or any intermediate point on this continuum. In the following case examples, the first patient, suffering from a depression, was treated primarily by supportive psychotherapy, although transference was recognized and partly interpreted. The second patient was also depressed, but early recognition of ego strengths and an oedipal conflict led to the choice of psychoanalytic treatment. The third patient, who had a psychoneurosis, was treated by psychoanalysis and was not only relieved of his neurosis but also had a change in sexual preference.

Case 1

Mr. L, a 60-year-old artist and art teacher, came for treatment with classic symptoms and signs of depression. His lover for the past 15 years, a man about 20 years younger, had recently left him for a younger man. At the same time, Mr. L felt that he was no longer appreciated in the art school where he had been esteemed for the past 30 years. He felt that he had lost his creativity and had no new ideas to express. Mr. L felt alienated from everyone in his family except one sister, who continued to be supportive. Although he had not been close to his mother at the time of her death years earlier, history revealed as the treatment developed that he had been her favorite child, in a large Italian family, and had had a clinging attachment from his earliest years through adolescence. It was only after his homosexuality became obvious and he began to openly have lovers that he had to move out of the family home. Mr. L was able to tolerate his family's rejection of himself and his sexual preference because one sister had become a mother substitute and remained close, and he had successfully formed close identifications as well as mother-child relationships with other homosexual men.

The first part of treatment involved listening sympathetically to Mr. L's tale of desertion and his feelings of hopelessness, despair, devastation, and unrelieved loneliness. All the while, I knew that the patient, in his desperation, would form a therapeutic attachment if given time, because of his propensity to find a substitute for the lost object. As the supportive therapeutic attachment developed, helpful external events began to occur.

His sister, worried by Mr. L's abject appearance, prevailed on other members of the family to become more accepting. He was invited to relatives' homes and treated with concern. At the art school, some of his colleagues began to talk of arranging a retrospective show of his work.

After some restoration of his narcissistic balance, the therapy was able to become more analytic. Mr. L became able to express more anger at the disloyal lover. He was also able to recall his positive relationship with his mother. Unconscious rage at her had interfered with the mourning process when she had died. He had left his mother not only because he had made new attachments but also because she was ashamed of him and had been exhorting him to find a girl and get married. Although Mr. L had remained outwardly fond of his mother and felt close to her, her expressed disappointment in him was a narcissistic blow that had resulted in unconscious rage at her. The negative part of his ambivalence had remained repressed and had to be resolved in the treatment.

It often occurs that the mother in this kind of relationship is ambivalent toward the pathologically bound son; although she needs him, he is also the target of her antagonism toward men. It is not unusual to find such a mother undermining her son's masculinity and then taunting him for not being a man. Although the son needs to cling to the mother, he unconsciously regrets the loss of his autonomy and masculinity, blames her for it, always fears being harmed by women, and is angry at them. This narcissistic damage must be gently and gradually explored in the treatment at a pace determined by the patient's tolerance for experiencing the pain.

It is also to be expected that the ambivalence toward the mother will eventually be expressed in the transference. The feminization resulting from his identification with his mother had been a blow to the patient's masculine narcissism, but was somewhat ameliorated by the availability of the male therapist as a masculine identificatory object. With a female therapist, the revival of heterosexual oedipal fantasies can also aid in the restoration of masculine narcissism.

Toward the end of treatment, the frustration of unfulfillable fantasies added to the negative transference. Mr. L was disappointed by my rejection of his homosexual desires. At the time of treatment, I was a few years younger than the patient and the patient's fantasy was that I would be a replacement for his lost lover. (With a female therapist, he might have experienced the same anger he had had against his mother.) He began to complain that I had really done nothing for him and could do nothing.

As is true with all depressed patients, the therapist's ability to tolerate the patient's recriminations without showing narcissistic injury is an important part of the treatment. Such negative feelings at the end of treatment had been made inevitable by the fostering of an anaclitic relationship at the beginning, which led to the later disappointment. However, it is not possible to begin treatment of a deprived and rejected patient without providing a sympathetic, listening attitude that promises the closeness the patient seeks. Tact and constant understanding are required to change the supportive therapeutic stance into an analytic one, and to help the patient accept the necessity for the therapist's different attitude in each phase of treatment. When this is successfully done in the termination phase of treatment, the recovery can be sustained even though the patient is separated from the therapist. In some cases, the need for a continuation of the supportive relationship cannot be completely resolved, and the patient may have to be seen in interminable therapy with a gradual lengthening of the intervals of separation.

In this case, the treatment began with sessions three times weekly for the first 2 weeks. The therapy was continued with twice-weekly visits for about 1 year and then once-weekly visits for another year. By that time, Mr. L had recovered from his depression and had new homosexual friends, although he had not found another monogamous relationship. The reunion with his family was sustained. He also became reconciled to the process of aging and to some displacement by younger faculty at the art college. He was seen every few months, at his request, over the next few years.

The case of Mr. L represents a depressive syndrome in a narcissistic homosexual patient who has lost a valued object. In many individuals, the symptoms are quickly relieved when another liaison is established. The patient may then find the treatment unnecessary and interrupt it. If the patient has gone through two or more therapeutic attempts following loss of a lover that are interrupted when another lover is found, he might be helped to see the value of continuing psychoanalytic treatment to solve the more basic causes of his difficulties.

The reader will note that nothing has been said about change of sexual orientation in this patient. Such a change would not be a therapeutic goal for a patient unless there was a connection between his character difficulties and his sexuality. It is a matter of therapeutic discernment in each individual case whether sexuality is a component of the treatment. In general, there are two powerful motivations for the patient to avoid the topic of his sexual activity: 1) it represents a successful form of gratification and he does not want to jeopardize his continued ability to have sensual pleasure, and 2) it represents a defense against unknown disturbances and, although the patient is not conscious of what these are, any prospect of character change produces severe anxiety. In this case example, the therapist's acceptance of Mr. L's homosexuality helped to counteract the traumatic fact of his family's rejection of it.

Case 2

Mr. M, a 35-year-old corporate executive, sought treatment because of episodes of feeling like crying and fear that his colleagues would see that something was wrong with him. In the first visit, he did not speak about his sexuality. He described loneliness and a general feeling of unhappiness, although he was doing very well in his career. Mr. M was becoming financially successful and had friends who he believed liked him. He cried during the session and said that showed what he meant, because he could not explain why it happened.

In the second session, held the following day, Mr. M was asked for more details about his friendships, which he had first said were satisfying. He revealed that he did not feel close to anyone. On further questioning about what he wanted from friends, he replied that he yearned to have a man he could feel close to and admitted that he had felt much better after our first session because I seemed to understand him. Mr. M's father lived on a farm about 100 miles from the city. He said that he would like to visit his father but was afraid that this would make his mother angry at him. His mother still lived in the town where he had been born and raised, not far from the father. His parents had separated and divorced when he was about 12 years old. He had stayed with his mother and she did not allow his father to see him. In his early 20s, when he wanted to look up his father, his mother said her feelings were hurt and warned him that she would never feel the same about him if he became friendly with his father. As a result, Mr. M had dropped the idea of contacting him.

Mr. M had a younger, married sister who was now pregnant with her first child. He had occasional contact with her, and she told him that she had told their father about the pregnancy and that the father had visited her. It was about that time that he had noticed the sadness that had brought him into treatment. I asked him how he felt about the father's apparent interest in his sister's pregnancy. Mr. M immediately denied that he was jealous of his sister, that he wanted their father to be interested in a baby of his, and that he ever wanted to have a baby of his own. Rather, he said he felt sad that he never expected to be married or father a child. When queried, he first became silent and then, with great difficulty, told me that he had known he was homosexual from about age 13. Part of his sadness was that he wanted to live a normal life but knew he would never be able to love a woman.

Mr. M was also sad because he had never been able to sustain a relationship with a man. He picked up men in bars and took them to his apartment for sex. Another practice was to have casual sex with men in the park, in the azalea gardens behind the art museum on summer evenings. Recently, there had been muggings of homosexuals in the park as well as arrests for indecency. He knew of stories in the newspapers of homosexuals being murdered by strangers they had taken into their homes. He was fearful not only of being injured or killed but also of being publicly exposed as a homosexual if he became a victim. Mr. M's fears had caused him to try to restrict his homosexual activity, but his attempts to stop it had made him more miserable.

It was now apparent why Mr. M had developed symptoms and had come into treatment at this particular time. He realized that he could neither be what he considered a "functioning male" nor have a baby like his sister. He wanted to be loved by his father but he feared that achieving this would have cost him his mother's love. Events had occurred that made Mr. M's homosexual practices dangerous, and the attempt to reduce his sexual activity for the sake of safety interfered with the defensive function of his homosexuality. He had other aspirations in life, such as career goals and a wish to be what he considered a "normal" man, which he feared were not compatible with his homosexuality.

Mr. M was a high-functioning individual with evidence of a considerably healthy ego. He was a college graduate with an MBA degree, a successful executive, and outwardly socially acceptable. He owned a home in a recently gentrified neighborhood as well as other properties, was respected by his neighbors, and was a leader in community affairs. The brief history obtained in the first few sessions indicated that he had unresolved oedipal conflicts. I offered to treat Mr. M with psychoanalysis and he readily agreed, after some exploration of what the treatment would consist of.

Mr. M had an air of sadness and loss as he lay on the couch and talked about his early life. His father had been drafted into the Army when the patient was about 2 months old. He was told by his mother that she worked as a bank teller in a small town and kept the patient with her during her working hours. He was a good baby who slept peacefully in his carriage and rarely interfered with her duties. In older infancy, he was the pet of other female employees of the bank and he had memories from the age of 3 or 4 of being the center of admiring women. He and his mother were an inseparable duo. When he was about 4 years old, his father returned from the war, but the closeness between Mr. M and his mother continued. He always felt that his mother cared for him much more than for her husband. His father had a farm and also worked intermittently in a local factory. Although his father tried to get him to do "boyish" things such as playing catch, he resisted these activities. His sister had been born the year following the father's return, but Mr. M felt that she had never replaced him as their mother's favorite child. (In his later conversations with his sister as the analysis progressed, she told him of her inability to attract her mother's interest and of her decision early in adolescence to give up the mother as a "hopeless case.")

Strangely enough, although he had not responded to his father's overtures for masculine activities, he became a sort of playmate for his mother, who had tomboyish tendencies. For example, they would play catch or race each other on ice skates. She encouraged him to have a newspaper delivery route by bicycle, and this was built up into a considerable business after the parents separated when he was 12. He felt like the man of the house, supporting his mother.

During the second year of the analysis, Mr. M told me something that had been on his mind for a long time but that he had been too ashamed to divulge. Between the ages of 10 and 12, perhaps earlier, his mother had taught him to wrestle! She taught him holds and they would wrestle together on the living room carpet. There was close body contact. In grasping her around the waist, he would manage to move up to her breasts. At times she would be holding him by the crotch as he was on his hands and knees in a standard position and she was over him. He recalled his mother's face, red with exertion, and her panting. He became aware of strange excitement, would have erections, and would later masturbate while thinking of the wrestling. The wrestling stopped when he was about 15.

In the meantime, Mr. M had begun to wrestle with male friends. He thought of doing this as a high school sport but was afraid of the sexual excitement that might become evident. He would induce younger boys to wrestle with him in private situations and tried to turn these sessions into mutual masturbation experiences. Although he found some submissive boys, other boys resented his seductions and passed word around that he was "queer." He was intensely ashamed and distressed that he was different from other boys. At this time, he believed that he was homosexual. He tried to controvert the public opinion of him by dating girls in high school. He had no difficulty obtaining girl friends: he was good-looking and a good dancer; in addition, he liked girls and preferred talking with them to talking with boys. He even tried to kiss and fondle them, but found that although it seemed interesting at first, he soon became very nervous; he would perspire, his heart would beat furiously, and he was afraid that he would faint. He liked to dance but might get the same symptoms and have to suddenly leave the floor. Because of these symptoms and group disdain, he became more and more reclusive. His mother would try to comfort him in his unhappiness, but he felt afraid to tell her how he really felt or anything about his sexuality. He took to the high school senior prom a girl who had confided in him that she knew what he was but it didn't matter because she couldn't like boys, and she proposed that they could go together to fool the others.

He looked forward to going away to college as an escape from an intolerable situation. There Mr. M carefully maintained a personal distance and a cool, superficial friendliness with classmates. He was thus able to do his work and get along without undue anxiety, although he often felt lonely and sad. By his sophomore year, he found that there were other men who acted seductively toward him. He occasionally had a partner for mutual masturbation but never felt attached to anybody.

Mr. M felt uncomfortable when around his mother; he had a fear of losing her affection and therefore was always afraid of offending her. He carefully tried to avoid contact but usually had to do whatever she wanted when he was with her and agree with her when speaking on the telephone. He had had no contact with his father since the parental separation, although the father lived only a few miles from the mother. The mother insisted that it was a choice without compromise: either her or him!

Mr. M had many long silences on the couch and finally confessed that he had fantasies during these periods. With great difficulty and after many attempted starts, he told me one day that the fantasy began with the wish that I would reach across the couch pillow and put my hand on the back of his neck. After considerable time and effort, I learned that his father would do that when, as a little boy, the patient was sitting in a chair doing his homework, and it would give him a comforting, peaceful sensation, followed by gooseflesh all over his body. He later disclosed that this could only happen if his mother were not in the room. The wish was also connected with being petted by his mother.

About this time in the analysis, Mr. M had begun to ask female business acquaintances and neighbors to dinner and entertainments. He was very gentlemanly and the ladies seemed to like him, but were disappointed when he showed no sexual interest in them. The analysis disclosed that he hoped to please me by showing an interest in women. He wanted to regain the respect of his father, who he felt had always disdained him for being a "mamma's boy" and a "sissy."

Attempts to please the therapist by seeming to become interested in women may occur in the treatment of homosexual men. It is important that the therapist recognize the countertransference component at such times and that the patient not be pushed toward heterosexuality in order to satisfy the therapists' narcissistic wishes or to support the therapists' defenses against his own homosexual conflicts.

As a result of the frustration of his transference wish to have the therapist for a friend, Mr. M began to seek out male friendships for purposes other than his previous brief sexual activity. He made friends among both gay and straight peers; for example, he joined a racquet club to which some of his business colleagues belonged and took lessons in squash and tennis. He met these colleagues in other social situations and escorted a woman friend to make up a couple with the men and their wives.

During this time, Mr. M also talked about his business activities and how he got along with men and women. There was much improvement in his ability to negotiate. Previously, his business tactic had been based on passivity and willingness to quickly surrender a position, but now he was becoming able to be assertive, even with women subordinates, whom he had always feared. He had always gotten along well with most men by being "the nice guy," but now he began to use his intelligence and experience with force and ingenuity and was planning better, reaching goals, and gaining more respect from his superiors.

Some external events occurred that had important effects on Mr. M's progress. His sister was giving a birthday party for her baby. Both children had always respected their mother's wish that they choose her over their father, although Mr. M's sister, unlike him, had remained in contact with their father over the years. During the previous year, Mr. M had become more friendly with his sister, visited often, and enjoyed seeing his little niece. His sister had been told by their mother in no uncertain terms not to invite their father to the party, but sister and brother discussed the problem among themselves. When Mr. M brought the problem into the analysis, I asked him why he and his sister considered the question to be primarily their problem and not their mother's. Did they still need their mother so much more than she needed them? Was it not the sister's privilege to invite whomever she pleased to the party and was it not the invitee's decision to accept or decline? One aim of my questions was to give Mr. M some support against his mother, which he had never had from his father. Subsequently he advised the sister to invite both parents to the party, which she did and, in fact, both parents came! His mother was cordial to both children and polite to her ex-husband. It was the first time Mr. M had seen his father since he was 12 years old. After that, he stayed in touch with his father and enjoyed visiting him on the farm. Somewhat to his surprise, his mother remained friendly to him and accepted his reunion with his father. The father occasionally came into the city to see sporting events and Mr. M began to accompany him. (Toward the end of the analysis, he was contemplating buying a piece of land adjacent to his father's farm that would be suitable as a vacation place.)

Mr. M began to speak about his mother in a more humorous fashion and to enjoy recounting her idiosyncrasies. He also recognized the sexual feelings he had had toward her in childhood and wondered if those experiences had made him afraid of having sexual feelings with a woman. He considered it paradoxical that getting acquainted with his father and liking him was not driving him to seek more sexual attention from other men. His homosexual activity had become less frequent, less frantic, and less dangerous, and was with men with whom he also shared interests and sustained friendships. Mr. M still had a fantasy that someday he might find a man with whom he could have a permanent, intimate, loving, monogamous relationship. At the end of the 3-year analysis, he said that he would like to try making love to a woman but not when he would have to talk to me about it. I told him that although he might have wanted to do this to please me, he also feared that I, as a forbidding father, would not permit it and might punish him for it. Mr. M said that he would think about that and time would tell. In retrospect, I think that he wanted to stop the analysis because he was afraid that it would interfere with his capacity for homosexual pleasure and he was not sure that he could function heterosexually. I now believe that I allowed the analysis to end prematurely and should have pushed further into the resolution of the Oedipus complex.

This analysis illustrates the importance of establishing an accepting, sympathetic therapeutic environment. The patient's identification with his father had been impaired both by events (the 4-year war separation) and by his mother's inability to allow him to separate normally from her. In the treatment, he was able to identify with the male analyst as well as to use the analyst as a substitute for the mother from whom he had become disattached. He reenacted both the loneliness of losing her and the rediscovery of that connection in the transference. His homosexuality was an attempt to restore the mother as well as to satisfy his yearnings for the father he had lost. He recovered from the depression that had brought him into treatment, and made considerable gains in character change and in interpersonal relations. His sexual patterns changed, especially in the regard that sexual activities became a part of object relations and were no longer potentially self-destructive. What about Mr. M's future sexual orientation? We do not know. We know only that his sexuality will be a part of his total person and he will be the better for it.

Case 3

Mr. N, a man in his mid-30s, sought treatment because of a street phobia that hindered his activities and interfered with his ability to go about his work. Several months before the phobia started, he had been arrested by a detective for exposing his penis in a public toilet, in a situation that looked like an entrapment. He had the choice of either paying blackmail to the detective or undergoing a public trial for indecent exposure and solicitation of sodomy. Mr. N had always carefully concealed his homosexuality and feared being disgraced before his family and the public if he followed his wish to actively fight the charges in court. He was afraid of being humiliated if he fought back openly, and resentful of "feeling screwed" repeatedly if he succumbed to the blackmail attempt. He felt that he had been put in a helpless position. His sexual proclivity had been to pick up another homosexual in a park, theater, or other public place and then go somewhere with him to quickly have fellatio. Mr. N was now afraid to be on the street looking for a homosexual partner, and that fear had spread to the general situation of being on the street for any reason. He was particularly afraid of crossing streets and feared being hit by a truck. Being hit by a truck was a metaphor he had used to describe his feeling when the detective showed his badge and arrested him.

Although Mr. N had come to treatment specifically for the treatment of the phobia and anxiety, he talked about his homosexuality at the second interview and said that he knew he was homosexual from his teens but always had a wish that he had been what he called "normal." He was willing to have psychoanalytic treatment because he wished to understand himself better and to have more control over his life. However, Mr. N also feared that the analyst would have too much control over him. He imagined that after he was helplessly embroiled in the analysis, his fee would be raised and he would be able to do nothing about it. He was afraid of being "screwed" by the analyst.

Mr. N was the youngest of five children and had a sister and three brothers. His mother had phlebitis when he was born and was thereafter chronically crippled by a painful, swollen leg. He believed that she blamed him for her illness and that he was supposed to make it up to her. He was her favorite child and she always kept him close to her. As a small child, he was frequently in her bed and remembered from an early age his revulsion at seeing her swollen, discolored leg. Later, he remembered seeing the discoloration to the top of her thigh and glimpses of her genitals under her nightgown, which to him looked even more horrible and disgusting. As a boy, Mr. N tried to help his mother around the house because she complained about the pain in her leg. He helped with the housework, and he felt that he was treated like a younger daughter. His older brothers were "macho" and had disdain for "the sissy."

As a schoolboy, Mr. N looked for opportunities to urinate with other boys and to engage in mutual masturbation. In his early teens, he tried to take out girls as he was expected to do, but found that he was both disinterested in and afraid of them. He remembered being disgusted when a more sexually aggressive girl put her tongue in his mouth when she kissed him. In college, Mr. N began to have mutual masturbation experiences with other men and particularly sought out such experiences if he felt anxious about anything. Later, the desired act became fellatio, and he developed a fantasy that was satisfying no matter which role he played. He imagined that if he took the other man's penis into his mouth, he was taking the masculine strength from him and the ejaculate was a transfusion of power. However, if the other man sucked his penis, he would be humiliating the other man and proving his own superiority as a man. In the time from the casual pickup to the act, he would be ruminating on which way he wanted it to go, but he had it worked out that he was the victor either way. Later in the analysis, Mr. N had a more permanent lover, a college professor. Sex with this lover was infrequent because the patient always felt guilty about taking advantage of his friend in his persistent fantasy of either stealing strength from or humiliating the other man.

If a sexual partner were insistent, Mr. N might have anal intercourse, but he liked it less than fellatio. If he penetrated, he would be bothered by getting feces on his penis, although he had the feeling that he had overcome the other man. If he were the recipient, he would fantasize that he had incorporated the strength of the other man as in fellatio, but he could not overcome a feeling of humiliation and powerlessness if he were penetrated, and he disliked the feeling of being used "like a woman." During the act, Mr. N would have visual images of his mother's "big behind." He believed that he had seen his parents have intercourse in this way.

There were several transference transactions that showed Mr. N's conflicts over feeling feminized by homosexuality. He often complained of a sore back, and his posture was usually upright and rigid. I noticed that his rigidity was maintained even while lying on the couch, and that at the end of each hour, his back seemed even more stiff as he arose from the couch. When this rigidity was called to his attention, he admitted that he kept his buttocks tightly held together as well as tightening his back muscles. He was trying to keep his anus closed so that the analyst could not penetrate it. He also felt that anything I might say or interpret would represent a kind of penetration. The sore back was relieved after these insights.

One day, as I was driving to our 8:00 A.M. appointment, my car was struck lightly in the back bumper by a delivery truck at a downtown stop sign. I got out, saw there was no damage, and proceeded to the garage. When he was on the couch that morning, Mr. N said that he was walking on the street to my office and had seen the accident. He was amazed that I did not seem upset, but instead acted very calmly, got back into my car, and drove away. He would have been enraged. He said that he wished he could have handled such a situation as I had done. The next day, Mr. N reported a dream in which he was driving his mother's car and it had been badly damaged from being struck from behind. The car was a big sedan that his mother had kept after his father had died, although she did not drive. He had used it before he had bought his own car. She still had this sedan and he occasionally drove her in it. Its big rear reminded him of his mother's "big behind." A few days later, Mr. N had gone to a business meeting at a hotel. The parking lot attendant offered to park his car for him, but he said he would park it himself. He misjudged the distance and damaged the rear of his car when he backed it forcefully into a wall. He felt humiliated and emasculated by the incident.

Continued discussion of the transference conflictual wish to be penetrated by the analyst led to a realization that an important part of Mr. N's homosexuality was an effort to restore his damaged masculinity and to have a good penis, but the homosexual acts that followed made him fear that he would become a woman. He had identified with his mother but did not want to be like her. Also, being a woman meant not having a penis, a condition that made him shudder. When I reminded him that he had expressed a wish to be able to act like I had when my car was struck from behind, Mr. N admitted that he admired me and wanted to be like me. I asked whether he had ever wanted to be like his father or brothers. At first he said that he had hated his father and had never wanted to be like him. He recalled that he thought his mother loved him more than she loved his father, and he feared that his father wanted to get rid of him because of this. There were many times when his father had carried him, against his protests, out of the mother's bed and then got into bed with her himself. The boy had greatly resented his father at those times.

Mr. N's father was a cabinetmaker with his own shop. All the sons were brought into the shop as preteens to work as apprentices. Mr. N said that he hated the work. He would be given the task of sanding a leg for a chair and his father would make him go over the work endlessly, and would be hard to please. He would sit sullenly in a corner, sanding and having fantasies of throwing the piece at his father. His older brothers would be doing more advanced work and were constantly teasing him about being a "weak sissy." He would rather have been at home helping his mother with the housework.

When Mr. N was in his second year of college, his father died. He recalled that he had been called out of a class and told to go to a hospital to which his father had been taken. When he arrived, he found that his father had already died of a heart attack. He was shocked and intensely angry that he had not been prepared for what had happened. He was surprised that he was disappointed at not seeing his father before he died, because he thought that he hated his father. Then he had cried and sobbed and was again puzzled by his emotions.

As memories of the wood shop were recalled in more detail, Mr. N admitted that he admired his father's artistry, skill, and strength. In his spare time, he used to go to furniture auctions. He said that he liked antiques and was interested in interior design. He was not looking for anything in particular when he went to these, and he seldom entered into the bidding. After the emergence of memories of his father's shop, Mr. N was at an auction and asked to examine a small chest with an inlaid pattern of interesting woods. He was delighted when he found his father's benchmark on the piece, and he successfully bid for it. After that, he went more frequently to antique shops and auctions, consciously looking to buy pieces that had his father's benchmark.

About this time, Mr. N decided to move out of his mother's home. His decision was supported by his sister, who promised to spend more of her time visiting their mother. He hired a part-time housekeeper for his mother and continued to go there to take care of the grounds for her. His new apartment building included an area where tenants could have their own space for a hobby. He cleaned up some of his father's tools that had been left in his mother's basement and bought new tools. He set up a woodworking shop and derived much satisfaction in the work. Mr. N could see that he was identifying with his father. Friends and relatives, to whom he gave the pieces he made, were admiring and appreciative. During this time, his casual homosexual activity was greatly reduced.

The legal case had been settled by an agreement between his lawyer and the prosecutor, and Mr. N had paid a small fine and been placed on probation without a public hearing or publicity. His phobic and anxiety symptoms had dissipated. He attributed this improvement to his relief over the cessation of the prosecution, but later acknowledged that the understanding and resolution of his conflicts had also been helpful. It was still difficult for Mr. N to admit that the analyst could do anything for him. His relationship with his friend was also losing its sexual aspects and he felt guilty, as if he had abandoned him. These feelings were related to the guilt of abandoning his mother and perhaps also his father.

Over the years, Mr. N's sister had often introduced him to her girlfriends and encouraged him to take them out, but he was reluctant. Now, he began to date one of her friends, but was not entirely comfortable. He thought that the woman was too close to his sister. About a month after a summer vacation period, Mr. N told me that he had attempted intercourse with a woman while I was away but had lost his erection. He had delayed telling me about it for two reasons: first, he felt emasculated if he had to admit his impotence, which meant sexual inferiority to me; and second, he feared that I would disapprove of his trying to take advantage of a woman and would in some way punish him for it. He said "How would you feel if she turned out to be someone in your family?" Mr. N had a dream in which a sexual offense against a woman had been discovered by her father. In the dream, the woman's father had had a beard. This was the summer when I had grown a beard on vacation and kept it when I returned to practice (see Freedman 1970). When I questioned him about his associations to the bearded man in the dream, he had none. When I asked him if it had anything to do with my beard, he said that that was ridiculous because I did not have a beard. He was astounded when he turned around on the couch and looked at me. He had not noticed my beard for the few weeks since the analysis had been resumed.

The oedipal transference situation resulted in many discussions and recall about his own Oedipus complex and led to the beginning of its resolution. Mr. N later met a woman who lived in a nearby city and did not know anyone in his family. He became engaged to marry her after dating her for about 6 months. He lost interest in further analysis, stating that there were too many other things to occupy his time, such as traveling to see his fiancee, and we terminated about a month before the marriage date. He said that he would contact me if there were any difficulties, but I never heard from him again.

In this patient, there was an early identification with the mother, but there was also an Oedipus complex with sexual wishes toward the mother and fear of a threatening father. The identification with the father had been repressed, and the oedipal conflict was left unresolved. Although the patient's defenses depended on the feminine identification, there was an unconscious masculine push that made this identification conflictual. The patient's homosexual activity had the defensive value of protecting against castration anxiety and restoring the damaged penis, as well as providing sexual satisfaction. The equilibrium was upset by the entrapment incident, which threatened Mr. N's homosexual defenses and stimulated the fears of emasculation and consequent humiliation.

In the analysis, the patient's identification with his mother was replaced by an identification with the analyst that did not interfere with the patient's autonomy. His conflicts over masculine and feminine strivings became conscious as they appeared in the transference, and his predominant choice was for masculinity. Also, his negative feelings toward his father gave way to an acknowledgment of his ambivalence and, finally, to a realization of his wish to identify with his father. As these changes occurred, he began having heterosexual wishes. The oedipal situation was revived in the transference and could now be resolved.

Summary

The case examples in this chapter have shown how preoedipal and oedipal psychosexual development can be reconstructed within the psychodynamic or psychoanalytic treatment of depressed homosexual patients, regardless of the presence of any other factors such as constitutional predisposition. Patients who have a preponderance of preoedipal psychopathology tend to have strong maternal identifications and a proneness to depression, as did Mr. L. Patients with a preponderance of oedipal psychopathology have more overt neurotic conflicts and symptoms like those seen in Mr. N. Finally, many patients have psychopathology derived from both sources, as was true for Mr. M. The transference can evoke the reenactment of the patient's earlier relations with each parent. Identification with a male therapist or revival of oedipal wishes with a female therapist occurs in the transference and can be therapeutically useful. The treatment can vary from supportive to analytic, depending on the nature of the patient and his psychopathology.

For Further Study

Freedman A: A psychoanalytic study of an unusual perversion. J Am Psychoanal Assoc 26:749–766, 1978

Freedman A, Slap J: A functional classification of identification. Bulletin of the Philadelphia Association for Psychoanalysis 10:37–49, 1960

Freud A: The Ego and the Mechanisms of Defense. London, Hogarth Press, 1937

Freud A: Some clinical remarks concerning the treatment of cases of male homosexuality. Int J Psychoanal 30:195–204, 1949

Freud A: Homosexuality. Bulletin of the Philadelphia Association for Psychoanalysis 7:117–118, 1952

Freud A: Studies in passivity (1949–1950), in The Writings of Anna Freud, Vol 4. New York, International Universities Press, 1952, pp 245–259

Freud S: Three essays on a theory of sexuality (1905), in The Standard Edition of the Complete Psychological Works of Sigmund Freud, Vol 7. Translated and edited by Strachey J. London, Hogarth Press, 1953, pp 125–245

Greenacre P: Pregenital patterning. Int J Psychoanal 33:410–415, 1952

Greenacre P: Perversions: general considerations regarding their genetic and dynamic background. Psychoanal Study Child 31:47–63, 1968

Isay RA: The development of sexual identity in homosexual men. Psychoanal Study Child 41:467–484, 1986

Lipton S: On the psychology of childhood tonsillectomy. Psychoanal Study Child 17:367–417, 1962

Lochstein LN: Female to Male Transsexualism. Boston, MA, Routledge & Kegan Paul, 1983

Morganthaler F: Homosexuality, heterosexuality, perversion. Hillsdale, NJ, Analytic Press, 1988

Ruse M: Homosexuality: A Philosophical Inquiry. New York, Basil Blackwell, 1988

Socarides C: Homosexuality. Northvale, NJ, Jason Aronson, 1978

Socarides C: The Preoedipal Origin and Psychoanalytic Therapy of Sexual Perversion. Madison, CT, International Universities Press, 1988

Socarides C: The Homosexualities and the Therapeutic Process. Madison, CT, International Universities Press, 1991

References

Freedman A: The effect of a change in the analyst's visage on transference. Bulletin of the Philadelphia Association for Psychoanalysis 2:117–130, 1970

Freud A: Some clinical remarks concerning the treatment of cases of male homosexuality. Int J Psychoanal 30:195–204, 1949

Freud A: Homosexuality. Bulletin of the Philadelphia Association for Psychoanalysis 7:117–118, 1952

Freud A: Studies in passivity (1949–1950), in The Writings of Anna Freud, Vol 4. New York, International Universities Press, 1952, pp 245–259

Freud S: Three essays on a theory of sexuality (1905), in The Standard Edition of the Complete Psychological Works of Sigmund Freud, Vol 7. Translated and edited by Strachey J. London, Hogarth Press, 1953, pp 125–245

Freud S: Hysterical fantasies and their relationship to bisexuality (1908), in The Standard Edition of the Complete Psychological Works of Sigmund Freud, Vol 9. Translated and edited by Strachey J. London, Hogarth Press, 1959, pp 155–167

Freud S: Analysis of a phobia in a five year old boy (1909), in The Standard Edition of the Complete Psychological Works of Sigmund Freud, Vol 10. Translated and edited by Strachey J. London, Hogarth Press, 1955, pp 1–149

Freud S: The infantile genital organization (1923), in The Standard Edition of the Complete Psychological Works of Sigmund Freud, Vol 19. Translated and edited by Strachey J. London, Hogarth Press, 1961, pp 141–147

Greenacre P: Pregenital patterning. Int J Psychoanal 33:410–415, 1952

Greenacre P: Perversions: general considerations regarding their genetic and dynamic background. Psychoanal Study Child 31:47–63, 1968

Ruse M: Homosexuality: A Philosophical Inquiry. New York, Basil Blackwell, 1988

Socarides C: Homosexuality. Northvale, NJ, Jason Aronson, 1978

Socarides C: The Preoedipal Origin and Psychoanalytic Therapy of Sexual Perversion. Madison, CT, International Universities Press, 1988

Socarides C: The Homosexualities and the Therapeutic Process. Madison, CT, International Universities Press, 1991

Stoller C: Sex and Gender. Northvale, NJ, Jason Aronson, 1968

Stoller C: Sex and Gender, Vol 2: The Transsexual Experiment. Northvale, NJ, Jason Aronson, 1975

Chapter 19

The Patient With a History of Childhood Sexual Abuse or Incest

Howard B. Levine, M.D.

Current Psychodynamic Perspectives

Childhood sexual abuse is defined as

> the involvement of dependent, developmentally immature children in sexual activity that they do not fully comprehend, without consideration for the child's stage of psychosocial sexual development. [This can occur in many forms and] at any age from infancy through adolescence with various family members, relatives or strangers. It can be a single, isolated incident or repeated frequently over many years. It may be homosexual or heterosexual with either girls or boys, and involve anything from fondling to full genital intercourse or variations of oral and anal contact. It may be done with some degree of love and gentleness or involve verbal threats and physical violence. All of these variables have a bearing on what the sexual experience means to the child and how it is woven into the child's psychic development and affects later behavior. . . . [T]he sexual events themselves are not the simple, direct cause of subsequent difficulties. . . . The trouble comes when the sexual activities are instigated by a person older than the child and are beyond the child's

---

Portions of this chapter were adapted from Levine HB (ed): *Adult Analysis and Childhood Sexual Abuse.* Hillsdale, NJ, Analytic Press, 1990.

> ability to truly understand or emotionally manage the affects and conflicts that are generated. The activity is not a consensual one between peers but is exploitative, more for the satisfaction of the perpetrator than the child victim. . . . [T]he degree of trauma is related to the discrepancy between the intensity of the noxious stimulae and the ability of the child's ego to cope. (Steele 1990, pp. 21–22)

The broad range of possible variables involved in childhood sexual trauma means that adults who were sexually abused as children are members of a heterogeneous group that defies simple categorization. Reports in the literature (e.g., Bernstein 1990; Bryer et al. 1987; Burland and Raskin 1990; Deblinger et al. 1989; Goodwin et al. 1979; Levine 1990; Lindberg and Distad 1985; Shengold 1989; Steele and Alexander 1981) document a wide variety of adult symptomatic consequences of childhood sexual trauma. These include depression, low self-esteem, phobias and anxiety states, impulsive or self-punitive behaviors, eating disorders, learning disabilities, cognitive dysfunctions, self-doubting and confusional states, promiscuity, seductive behavior, sexual inhibitions and dysfunctions, distrust of others, depersonalization, dissociative phenomena, psychosomatic symptoms, and self-destructive or self-mutilating reactions.

Many of the symptoms encountered are related to the patients' reliance upon a repertoire of dissociative defense mechanisms, such as ego splitting, denial, and dissociation, which follow from the injured child's attempts to control or eliminate the overwhelming, traumatic stimulation by averting their attention, both at the time of the injury and subsequently at such moments when the trauma might be recalled. The long-term effects of these defenses may range from a true forgetting (repression) of the trauma to a failure to take its emotional consequences into account (disavowal, denial, or splitting). At times, the neglected or forgotten memories may return in dissociated or symbolic forms, contributing to such phenomena as psychosomatic symptoms, sexual dysfunctions, nightmares, panic attacks, and impulsive behaviors. Many of these phenomena contribute to or constitute some of the familiar "flashback" experiences described in the literature on posttraumatic stress disorder (PTSD).

The effect of repressed or dissociated memories of childhood sexual trauma on adult sexual functioning may be particularly striking. Often, the memories "return" during foreplay, intromission, or coitus in the form of disturbed bodily sensations. The latter may range from displeasure, aversion, or physical pain to muted feelings, frigidity, and anorgasmia, or patients may report feeling incomprehensibly furious during lovemaking, even when they had initiated or consented to the sexual act.

Kramer (1990) called these physical sensations—which can persist throughout adulthood and which she believed often followed from childhood incestuous contact with either father or mother—"somatic memories."

In the contemporary psychoanalytic view, the ways in which individuals experience, adapt to, remember, and transform their memories of significant childhood events in the course of their development are complex and multidetermined (Kris 1956). The ultimate meaning that a childhood traumatic experience—sexual or otherwise—will come to have for an adult extends beyond the details of the actual trauma itself to include 1) how the trauma was experienced by the child in line with pretraumatic and ongoing developmental issues and conflicts; 2) elements of the various ways in which the trauma was responded to by the child and its network of supportive objects—that is, the ways in which the trauma was elaborated in the child's fantasy and play, how the trauma was connected with the child's character and symptom formation (including the regressive reversal of previously obtained levels of development), and whether or not the child was believed by others or helped by them to deal with the trauma; 3) contributions of the trauma to subsequent developmental disturbances; and 4) how the affects and memory traces connected with the trauma underwent repression, distortion, and symbolic elaboration.[1] Consequently, a positive history of a childhood sexual trauma is not correlated with any one particular type of character structure, but rather may be associated with neurotic, borderline, or psychotic features. In therapy, the childhood trauma may be reported, repressed, or knowingly withheld by a patient in the course of an evaluation or even a lengthy treatment. Given this wide range of possibilities, it is particularly important not to prejudge the meaning or impact of a given traumatic experience on an individual patient. Rather, one must try to understand each patient's uniquely subjective response to his or her own life experiences.

Despite the extraordinary degree of symptomatic variation noted in adults who were sexually abused in childhood, a broad area of common dynamic issues exists that unites these patients, determines the kinds of clinical challenges that they may present to the psychotherapist, and warrants their being studied as a group. The most significant common feature among these patients is the way in which the memory of the trauma and its associated events seems to unconsciously organize and inform their experience of virtually every relationship of any import. This is particularly true of the transference relationship, wherein patients who were sexually traumatized in childhood can encounter an enormous pressure to reexperience and relive aspects of the sexual abuse in ways that range from the symbolic (e.g., a fantasy that a therapist is being manipulative and dishonest for his or her own purposes) to the literal and concrete (e.g., attempts to seduce the therapist or other people in the patient's life or to engage them in corrupt or shady dealings). Often, elements of symbolic repetition are noted to occur around boundary issues that may arise either in the therapy (e.g., in the handling of insurance payments, clinic fees, or negotiations around hours) or in the patient's outside life (e.g., a special sensitivity to ferreting out or accusing others of perverse, corrupt, or abusive behavior).

The strong pressure to repeat—coupled with a tendency to reenact rather than remember (Freud 1914/1958)—may leave these patients particularly vul-

---

[1]For an illustration and discussion of these complex developmental issues, see Levine (1990), especially pp. 11–17.

nerable to becoming sexually involved with their therapist (Smith 1984) or to becoming masochistically enthralled by a charismatic therapist, who may use them in a narcissistically appropriating, self-gratifying manner. Although this latter kind of exploitation may not go so far as to include actual physical or sexual relations between therapist and patient, the elements of transgression of boundaries and symbolic reenactment of the trauma are evident.

At times, the compulsion to repeat the trauma may be so powerful and the line between reality and fantasy so tenuously drawn that the "as if," illusory quality of the transference may disappear (Levine 1982). At that point, for the patient, *the experience of the therapy situation may feel like or even become the trauma.* Patients may, either consciously or unconsciously, fail to distinguish between the therapist's attempts to help them talk about the past trauma and the trauma itself. Thus, they may believe that the therapist is hurting them, intruding on their privacy, becoming voyeuristically invested in the gruesome or exciting details of their childhood sexual experiences, using them for his or her own pleasure, or failing to protect them from the pain of remembering. In this regard, the quality of the transferences that develop in these cases can, at times, be more akin to transference psychoses than to the usual neurotic transferences.

A brief summary of 2 hours from the treatment of a patient who had been incestuously involved with both parents may further illustrate these phenomena:

> The patient, Ms. O, a woman in her mid-30s, began the hour by expressing concerns about a relative's behavior at a family party. Elements of this behavior led associatively to memories of how, when the patient was between 3 and 5 years old, her mother would use the patient's body to masturbate herself. Further thoughts led to pleasant memories of childhood visits to the rodeo with her family and of her pleasure and excitement at watching the calf roping. Next, Ms. O thought of how "tied" she still was to her parents and her traumatic past—how both parents had tied her to them, greedily appropriating her childhood for their own sexual and narcissistic pleasure. The image of the calves with their legs tied up then gave way to the image of her father holding down her hands and arms as he molested her. As she talked, she became quite anxious and upset, unconsciously assuming on the couch the posture she was describing—writhing while holding her hands behind her over her head.
>
> In the next hour, Ms. O was afraid to go further. She reported that following the previous hour, she had been terribly anxious and depressed all day. The memories of the incest had disorganized her thinking. She feared seducing the analyst or being seduced or taken advantage of by him. She worried that the material of the last hour—or the dialogue taking place at that very moment—might be the prelude to a seduction.

For each belief about the therapist's motivations that the patient develops as part of the transference, the therapist is susceptible to parallel feelings (countertransference). Thus, it is not unusual for the therapist to find him- or herself at various times feeling stimulated, tempted, repelled, judgmental, identified with, or protective toward the patient. Although such feelings are better recognized and attended to by the therapist alone in the privacy of his or her own personal treatment, self-reflection, or supervision, the fact of their being engendered and felt, often as an impulse to reciprocal action, is an expectable, almost inevitable part of the treatment process.[2] The expectation that such countertransference feelings will be a normative part of the therapy experience can alert the therapist to the likelihood of their appearance and allow him or her to judiciously use their presence as further data about the quality and meaning of the patient's transference relatedness.

It is important to recognize that no matter how great the pressure that a patient may feel internally or attempt to mobilize in the therapist to literally or symbolically reenact the transgression of a childhood sexual trauma, *under no circumstances is it appropriate for the therapist to offer direct gratification of the patient's wishes for a symbolically or literally corrupt or physically gratifying relationship.* To do so not only would repeat the traumatic past in the therapy but also would constitute a violation of the patient's rights in the present and a breach of therapeutic ethics and responsibility.

It is not yet clear why childhood sexual traumata exert this almost magnetlike effect on the unconscious minds of some patients and not others. A similar phenomenon has been observed in other, nonsexual, situations of significant early childhood trauma, such as early parent loss and, to a lesser extent, in the analysis of children of survivors of the Holocaust (Levine 1982). One suggested explanation for its occurrence (Levine 1990) is that it follows in part from the child's traumatic loss of the sense of an omnipotent, protective parent in situations of severe early childhood trauma. This feeling of loss of parental protection, which is an important part of the "basic trust" (Erikson 1954) or "background of safety" (Sandler 1960) on which the unfolding of the psychotherapeutic process depends, is an important concomitant of severe childhood sexual trauma. Its appearance is particularly striking among those adults who experienced parental incest or repeated or violent sexual abuse in childhood.

The feelings of lost protection often become connected in the patient's inner world with intense conflicts over abandonment and separation. In such instances, patients may be so vulnerable to feeling abandoned that they cling desperately and masochistically to an intrusive, cruel, seductive, or neglectful relationship (see Valenstein 1973). As noted by Steele (1990), many victims of paternal incest have suffered pretraumatic deprivations in the mother-child relationship, making the overtly incestuous object tie with the father their best or only source of comfort or warmth. The fact that so many of these patients seem particularly vulnerable to feeling abandoned in times of separation and loss emphasizes the need for careful working through of such issues in the transference.

In instances of parental incest, the roots of the trust issue are further complicated by the central role that the parents play in the development and mainte-

---

[2]See Sandler's (1976) discussion of the therapist's "role responsiveness."

nance of the child's sense of morality and reality (see Ferenczi 1933). It is important for therapists to bear in mind that, although it has been reported with a lesser frequency, mothers may also be the perpetrators of childhood sexual abuse.[3] When they are, maternal overstimulation (Shengold 1989) and narcissistic appropriation of the child for the mother's gratification, even in the absence of cruelty and neglect, may simultaneously be experienced by the child as a traumatic abandonment and a loss of parental protection.

Many times, paternal incest occurs in the setting of a preexisting state of relative maternal deprivation; that is, a maternally deprived child may turn to a father as a compensatory substitute for warmth, gratification, and protection. The father may also feel deprived—in his relationship with his wife and/or in his own childhood relation to his mother. The result is a father-child pair in which the prospect of closeness can readily stimulate intense, frustrated archaic needs for closeness. In such a pair, if these needs become erotized and the adult's controls are weakened by psychosis, alcoholism, psychopathy, impulsiveness, or the like, the danger of incestuous action becomes heightened. Then, should the incestuous breach occur, it may carry with it for the child the important intrapsychic meanings of the repetition of the loss of the protecting, nurturing mother and the loss or destruction of the father as a life-giving object and a substitute source of nurturance, protection, and attachment.

This possibility of a preexisting maternal deprivation makes it difficult to separate the extent to which such findings as mistrust, fear of closeness, and difficulties in reality testing or in establishing a conviction about what one knows to be true are functions of a childhood sexual trauma per se or are related to pretraumatic events within a disordered mother-infant relationship. The importance of this issue in the treatment of adults who as children were involved in incestuous relationships with their parents is, however, attested to by the fact that the exploration and affective reliving of the incest trauma often becomes engaged around an actual separation from the therapist in the context of the patient's experiencing a sense of safety in the therapeutic relationship. That is, even in those instances in which a consciously recalled memory of incest is part of the patient's presentation in the therapy, the issue may not be affectively engaged in the therapy until the patient experiences a bond of security, safety, or trust in the therapeutic relationship and that bond is threatened by an interruption, such as a vacation or other extended absence. It is at this point—on the brink of feeling "abandoned" during the period of impending separation—that the patient may begin to painfully and affectfully recall aspects of the childhood trauma or even initiate a precipitous action related to that trauma, such as the decision to confront his or her parents about its occurrence. The result of either course of action may be to inadvertently and unconsciously create a situation in which the patient feels overwrought and unprotected by the therapist, much as the patient must have felt during the original traumatic episode.

---

[3]See Kramer (1983, 1990) and Margolis (1991) for a further discussion of maternal incest.

The mode of organizing one's psyche around conflicts and derivatives of the childhood sexual trauma has enormous implications not only for the nature of the transference that unfolds but also for the difficulties encountered in the development of a therapeutic alliance. As Raphling (1990) has described, these patients are liable to demonstrate a fierce resistance to the formation of a therapeutic alliance. This resistance is partly based on the intense pressure to repeat or to reexperience the trauma that arises whenever a close relationship is at hand. Patients cannot trust themselves or their therapists not to engage in illicit, symbolic, or actual traumatic repetitions of the childhood abuse. The patient's distinctions between fantasy and reality, past and present, and remembering and reliving may be either threatened or lost. Adult, cooperative parts of the patient's ego, including the capacities for self-observation and the formation of a therapeutic split, are often overwhelmed by the intrusion of powerful negative and/or erotic transferences.

The formation of a therapeutic alliance not only necessitates the patient's emotional investment in and recognition of the presence of another object, with all of the dangers of injury, seduction, and betrayal that that entails, but also ultimately requires an acknowledgment of previously unacceptable sexual and angry feelings and a relinquishment of characteristic defensive stances against these, such as entitlement, projection, blaming the abusers, and clinging to a self-definition as victim.

It is not unusual for patients who were sexually abused as children to maintain a relationship to the therapist that is marked by a defensive counterdependency and self-sufficiency for very long periods of time or to defensively rely on a self-defined—and socially supported—role as "victim." The exploration of this position must be handled with particular sensitivity. The sexually traumatized child *was* victimized by the adult—and, in today's society, there is enormous cultural support for viewing adults who were sexually abused as children only as "victims." (Note the commonly used term "survivors" of incest.) In attempting to explore the defensive uses to which a patient may be trying to put the childhood sexual abuse in the current treatment, a therapist must be sensitive to these cultural forces and take care not to fall into the stereotyped role of blaming the victim.

From a *moral* point of view, in the adult-child relationship, the burden of restraint lies with the adult, who has a clear responsibility to care for and protect the child. In this sense, these patients were the victims of their seducers. At the same time, from an *analytic* point of view, we must not lose sight of either the defensive uses to which a patient may put the victim status or the wishful components that may have been unconscious motivational factors in the childhood sexual encounter (e.g., see Greenacre 1950). Alternatively, some patients may attempt to protect their emotional attachment to an abusing parent by denying the extent of the damage done by the inappropriate sexual behavior. (Such denial is easier to maintain if the sexual aspects of the approach were attenuated—for example, overstimulation without penetration or invasive fondling—and were made in a warm and "loving" manner.) For these patients, acknowledging their victimhood may be an important first step in a therapeutic process that will weaken the protective denial and lead to a more balanced view of their past and present psychic realities.

A patient who defensively clings to the victim role may do so in the service of limiting the scope of what is available for self-observation and therefore for exploration within the treatment. In many instances, early childhood seductions become the basis—by way of identification with the aggressor—for later seductive behavior in early adolescence or adulthood (see Bigras 1990). For example, one patient who had been sexually abused by both parents in early childhood and latency reported that during adolescence, she actively sought out her father for sexual contact and attempted to seduce other older male acquaintances. Although the reconstruction and understanding of these events was leavened by the recognition of the role played by the earlier seductions and her identification with her aggressors, it would have been a serious omission not to address the guilt that followed from her subsequent active, sexual provocations or to consider her only to be a "victim" or "survivor" of incest.

The definition of self as victim can also have important consequences for a patient's attitude toward his or her activity, assertiveness, adult responsibility, and desire. Ehrenberg (1987) noted that incestuous and sexually abusive relationships in childhood can have

> [a] profound impact on the nature of the [adult] individual's patterns of relation to desire [in both a sexual and a more general sense]. . . . To the degree that arousal of the victim's own desire is experienced as the basis for the vulnerability [to the trauma], the relation to desire becomes quite problematic. This is particularly so when the relationships in question endured over considerable periods of time. In such instances, it is clear that unless the child had been a cooperative participant, and derived some gratification from the involvement, the relationship could not have been possible. The individual's coming to terms with his or her own participation in these early relationships, . . . constitutes one of the pivotal issues in treatment. (pp. 593–594)

Needless to say, these are issues that can be taken up only with the greatest tact and care, after the basis for the protective security of the therapeutic relationship has been carefully established.

When patients who suffered childhood sexual abuse do relate memories of the abuse experience, it is often with a great deal of doubt and uncertainty about what actually happened. This may be as true for those patients who enter therapy aware that a sexual trauma took place in childhood as it is for those whose memories of the abuse emerge from repression or are reconstructed during the course of treatment. The intensity of the doubting may surprise an unsuspecting therapist, especially when the patient is dealing with memories rather than attempts at reconstruction and these memories relate to a time in childhood when the patient would ordinarily be expected to have a clear sense of whether the memory was real or fantasy. Kramer (1983) described one aspect of this problem as "object-coercive doubting" and related this aspect to maternal incest. Such doubting, however, may occur in any case of parental incest, regardless of the sex of the parent involved, and in many instances of non–parental-involved childhood sexual trauma as well (Levine 1990). The doubting and confusion, coupled with a reliance on dissociative defenses, may even evolve into a global cognitive style that leads to generalized difficulties in learning (Bernstein 1990; Kramer 1990).

At some point in the treatment, the doubting and uncertainty about "What really happened?" and "Was it real or fantasy?" may assume center stage for the patient and produce difficult technical challenges for the therapist. Patients may beseech the therapist to offer them help, certainty, or confirmation in knowing what took place, or demand that the therapist express belief in their doubt-ridden accounts. At one level, this phenomenon may represent a transference repetition—that is, the patient is asking, "Will you recognize and identify for/with me what is really going on, as I wished my parents or other significant adults to do? Or will you turn away and pretend not to notice or even covertly foster the continuation of the incest, as my parents did?"

Simultaneously, the doubting may unconsciously repeat the trauma—that is, the patient, in the unconscious role of the incestuous parent, may be angrily or seductively attempting to make the therapist do something to relieve the patient's distress. Alternatively, the angry doubting and cranky demands may reenact feelings of undischarged sexual tension, which were an important part of the abuse experience (Shengold 1989). In relation to the therapist's proper role in the treatment, the elements of the narcissistic use of the object and the demand for transgression of boundaries inherent in this transaction are readily apparent to the observer. These meanings, however, are apt to be much less apparent for the patient. The result is often some of the most complex and difficult moments in the therapy. Regression, a weakened alliance, hypersensitivity, and confusion on the part of the patient can run headlong into the therapist's countertransference strain. The latter arises because the therapist is under attack and is being forced by the patient to take sides, to know omnisciently what was or was not real, or to otherwise abandon a position of abstinence, neutrality, and optimum analytic effectiveness.

In trying to find a way through this complex and demanding set of problems, a therapist must assess the extent to which some active support for the patient's reality testing is necessary or possible. In childhood, many of these patients did not have relationships with adequately protective or reality-supporting figures who would affirm that the seduction of children was wrong and not the fault of the child or to whom they could "report" their abusers. For many patients, the limitations of the adults in their world were compounded by their own childhood feelings of guilt or by threats or enticements not to tell. One patient reported that her father, with whom she had had an incestuous sexual relationship for many years, would always say, "A person is always free to choose what they want." The contribution of such a pronouncement to later doubts and confusion about what is real is devastatingly apparent.

Clearly, then, some patients in this most difficult moment in treatment seek to enact the wish that the analyst function in a longed-for, but never provided, protective parental role. But what are the consequences of the therapist's attempting to satisfy this need for the patient? Will doing so prove helpful or will it unconsciously reenact some component of the sexual trauma? Will it foster regression by attempting to fulfill a universal childhood longing for an omniscient object? Will it encourage a sense of entitlement to be compensated for the sexual trauma or reinforce a patient's view of him- or herself as victim and thereby contribute to a suppression of either fears or perceptions of assertive or seductive behavior?

These are difficult questions, and their answers must be determined individually in each instance. Therapeutic technique at such moments of strain must be guided by the therapist's assessment of the extent to which the patient is able to bear the existential burden of not knowing and can accept the necessary uncertainty that surrounds almost any "truth" that derives from the subjective realm of psychic reality. To what extent can a therapist ever really know what happened? As Freud (1899/1958) said in his paper on screen memories, we may not have memories from childhood, but only memories *about* childhood—that is, the best that we may be able to do is to reconstruct what is "likely" rather than what was "true" (Sherkow 1990).

From this perspective, as well as that of technique, the therapist does not have to decide whether something was actually real or not. Instead, he or she need only recognize and acknowledge the tremendous importance that the wish for certainty holds for the patient, explore the fact and consequences of the patient's uncertainty and doubting, examine the ways in which doubting the experience may have been reinforced by the child's own guilt and by the action of the parents, explore the meanings that the doubting assumes and the uses to which it is put in the transference, and try to follow the evolution of the material within the therapeutic process.

Historical Review

In his first attempts to understand neurosis, Freud (1896/1958) formulated a theory that proposed an actual childhood sexual seduction as the causal factor in neurosogenesis. Although he no doubt did so under the influence of actual reports of childhood seductions by *some* of his patients, there is much data to conclude that the evidence Freud used for the reconstruction and interpretation of childhood sexual trauma in the majority of his patients during this early phase of his work was highly speculative. Schimek (1987), in a thorough review of the evolution of Freud's "seduction theory" and its evidentiary basis, concludes that Freud did not turn his back on firm evidence of actual childhood trauma, as Masson (1984) has claimed. Rather, Schimek suggests that Freud was an overzealous interpreter of childhood sexual injuries at this point in his career—that is, Freud would take this or that current symptom and find a way of forcibly insisting to his patients that it must be the remnant or consequence of a childhood sexual trauma.

Freud himself came to recognize the limitations of this early theory when his broadening clinical work and his own self-analysis led him to implicate as seducers of children men whom he knew to be of impeccable integrity, including his own father! The resulting crisis in his thinking led Freud to appreciate the central importance of unconscious fantasy in human mental life and gave birth to psychoanalysis as we know it today.

The exploration of unconscious fantasies that followed Freud's revision of his seduction theory and his emphasis instead on a theory of innate sexual and aggressive drives as a continual influence on development and mental functioning led to a relative deemphasis of external factors in the elaboration of psychoanalytic theory. However, in his own writings, Freud never lost sight of the importance of actual childhood trauma, including actual sexual trauma, as a factor in pathogenesis.[4]

Indeed, as clinicians, psychoanalysts have always been alert to and dealt with the adverse impacts of actual childhood traumatic situations on emotional development. What changed in regard to the early seduction hypothesis was that in Freud's revised theory, the reality and consequences of actual trauma were seen in relation to a far more complex view of development and mental functioning. The latter took into account intrinsic factors that resulted from constitutional givens (e.g., strength of drives or innate capacities for the development of ego functions) and studied their interrelationship with actual events. In fairness to many critics of psychoanalysis, the emphasis on internal factors did lead to a relative neglect in recognizing the extent and consequences of actual childhood sexual trauma and incest. This neglect mirrored and was part of the more general denial of childhood sexual traumata and incest that existed in our society at large. With the increasing awareness in recent years of childhood sexual abuse as a problem within our culture, analysts have joined in the vigorous pursuit and investigation of the problems that the treatments of these patients present.

Differential Dynamic Diagnosis

Given the protean manifestations of the adult consequences of childhood sexual abuse, these patients may present within any conceivable diagnostic category. Most commonly, they show some combination of depression and low self-esteem, problems in intimate relationships, impulsiveness or extreme constriction, phobias and anxiety phenomena, sexual dysfunctions, or psychosomatic disturbances. As noted above, a history of childhood sexual trauma may be consistent with neurotic, psychotic, or borderline character structures. Thus, differential diagnostic considerations will center on separating any given patient who

---

[4]See Levine 1990, especially pp. 5–10, for a more detailed discussion of these issues.

was sexually abused in childhood from other patients with depressive, hysterical, schizoid, borderline, or narcissistic symptoms who were not.

Summary

From a clinical perspective, the diagnostic question "How do I know if a patient has had a childhood sexual trauma?" is best answered by studying the patient's response to the treatment setting, including the patient's reactions to the therapist's tentative and judicious attempts to reconstruct the existence and consequences of presumed childhood trauma. As noted above, the form and content of the transference relationship that develops over time will often revolve around fears of repetition and pressures to repeat elements of the childhood sexual trauma and its consequences. The traumatic aspects of the original events can include not only components of the actual trauma (e.g., overstimulation, fear, invasion, pain, guilt) but also feelings of being narcissistically appropriated for the gratification of the other or of being abandoned by the omnipotent, protecting parent. The ways in which these elements of the original trauma are remembered and repeated in the treatment will be influenced by the level of development that the child had attained prior to the onset of the trauma, by subsequent posttraumatic events, and by the elaborations in fantasy to which the child resorted in attempts to deal with the original trauma.

For each position that the patient assumes in the transference, the therapist is susceptible to feeling pressure to adopt the same or a complementary role in the countertransference. The therapist's tendency toward countertransference enactment (role responsiveness) can offer important clues about what is being unconsciously mobilized in the therapeutic relationship. However, no matter how powerful or how well rationalized these impulses toward the patient may be, it is essential that the therapist not act upon them. Rather, the therapist should attempt to use his or her awareness of these impulses as further data about the patient that is being communicated via the countertransference (Heimann 1950). To effectively do so, a therapist must have considerable familiarity with and objectivity toward his or her own personal conflicts, as well as the capacity to bear them without acting upon them. The attainment of these capacities may require personal therapy and a commitment to continued self-scrutiny. However, the therapeutic advantage that such an endeavor can offer is well worth the time and effort that it requires. The therapist's countertransference responses, when taken together with the patient's history and the developments within the transference relationship, can serve to guide the therapist toward a sense of conviction about what may or may not have happened in the patient's childhood. This conviction may then be offered to the patient in the form of tentative reconstructions. As with any other interpretive intervention, the therapist must then follow and explore the patient's response to these proposed reconstructions in the continued elaboration and working out of the therapeutic process.

For Further Study

Bird B: Notes on transference: universal phenomenon and hardest part of analysis. J Am Psychoanal Assoc 20:267–301, 1972

Boesky D: Acting out: a reconsideration of the concept. Int J Psychoanal 63:39–55, 1982

Gill M: Analysis of Transference, Vol 1. New York, International Universities Press, 1982

Herman J: Father-Daughter Incest. Cambridge, MA, Harvard University Press, 1981

Jacobs T: Countertransference enactments. J Am Psychoanal Assoc 34:289–308, 1986

Joseph B: Transference: the total situation. Int J Psychoanal 66:447–454, 1985

Katan A: Children who were raped, in The Psychoanalytic Study of the Child, Vol 28. New Haven, CT, Yale University Press, 1973, pp 208–224

Kluft R (ed): Childhood Antecedents of Multiple Personality. Washington, DC, American Psychiatric Press, 1985

Margolis M: Parent-child incest: analytic experiences with follow-up data, in The Trauma of Transgression. Edited by Kramer S, Akhtar S. Northvale, NJ, Jason Aronson, 1991, pp 57–92

Meiselman KC: Incest. San Francisco, CA, Jossey-Bass, 1978

O'Brien JD: The effects of incest on female adolescent development, J Am Acad Psychoanal 15:83–92, 1987

Schafer R: The Analytic Attitude. New York, Basic Books, 1983

Sherkow S: The evaluation and diagnosis of sexual abuse in little girls. J Am Psychoanal Assoc 38:305–327, 1990

Silber A: Childhood seduction, parental pathology and hysterical symptoms. Int J Psychoanal 60:109–116, 1979

Terr LC: Childhood traumas: an outline and overview. Am J Psychiatry 148:10–20, 1991

Williams M: Reconstruction of an early seduction and its aftereffects. J Am Psychoanal Assoc 35:145–163, 1987

Wolf EK, Alpert JL: Psychoanalysis and child sexual abuse: a review of the post-Freudian literature. Psychoanalytic Psychology 8:305–327, 1991

Zetzel ER: Therapeutic alliance in the analysis of hysteria (1958), in The Capacity for Emotional Growth. New York, International Universities Press, 1970, pp 182–196

References

Bernstein AE: The impact of incest trauma on ego development, in Adult Analysis and Childhood Sexual Abuse. Edited by Levine HB. Hillsdale, NJ, Analytic Press, 1990, pp 65–91

Bigras J: Psychoanalysis as incestuous repetition: some technical considerations, in Adult Analysis and Childhood Sexual Abuse. Edited by Levine HB. Hillsdale, NJ, Analytic Press, 1990, pp 173–196

Bryer JB, Nelson BA, Miler JB, et al: Childhood sexual and physical abuse as factors in adult psychiatric illness. Am J Psychiatry 144:1426–1430, 1987

Burland JA, Raskin JA: The psychoanalysis of adults who were sexually abused in childhood: a preliminary report from the discussion group of the American Psychoanalytic Association, in Adult Analysis and Childhood Sexual Abuse. Edited by Levine HB. Hillsdale, NJ, Analytic Press, 1990, pp 35–41

Deblinger E, McLeer S, Atkins M, et al: Post-traumatic stress in sexually abused, physically abused and non-abused children. Child Abuse Negl 13:403–408, 1989

Ehrenberg DB: Abuse and desire: a case of father-daughter incest. Contemporary Psychoanalysis 23:593–604, 1987

Erikson E: Childhood and Society. New York, WW Norton, 1954

Ferenczi S: The confusion of tongues between the adult and the child. Int J Psychoanal 30:225–230, 1933

Freud S: The aetiology of hysteria (1896), in The Standard Edition of the Complete Psychological Works of Sigmund Freud, Vol 3. Translated and edited by Strachey J. London, Hogarth Press, 1958, pp 191–221

Freud S: Screen memories (1899), in The Standard Edition of the Complete Psychological Works of Sigmund Freud, Vol 3. Translated and edited by Strachey J. London, Hogarth Press, 1958, pp 299–322

Freud S: Remembering, repeating and working through (1914), in The Standard Edition of the Complete Psychological Works of Sigmund Freud, Vol 12. Translated and edited by Strachey J. London, Hogarth Press, 1958, pp 145–156

Goodwin J, Simms M, Bergman R: Hysterical seizures: a sequel to incest. Am J Orthopsychiatry 49:698–703, 1979

Greenacre P: The prepuberty trauma in girls. Psychoanal Q 19:298–317, 1950

Heimann P: On countertransference. Int J Psychoanal 31:81–4, 1950

Kramer S: Object-coercive doubting: a pathological defensive response to maternal incest. J Am Psychoanal Assoc 31 (suppl):325–351, 1983

Kramer S: Residues of incest, in Adult Analysis and Childhood Sexual Abuse. Edited by Levine HB. Hillsdale, NJ, Analytic Press, 1990, pp 149–170

Kris E: The recovery of childhood memories. Psychoanal Study Child 11:54–88, 1956

Levine HB: Toward a psychoanalytic understanding of children of survivors of the Holocaust. Psychoanal Q 51:70–92, 1982

Levine HB (ed): Adult Analysis and Childhood Sexual Abuse. Hillsdale, NJ, Analytic Press, 1990

Lindberg F, Distad L: Post-traumatic stress disorders in women who experienced childhood incest. Child Abuse Negl 9:329–334, 1985

Margolis M: Parent-child incest: analytic experiences with follow-up data, in The Trauma of Transgression. Edited by Kramer S, Akhtar S. Northvale, NJ, Jason Aronson, 1991, pp 57–92

Masson JM: The Assault on Truth. New York, Farrar, Strauss, Giroux, 1984
Raphling D: Technical issues of the opening phase, in Adult Analysis and Childhood Sexual Abuse. Edited by Levine HB. Hillsdale, NJ, Analytic Press, 1990, pp 45–64
Sandler J: The background of safety. Int J Psychoanal 41:352–356, 1960
Sandler J: Countertransference and role responsiveness. International Review of Psycho-Analysis 3:43–48, 1976
Schimek JG: Fact and fantasy in the seduction theory: a historical review. J Am Psychoanal Assoc 35:937–966, 1987
Shengold L: Soul Murder: The Effects of Childhood Abuse and Deprivation. New Haven, CT, Yale University Press, 1989
Sherkow S: Consequences of childhood sexual abuse on the development of ego structure: a comparison of child and adult cases, in Adult Analysis and Childhood Sexual Abuse. Edited by Levine HB. Hillsdale, NJ, Analytic Press, 1990, pp 93–115
Smith S: The sexually abused patient and the abusing therapist: a study in sadomasochistic relationships. Psychoanalytic Psychology 1:89–98, 1984
Steele BF: Some sequelae of the sexual maltreatment of children, in Adult Analysis and Childhood Sexual Abuse. Edited by Levine HB. Hillsdale, NJ, Analytic Press, 1990, pp 121–34
Steele BF, Alexander H: Long term effects of sexual abuse in childhood, in Sexually Abused Children and Their Families. Edited by Mrazek PB, Kempe CH. New York, Pergamon, 1981, pp 233–234
Valenstein A: On attachment to painful feelings and the negative therapeutic reaction, in The Psychoanalytic Study of the Child, Vol 28. New Haven, CT, Yale University Press, 1973, pp 305–392

Chapter 20

The Psychosomatic Patient

Ira L. Mintz, M.D.

Current Psychodynamic Perspectives

Current views on psychosomatic disease suggest that psychosomatic symptoms develop in biologically and socially predisposed individuals whose early developmental vulnerability sets the stage for later psychosomatic decompensation (L. Deutsch 1980; Pollock 1977). Discussing this concept further in his paper on asthma, L. Deutsch (1987) noted that complex psychological factors such as the quality of ego functioning, early childhood experience, sexual and aggressive stimulation, and the quality and degree of rejection can all play a role in the ultimate development of asthma.

Sperling (1978a), Wilson (1989), Hogan (1989), and Mushatt (1989) view psychosomatic patients as having primarily oral and anal fixations, with an inability to tolerate frustrations and a need for immediate gratification of aggressive, sexual, and dependency needs. These impulses are usually not conscious and are not acted out, so that the patient does not typically have overt difficulties with people. Instead, the desires are discharged as psychosomatic symptoms. Although preoedipal conflicts predominate, additional oedipal turmoil adds to the burden.

Following birth, an infant passes through the first 5-month symbiotic stage, during which the infant is fused with the mother as if it were a part of her.

The subsequent gradually unfolding separation-individuation phase (from 5 to 36 months) ushers in the infant child's gradual awareness of his or her own body separate from that of the mother, who initially stands for the world. Both the symbiotic attachment and the separation-individuation reflect an intrapsychic state of mind (Mahler 1952, 1975). The individuation component refers to the child's developing increasing awareness, both of its own being and of the developing characteristics of its own essence: the ability to walk and talk, the sound of its own voice, awareness of its own thoughts, and the boundaries of its own body. Disturbances in the mother-child relationship that interfere with this early, crucial intrapsychic achievement can damage the evolving personality structure and compromise its capacity to effectively cope with life's pressures, predisposing these individuals to neurotic, psychosomatic, borderline, and psychotic decompensation.

At a more clinical level, the very young child's helplessness in terms of being unable to exercise any control over the world and the people who populate it results in the ultimate awareness that what can be controlled best is parts of one's own body. Most early and prominently recognized is the ability to control body sphincters such as the mouth and anus. Pressured by an oversolicitous mother concerned about its nourishment, the infant child can close its mouth or—as a last resort—swallow but then vomit back. Withholding feces can also provide the child with a satisfying sense of control over its own body. The control over the mouth and rectum can ultimately be extended to control over part of the external world via the parent, who desperately attempts to get food into one orifice and feces out of the other.

In both cases an element of self-punishment results, because the child may require the food or feel better with the evacuation. Responding to the mother's frustration, the child ultimately recognizes that by misusing its bodily functioning it can exercise an upsetting and negative effect upon the mother. Thus, the need to control the parent-environment may ultimately supersede the need for the food or the evacuation, because both eating and evacuation provide a discharge of pent-up aggression and the need for ego control as an alternative to helplessness, as well as mastery over a symbolic situation that represents the original uncontrollable one. In an overly simplified fashion, the psychosomatic symptom in adolescence or later life in part represents a regressive reenactment of this earlier type of experience.

Crucial in most cases to implementing this set of circumstances is the presence of a strict, primitive, and punitive superego demanding perfection and requiring punishment through suffering. The guilt emanating from a presumed transgression is mainly related to unresolved aggressive, sexual, and dependency conflicts. Complementing the primitive superego are other, similar primitive aspects of the personality: frequently present are an undue degree of narcissism, omnipotence, magical thinking, and borderline defenses, as described by Boyer and Giovacchini (1975, 1980), Giovacchini (1977), Kernberg (1980), and Volkan (1976).

Mushatt (1975) emphasized that in vulnerable patients separation can initiate and perpetuate psychosomatic illness. He cited a patient whose ulcerative colitis was reactivated when his mother was dying. This patient fantasized pulling off the mother's breasts and pushing them under the skin of his chest in an unconscious attempt to deny her loss and maintain a symbolic nurturing. Crying, the patient revealed the additional fantasy of putting his mother's heart into his chest: "Then I would have my mother with me." Mushatt concluded that the intensity of the patient's loss, and his associations to childhood and the empty house, reflected his inability to deal with the earlier loss. Ultimately, the love and the loss were followed by anger toward the mother because of her abandonment.

In earlier papers (1954, 1975), Mushatt described how bodily secretions and excretions can, at a primitive level, symbolize separating and destroying. His patient, a scientist with asthma, for years refused to clean his suit so that he would not lose his sweat in the clothing. Mushatt cited F. Deutsch (personal communication, December 1953) as having told him that inspiration can be perceived as symbolically taking in part of the world, and expiration as restoring internalized objects back into the world. This concept is graphically illustrated by the asthmatic patient described later in this chapter.

Sperling (1978a, 1978b), discussing the treatment of psychosomatic diseases in children, cited the crucial role of the mother-child relationship. She postulated that the psychosomatic symptoms are the result of an "insoluble conflict" with the mother—that the mother tends to reward the child when it is sick and helpless and to reject it when it is healthy and attempting to separate, because she unconsciously needs a sick, helpless child to help her deal with her own unresolved conflicts and feels threatened by the loss of this crutch in maintaining her own ego homeostasis.

Sperling viewed ulcerative colitis as a disease that develops in early childhood but is not necessarily manifested until later in life, when it is set off by a specific emotional trauma, often a separation or a loss.

Sperling (1978c) cited a case of an 8-year-old girl with ulcerative colitis whose mother would feed her in the bathroom during a colitis attack. The mother needed the child to be sick and to stay home because the mother was afraid to be home alone when she had to use the toilet. Sperling added that the symptoms of bloody diarrhea and soiling permitted the child to express aggression toward the mother without fearing repercussions because she would be seen as sick, not willful. H. Shinya (personal communication, September 1986), who has conducted colonoscopic studies with a very large number of patients with ulcerative colitis, noted that he could often recognize adult colitis patients during the initial interview because they arrive with their mothers. That diagnosis is further confirmed when he asks the patient a question and the patient's mother replies. Sperling (1978b) considers the prognosis for ulcerative colitis to depend on the pathology in the patient's personality as well as in the mother's. She also believes that the amount of bleeding is determined by the intensity of the unconscious hatred.

Wilson (1989) emphasized that as the psychosomatic symptoms begin to subside during the course of treatment, they are replaced by other symptoms associated with the same underlying conflict, especially the symptom of depression. The aggressive component of the psychosomatic symptom can be replaced by the aggressive component of the psychological symptom.

According to Wilson (1989), psychosomatic patients are fearful of the eruption of long-repressed, unsublimated, primitive aggressive and sexual impulses, and their anxiety centers on the feared loss of control. He emphasized that "loss of control is the primary fear of all psychosomatic patients" (p. 15), and that this fear hides such wishes. Thus, the fear of giving in to these forbidden impulses is expressed in regressed, symbolic, somatic symptoms.

In some illustrations from my own practice, the patient with spastic colitis can deal with his conflict over symbolically releasing or controlling the aggression with diarrhea or constipation. With ulcerative colitis, the bloody stool is a symbol of the patient's bloody, deadly feelings of hatred. The asthmatic patient who wheezes expresses the impulse to choke others and, filled with guilt, chokes herself. Migraine headaches can symbolize the impulse to attack and destroy the ideas—or the actual head—of a hated individual. The anorexic patient's starving can symbolize the need to be weak and to be unable to destroy hated others, while avoiding the use of the destructive teeth. Like a carnivorous animal, the bulimic patient rips and tears at food, which symbolizes people (Mintz 1992).

The choice of the specific meaning of the symptoms is overdetermined and multiply determined by specific unconscious fantasies, impulses, and feelings derived from associative linkages to past life experiences. Therefore, each symptom can have a number of dynamic meanings.

Hogan (1989) emphasized the special problem with potentially fatal psychosomatic diseases (anorexia, asthma, ulcerative colitis), and warned that it is essential to quickly interfere with the downhill course of the disease by focusing on the self-destructive aspects of the symptoms that can result in the patient's death. Early in the treatment, patients will usually tolerate the therapist's pointing out that they do not treat themselves with consideration, that they have a need to hurt themselves and to suffer, and that unconsciously they are trying to kill themselves. Patients will likewise accept without undue objection the therapist's attempts to get them to recognize the existence of and the necessity for changing their strict, punitive conscience—although, of course, such change is not easily achieved. As regards the many manifestations of unrealistic guilt and self-destructiveness, modifying the damaging perfectionism is necessary for ultimate change. After patients become more aware of their excessively self-castigating attitudes, their unconscious hatred toward others can be addressed. To do so precipitously, however, can set off intense guilt that requires intensified self-punishment in the form of increased psychosomatic symptoms and/or depression rather than the subsidence of these symptoms.

Historical Review

The dynamic study of psychosomatic disease essentially began with the pioneers Alexander (1950), Daniels (1940), F. Deutsch (1953), Dunbar (1943), Engel (1952), Gerard (1946), Grinker (1953), Knapp and Nemetz (1957), Lindemann (1945), Sperling (1946), and Weiss and English (1957).

Dunbar (1943) believed that personality traits played a role in the development of psychosomatic disease. Selinsky (1939) considered anger and resentment to be the primary features in migraine attacks, whereas Fromm-Reichmann (1937) emphasized the importance of aggression against an ambivalently perceived individual.

Daniels (1940) noted that ulcerative colitis symptoms frequently covered up a depression, and that the illness represented an "organic suicide." He also felt that the more severe the symptoms, the more pathological the underlying psychiatric illness. Lindemann (1945) found that the death of someone close preceded the onset of ulcerative colitis in a high percentage of his cases. Sperling (1946), focusing on the underlying aggression, concluded that the bloody diarrhea in ulcerative colitis was a somatic discharge of this aggression, and that the patient had an unconscious wish to rid him- or herself of a hated internalized individual, symbolized by the bloody stool.

Engel (1955, 1956) noted that bleeding and constipation were early signs of ulcerative colitis, and that headaches were a frequent coexisting symptom. In addition, he recognized preoedipal conflicts, pathological interactions between mother and child, onset and exacerbations related to loss and separation, pathological dependency, and the importance of destructive impulses. Karush and Daniels (1953) attempted to evaluate the effectiveness of psychotherapy for ulcerative colitis.

Alexander (1950) believed that specific unconscious emotional conflicts associated with anxiety, anger, and other emotions played a role in the development of psychosomatic illness. He considered that physiological factors might also contribute to the psychological features and personality traits seen in Graves' disease.

French and Alexander (1941) described the basic problem in asthma as a conflict between the desire to be close to the mother and the wish to separate. However, they did not feel that this conflict was specific for asthma. Gerard (1946) observed that asthmatic children with allergies who were treated for the allergy became free of asthma and remained so even if exposed to allergens, although they continued to test positive. Knapp and Nemetz (1957) characterized asthmatic patients as passive and dependent, requiring reassurance and support from important people in their lives. Knapp et al. (1970) found that when asthmatic patients began to reveal feelings of hostility, a reaction of guilt and depression often followed. On occasion, such reactions resulted in an intensification of the asthmatic condition.

Wilson (1968) pointed out the pregenital, excessively dependent and demanding needs of psychosomatic patients and their acting out of these yearnings in the transference. He cautioned against gratifying these unrealistic, immature needs, emphasizing, rather, the necessity to interpret them and to advise patients that indulging such demands is at the expense of healthy self-esteem and mature interpersonal relationships. In discussing psychosomatic patients, Wilson (1971) emphasized that in addition to analyzing the transference, the therapist functions as a new and real individual with whom the patient must learn to interact; thus, the therapist-patient relationship models healthy relationships and contributes to the patient's maturation.

One of the most concise and cogent historical reviews of changing research in psychosomatic disease was provided by L. Deutsch (1980), who observed that "historically, psychosomatic medicine was intimately tied to psychoanalysis" (p. 654) and to the work of Franz Alexander (Alexander 1950; Alexander et al. 1968). Deutsch noted that although Alexander was aware of organic and developmental predisposing factors, he hypothesized that psychosomatic diseases were intimately related to unconscious intrapsychic conflict, and that each illness corresponded to a specific personality disorder. When further study did not validate this conclusion, the disappointment contributed to a decrease of interest in the role of unconscious conflict as a major factor in the cause, development, and maintenance of psychosomatic disease. The importance of unconscious conflict, however, has never been disproven.

Differential Dynamic Diagnosis

Psychosomatic patients can have an underlying neurotic, borderline, or psychotic personality structure. The healthier the personality, the more positive the prognosis with the use of dynamic psychotherapy or analysis. The healthier person has more resources available for dealing with and solving problems.

From the view of the ego, the healthier individual's thinking is more realistic and more creative; he or she is more capable of generating healthy and rewarding solutions and more willing to tolerate frustration and postponement while retaining the patience needed to work toward possible long-term goals. In general, the healthier person's quality of life is better, with more successes and enjoyment to balance the distress experienced from the psychosomatic illness. Family, friendships, and work situations provide more satisfaction and feelings of success. All of these factors contribute to the individual's sense of reasonable optimism toward resolving his or her current illness based on the awareness of past successes in dealing with adversity.

From the side of the impulses, the healthier patient is better able to deal with feelings of aggression, sexuality, and dependency, and thus experiences a greater sense of being in control. Finally, the strict and punitive conscience found in most patients with psychosomatic diseases is less primitive and rigid in the healthier patient and therefore more modifiable. Conversely, the sicker the patient, the fewer the positive assets, with less successful experiences in work, friendship, and family, and the more failures in life, leading to low self-esteem, needs for immediate gratification, unrealistic expectations, poor judgment in dealing with people and circumstances, meager support groups, difficulty controlling more primitive aggression, and sexual feelings mixed with marked dependency needs. Further complicating the situation is the aforementioned rigid, primitive conscience that continues to extract endless, severe punishment for imagined "defects" and failures to achieve unrealistic standards of perfection.

As "talking" treatments, dynamic psychotherapy and analysis require the ability to verbally communicate as well as the intelligence to understand ideas, symbolic concepts, causality, and conflict. Basically, exercising this ability results in changing physical symptoms into psychological ones with their attendant anxieties, depression, and phobias, requiring the patient to cope with the changed form of conflict without severe regression or decompensation. In addition, the close relationship between therapist and patient requires the patient to ultimately trust the therapist, to recount relevant experiences, and to be able to transfer onto the psychiatrist those earlier feelings, attitudes, and behaviors that facilitate an analysis of the transference.

Two treatment examples may help clarify these concepts.

> I saw a very bright, insightful 35-year-old lawyer who had been treated medically with drugs for severe weekend migraines for 12 years without any change in frequency or intensity of symptoms. After 1 year in psychotherapy the patient's migraine symptoms had subsided, although he continued in treatment to deal with his unresolved conflicts. This patient was a good candidate for dynamic treatment.

> By contrast, a resident presented a 24-year-old clinic patient with ulcerative colitis in treatment for 6 months, who then decompensated and had to be hospitalized for increasing depression and auditory hallucinations. Reviewing the history, the resident stated that in the initial evaluation, the patient had been depressed, with suicidal thoughts intermittently since the age of 12, had two previous hospitalizations for depression, had few friends, and had not worked in 2 years. This patient was a poor choice for dynamic psychotherapy because of his limited resources, two previous decompensations, and current inability to work. This patient should have been treated with medication.

Although certainly necessary and often lifesaving, medical treatment is usually directed toward eliminating the symptoms. Analytic treatment, on the other hand, is directed toward resolving both the symptoms and their underlying cause. At a chance meeting, a former patient who had had severe spastic colitis informed me that since ending her twice-weekly psychotherapy 18 years earlier, she had not had "one single attack of colitis." Another very anorexic patient completed her treatment symptom-free after resolving her conflicts during the treatment. I received yearly Christmas cards from her for 10 years after her termination in which she informed me of her subsequent marriage and increasingly successful employment, and the development of her two children.

Case Examples

Asthma

Initial contact. Twelve-year-old P was sent for treatment because of the increasing severity of her asthma despite years of medical treatment. The asthma had begun following her brother's birth when she was 18 months of age. At the time of referral, she was often unable to climb the bedroom stairs and had to be carried. She slept wrapped in a blanket and propped up by pillows to minimize her wheezing.

Salient features in the past history were a history of asthma in her mother and grandmother but none in the patient's two other sisters or younger brother. Conscious resentment toward the younger brother began almost at his birth, with her mother remembering pictures taken when P was 6, standing behind the brother holding him and gritting her teeth, and another with her clenched hands behind and close to his neck.

Seen in consultation, P was a tall, trim, verbal adolescent, sad and wistful in appearance, who described her symptoms matter-of-factly. A description of her allergies included being "allergic to her brother." She revealed ambivalent feelings toward both her mother and her father.

Bird identification. P was preoccupied with birds. She spoke sadly about birds in the pet store whose wings were clipped and couldn't fly. She had a bird who bit her and had to be given away. Her current bird begins talking too early in the morning and she'd like to "choke it." It has a sharp beak, long claws, and hangs upside down.

The birds seemed to be a projection of herself. She was the bird who had its wings clipped by the asthmatic disease and couldn't move about, and had to be carried upside down by her father. The first bird was too aggressive with its mouth, and was rejected—given away. The second bird had a sharp beak and long claws. P's incessant nail biting seemed to keep her claws sheathed. She choked her bird-self with asthmatic attacks to contain her explosive rage, repressing her anger out of fear of abandonment.

Reaction to grandmother's death. After she had been in treatment for a few months, P's father phoned to state that her beloved grandmother was dying of cancer. When he told the children, they all got very upset, with a great deal of crying, but P remained unconcerned and dry eyed. That afternoon she casually mentioned to me that her grandmother was ill but appeared unaffected. She pulled at her stocking, complaining that it was too tight and her leg couldn't breathe. The ring on her finger was too tight and it couldn't breathe. Her shoe was also too tight and the foot couldn't breathe. "I can't get the fresh air in there."

Repressing the trauma of the grandmother's impending death, she displaced the usual asthmatic attack from the bronchi to different outside parts of her body that "can't breathe," just as she projected her internal feelings out onto the birds.

Subsequently informed that the grandmother's death was imminent, P had a severe asthma attack that night, wheezing and choking so badly that she was unable to sleep or to go to school the following morning. That afternoon, she arrived at the session "totally unconcerned." The patient clearly demonstrated a need to suppress and repress thoughts and feelings. Despite being up all night and not well enough to go to school, she made no reference to the event at all. The conflict was absorbed by the asthmatic attack. This lack of appropriate response illustrates how somatizing deals with all kinds of distress, including loss, and creates the mistaken impression to the casual observer that the psychosomatic patient is not in conflict—not anxious, upset, depressed, or angry—and therefore does not warrant psychiatric intervention. Symptom removal releases the buried, hidden emotional anguish.

The session after the grandmother's death, P appeared nonchalant and wore roller skates into the office. After a while, I mentioned that her father had phoned to inform me of her grandmother's death. She said yes and began twirling her bracelet, while talking about a tornado and making sucking sounds as she described how the tornado sucks up and destroys the people, houses, and trees. Although she clearly identified with the tornado, I said that I was puzzled that she had not spoken about her grandmother's death. "Why should I?" she asked, as she continued twirling her bracelet. I attempted to encourage her to discuss it openly, because I was concerned that the continued denial of her feelings of anguish and loss might precipitate a severe asthmatic attack.

Volcanoes and tornadoes: unconscious symbolic displacements. P dealt with her grandmother's death by repressing any feelings about it and avoiding any discussion. Her response was to begin twirling a bracelet that she controlled, producing a movement of air that she described as volcanoes and tornadoes. These tornadoes suck houses loose and destroy them. Illustrated by pictures, the volcanoes erupt, pouring out pumice rock and dust with amoebas in the rock and dust. Drawings labeled the amoebas with "father pseudopods," "mother pseudopods," and "baby brother pseudopods." Accompanying bacteria in the dust had nuclei that looked like eyes wearing glasses and a large mouth. Both bacteria resembled human heads.

It appears reasonable to assume that the violent movement of air during her asthmatic attacks clearly represents her tornado and volcano self that sucks in and belches out objects: microscopic houses, trees, and people hidden in the dust and pumice rock. These objects can be retained inside her forever like the "loving" grandmother, or can be destructively sucked in by her tornado self or be exploded out by her volcano self, thus destroying her "hated" grandmother who had left her, her mother and father who had disappointed her, or her brother who just existed. Conversely, she can be destroyed from within by the dangerous, hostile introjects that she sucks in, and must therefore rid herself of them by expelling them from the lungs or the anus.

A further expansion of this concept relating to the unconscious symbolic meaning of nebulizers, air, steam, dust, smoke, infection, and exercise is described elsewhere (Mintz 1989a).

Transference and countertransference. Almost 18 months of the patient's analysis were filled with uncooperativeness and vituperative attacks upon the analyst. However, hidden in the attacks were signs of ambivalent feeling and attachment, in part reflecting her increasing awareness that her asthmatic symptoms were subsiding. Management of the hostile transference required great care and self-reflection. Listening to an endless stream of cursing, threats, and insults four sessions a week for many months mandated my having to repeatedly remind myself that this was a strong transference in a very sick child, whose hatred was originally directed toward herself by choking and now was being externalized and transferred onto me. It was my job to accept it and to search through it to facilitate this child's understanding and progress, not to respond to it as a personal attack upon me.

Her behavior varied from total silence to bringing in a tape deck and attempting to spend the session playing it at full volume—perhaps hoping to deafen me or to drown out my voice. Acting out also took the form of threatening to deliberately spill soda on my couch. My quick comment that if that happened, her next month's bill would include the cost for a new sofa resulted in her rapidly putting down the soda; she also acknowledged that her parents didn't know how she behaved here, and that if she behaved this way at home, "they'd kill me."

The preoccupation with symbolic asthmatic choking was almost always present, reflected in her continual play with the Rubik's Cube, twisting it incessantly. Empty soda cans were also twisted back and forth until they snapped and were destroyed. Interpretations that her hand-twisting was what she did to her neck with the asthma were met with hostile epithets, scorn, disbelief, and disgust.

Verbal assaults were endless: "I really hate you. I never ever hated anyone this much in my life. I wish you would die and then I wouldn't have to come here"—and ultimately: "I'd like to kill you" (with intense feeling). This was an opportunity. "How would you like to kill me?" I asked. Her immediate response, "I'd like to take a tennis ball and shove it down your throat." "Then I would choke, and not be able to breathe, like you," I replied. "You must feel so guilty about how angry you feel . . . that you need to punish yourself by choking yourself with asthma." The repressed aggression had been emerging in various forms, with most reflecting respiratory symbolism: tornadoes, volcanoes, earthquakes, blowing scraps of paper all over the floor upon leaving, wanting to "blow my brains out." Finally, it emerged as more dynamically meaningful—the wish to choke me.

Months later, after voicing a desire to kill me with a dagger, she added, "if I blow on you, you die." The latter followed an interpretation that her constant gum chewing and bubble blowing reflected an exhaling of air without words. She then revealed what the hidden words were, carried in the exhaled air—that they were lethal and could kill. She was the destructive tornado-volcano symbolized by the asthmatic attack. During the many months in which this volcanic child spewed out her aggression, she began to understand its meaning.

By now 90% of the asthma had abated. "I feel OK, but if I don't yell at you, what shall I do? I realize that when I scream at you, I don't wheeze, but when I don't scream, I start wheezing and I'm afraid to stop screaming." At this point, rather than behaving aggressively, her reply was more plaintive and anxious. Again attempting to clarify what I thought was her difficulty, I pointed out that it was difficult for her to find another way to deal with her aggression, and that's what we could discuss. I knew that she was very upset about her grandmother's death and couldn't discuss it. "That's the first time you ever said anything correct." Although the interpretation had been made innumerable times, and consciously ignored, or repressed, this time it was acknowledged as if she had heard it for the first time. By this time she was also aware of the family members she disliked.

An interesting aspect of the gum chewing and bubble blowing is that in addition to her asthma, P also had a subclinical anorexia—a not-uncommon combination. The gum chewing and the desire to kill me with a knife both have specific dynamic relevance for anorexia and are discussed elsewhere (Mintz 1992), as is the case of P (Mintz 1989a).

Ulcerative Colitis

The initial confrontation. I was asked to see Q, a 14-year-old girl who was hospitalized with ulcerative colitis following a decision by surgeons not to operate because her hemoglobin was 6 grams after 12 pints of blood. Q appeared wan, weak, and extremely pale. She summoned a surge of energy in response to my arrival, however, as she told me that she did not wish to see me. She was advised that her illness was physical. She rolled over, became silent, and faced me with her back. This degree of "cooperation" persisted for the next 2 weeks. At each visit during the week, she rolled over and remained uncommunicative apart from repeating her decision not to see a psychiatrist because she had no worries. I spent the time pointing out that she was very sick, had lost a great deal of blood, and could die. Certainly, no harm could be done by talking to me. I indicated that often, inner worries could contribute to attacks of ulcerative colitis, and that she might not be consciously aware of what might be bothering her. Silence. I added that sometimes people unwittingly push away painful thoughts and feelings, which get replaced by physical symptoms. Silence. I acknowledged that I was aware that it might not be easy for a person to talk about very personal problems to a total stranger. I knew that I could not expect her to trust me without having some evidence that I was trustworthy, and that might take some time. These sessions were spent with my talking and her silence, occasionally punctuated by her denial of psychological illness, attacks upon my being there, and vituperative outbursts at my continually bothering her and not listening to her insistence that she did not need me.

I used the time helping her to get to know me professionally and establishing a therapeutic relationship. I attempted to get across that I was neither discouraged nor put off by her resistance, that I was patient and listened carefully to what she said, and that although I was not put off by her attacks upon me, I took what she said seriously. It was especially important to get across in my attitude that I knew that she was troubled, in spite of her protestations. The therapist's attitude and sense of conviction can often be as important as what is said. In essence, through word and behavior I attempted to convey my acceptance of her behavior without being discouraged by or responding negatively to it. I was patient, attentive, and considerate, and I discussed the nature of ulcerative colitis in general terms, with limited comments about the dynamics. I focused primarily upon the self-punishing behavior and the fact that it was difficult for her to trust me. (Interestingly, I have also observed this kind of silence in an anorexic patient who kept a secret diary in which she clarified a great deal of her feelings and behavior [see Mintz 1992].)

In the third week, Q began to respond. She spoke about the loss of her best friend because of a disagreement, and how devastated she felt. Feelings of anguish accompanied her detailed description of her loss. Concomitantly, tears began to pour out of her with an intensity that literally soaked her bathrobe. Once the floodgates were opened, she was unable to contain them.

As the session ended, she kept crying and talking. I suggested that we could continue at the next session, but she kept talking. After allowing 10 extra minutes and telling her I had a patient waiting in the office, I got up to leave, but she was still talking as I reached the door. Q kept talking during the week with the same emotional intensity. I was able to point out that all the inner feelings that had been pouring into her colon in the form of fluid, cramps, diarrhea, and blood were now pouring out her mouth and eyes in the form of sadness, tears, and anger. By the end of the week, the cramps and diarrhea had abated markedly and the bleeding stopped. Her hemoglobin improved and she was well enough to be discharged. (Cullinan [1938], Sperling [1946], and Hogan [1989] noted that severe ulcerative colitis can develop rapidly and subside just as quickly.) For the next 2 months, she was seen six to seven times a week, and subsequently five times a week in analysis.

What was most striking, just as with P's asthma, was the total repression and suppression of all aspects of anxiety and conflict. Q's appearance, similar to that of P, was one of no emotion at all: a flattening of affect with overcompensation to defensively ensure containment of the strong emotions that ultimately burst forth. Superficial observation might again conclude that this girl showed no signs of psychological problems. True; except for the blunted affect, they were all absorbed by the psychosomatic symptoms. Conversely, opening the emotional floodgates meant that the symptoms of the ulcerative colitis were no longer required. As a consequence, one can then recognize that when any psychosomatic symptoms are left unanalyzed, they remain as an emotional repository of conflict.

Conflict and symptomatic response: cramps during sessions. During the course of treatment, it became evident that whenever Q began thinking of a painful experience or a comment of mine set off a distressing memory, her perceived inability to deal with the conflict caused an instant regression, with somatizing and abdominal cramps. Initially, I was not aware of this reaction because she did not reveal the conflict or the subsequent onset of cramps. When I became aware of the cramps from the distress on her face, her unwillingness to confide in me about the conflict was patently evident as she denied any worry. As I grew increasingly familiar with her problems, I was occasionally able to interpret what I thought was the difficulty, and noted the relaxation in her face with the subsiding of the cramps. This reaction was not happily volunteered, but sullenly acknowledged.

Because of Q's tremendous need to control situations to satisfy immature, narcissistic, and magical fantasies and needs, she perceived any accurate interpretation that helped her as a manifestation of my increasing control over her in spite of my repeated disclaimer of wanting to be in that position. This accounted for her not revealing the symptom or acknowledging its relief with insight. It was very difficult for her to consider treatment as a trusting relationship in a joint venture.

Symptoms arising during the analytic session were frequently of a transference nature. Discussions or associations leading to awareness of a painful experience that Q was reluctant to face resulted in cramps, with blame and anger toward me because of her perception that the pain was my contribution. This anger is somatized as the cramps. With other patients, headache, backache, and diarrhea are not uncommon symptoms that emerge in a similar setting.

During one of the sessions, Q acknowledged having severe abdominal cramps. In response to being encouraged to discuss what might have precipitated them, she could think of nothing. I pointed out how much she was suffering, and that I would try to understand whatever it was that troubled her. She protested that she had no thoughts and then fell silent, although she watched me carefully. I reminded Q that she had been able to figure it out on other occasions. At last she slowly, hesitatingly, and with obvious embarrassment revealed that just before she experienced the cramp, she had had the fantasy that she felt like a little girl and had the urge to sit on the floor next to my feet and to put her head on my knees and just hold on to them. This poignant fantasy revealed a regressive, childlike impulse to sit next to a parent's knee, seeking closeness, intimacy, and affection.

Now 17 years old, Q felt that she could not reveal these infantile wishes and needs, anticipating scorn, rejection, and mockery. I attempted to clarify to her that such fantasies are not to be scorned but understood—that they reveal the reliving of earlier memories of past significant experiences. The cramps subsided during this discussion. These types of cramps developed many times during the analysis.

Transference and countertransference. One of my reasons for presenting this ulcerative colitis patient is related to a countertransference problem that arose at a point in the fourth year when her ulcerative colitis was much improved. Early in the treatment of these psychosomatic patients I was very much aware of how it feels to attempt to treat a patient with colitis who can bleed to death while you interpret, or an asthmatic patient who can choke while you analyze, or an anorexic patient who insists on starving and ignoring the possibility of cachectic death (Hogan 1985; Mintz 1989b).

Although by the fourth year of analysis, Q's severe episodes of bleeding had stopped, a small amount of bleeding persisted along with the cramps and diarrhea. This puzzled me because the treatment was progressing satisfactorily.

From the very beginning, I was acutely aware that the severe bleeding was life-threatening because she could reactivate it at any time to self-destructively achieve a regressive symbolic solution to circumstances that appeared overwhelming, to gratify a need to discharge infantile sadistic aggression, or to attempt to control me by threatening to die. As a consequence, I had remained watchful for her possible attempts to control me by her bleeding. I felt that if she unconsciously perceived that she could control me by creating anxiety in me by her bleeding, she might continue to bleed, unmindful of the deleterious consequences to herself. It was now a number of years later, and I wondered why the bleeding persisted.

In reviewing the situation with a colleague, it occurred to me that the persistent bleeding might be related to my excessive concern, of which I had lost sight. Preoccupied with her endless aggressive outbursts, changing symptoms, withholding of important information, silences and manipulations, and other issues, I might have been less concerned with her attempts at controlling me with bleeding and the threat to die. Considering that possibility, I awaited the next session.

When she arrived, I greeted her as usual. As she walked in, she glanced at me, sat down, and asked "What's the matter with you? You look different." She had immediately sensed a difference in my attitude. In reply to my query about what she meant, she replied, "There's something different about you. . . . You don't seem as interested and concerned. You seem aloof."

My absent anxiety was instantly perceived and described as aloofness and lack of concern. This interchange serves to highlight the presence of unconscious nonverbal communication between patient and therapist and between therapist and patient: that demeanor, attitude, and other types of unspoken behavior can have a very significant conscious and unconscious effect on the patient's behavior, symptoms, and verbal productions. Repeated interpretations were made at appropriate times about her attempts to control my reactions by her bleeding. In about 5 months, the bleeding stopped completely.

Intimately linked with these psychosomatic illnesses were other symptoms of conflict: severe depression and self-destructive acting out, with accidents and alienation of friends and teachers. Thus, we see a trajectory of self-punishing behavior ranging from the series of psychosomatic diseases that intermingled with one another and were infused with depression and self-destructive acting out (Mintz 1980–1981).

Q's ability to control her psychosomatic bleeding is not unusual. Elsewhere (Mintz 1989b), I have described four cases (including Q's) in which the patients' analytic insight was almost immediately followed by a cessation of the bleeding. When seen 14 years later, Q had no symptoms of ulcerative colitis.

Alexithymia

Alexithymia is primarily viewed as an inability to express appropriate emotions. These patients appear wooden, not upset by anything. The presumed inability of such patients to express their emotions markedly interferes with their capacity to experience insight because they cannot perceive their painful and upsetting inner feelings. What is not recognized is that these "emotionless" patients who "do not have the capacity to experience their feelings" actually maintain those emotions in a repressed state, which then contributes to symptom formation.

I have presented the series of emotionally charged fantasies of P, the asthmatic patient, to illustrate, emphasize, and clarify both the existence of these feelings and the underlying repression that keeps them from conscious expression. I have likewise illustrated the "presumed existence of the early alexithymia" in P's "emotionless state"—her "unconcern" in response to learning of her grandmother's imminent death. Her feelings were expressed in the subsequent asthmatic attack. The "emotionlessness" reappeared the session following her grandmother's death, when she arrived nonchalant and wearing roller skates. Her feelings began to emerge in the tornado and volcano fantasies, and finally erupted into the atmosphere in a violent, toxic cloud of emotions and words—she hated me, wished me dead, and wanted to kill me.

A similar situation existed in Q, the ulcerative colitis patient, who insisted that nothing bothered her. She ignored me and was almost totally silent except to point out that she didn't wish to see me. In the third week, she spoke about what bothered her, and the tears poured out, literally soaking her bathrobe and pajamas. I have rarely witnessed such a torrent of tears.

What was technically helpful—not only for these but for all psychosomatic patients—was the therapist's knowledge and sense of conviction that the feelings are truly there but repressed. This attitude can ultimately be communicated to the patient in addition to the therapist's verbal interpretations and can contribute to the ultimate emergence of feelings. Other analysts experienced in working with psychosomatic patients have drawn similar conclusions (L. Deutsch 1987; Hogan 1989; Mushatt 1989; Sperling 1978a, 1978b, 1978c; Wilson 1989).

Knapp (1960, 1989; Knapp et al. 1963) described a very sick asthmatic patient whose asthma was so severe that she required large doses of steroids and repeated hospitalizations, and almost died. He emphasized this patient's strong emotional reactions and her extremely well-defended primitive defenses, in which she would be "living out violent emotions toward key persons within the body itself . . . There were no traces of 'alexithymia' (and indeed never had been)" (Knapp 1989, p. 837).

Psychosomatic Symptom Shift

One of the interesting features in Q's 7-year analysis was the presence of symptom shift. The ulcerative colitis was the most serious symptom: a lethal, deeply entrenched disease that lasted 4 years. As its seriousness and intensity began to abate, it was replaced by severe asthma. Both diseases coexisted until the asthma took over. The asthma was the only other potentially deadly disease.

The third disease was severe migraine, painful but not lethal. This was followed by angioneurotic edema, aseptic monoarticular arthritis of the knee, nasorhinitis, and hives. With this type of symptom shift, progress is usually evident if the shift in illness moves in the direction of a less-serious disease, suggesting that the intensity of the aggression has lessened and the primitive, punitive superego is being modified.

Anniversary Reactions

The anniversary reaction is a time-specific psychological response arising on an anniversary of a psychologically significant experience that the individual attempts to master through reliving rather than through remembering. It can take the form of psychosomatic or psychiatric symptoms, dreams, behavior, accidents, suicide, or associations during a treatment session (Mintz 1971; Pollock 1970, 1989). Psychosomatic illness has been reported on anniversaries (Engel 1955; M. Sperling, personal communication, September 1967). I have seen many such episodes.

> Ms. R, a 36-year-old woman, began treatment because of chronic obesity (Mintz 1971). She had been depressed over the past week, precipitating the consultation at that point in time. Linked to the depression was an inexplicable worry that her husband might become very ill, resulting in her phoning him frequently all week. She associated to her strong attachment to her father, remembering his death when she was 14. In reply to my query, Ms. R revealed that her father's death had occurred on October 11th, 22 years earlier. Because the first consultation was the 9th of October, the patient seemed to be reliving the experience of her father's death, with the worry displaced onto her husband and the anticipation of his death.
>
> In the next few weeks, Ms. R mentioned having become pregnant before her marriage and the guilt that the pregnancy created. On her father's deathbed, he had told the priest that he wanted his children to be an honor to his memory and to never disgrace his name. Had he been alive when she had become pregnant, she thought that she would have felt forced to kill herself.
>
> Ms. R's obesity had begun with that first pregnancy, arising out of her conscious fantasy that obesity can cause toxemia and possible abortion. Her weight fluctuated in a curious cycle. Her due date was between October 12th and 15th, very close to the date of her father's death. Every fall she went on a diet, and every spring she gained weight. The cyclical weight changes of eating and dieting closely corresponded to the dates of that first onset of pregnancy, and to the date of delivery.

Thus, one can appreciate the complex, multidetermined features in this patient's weight problem:

1. It was related to reliving continuous feelings of guilt over a pregnancy 22 years earlier.
2. The weight gain also relived an unconscious wish to abort that pregnancy.

3. The time cycle was identical to that of this first pregnancy, although the patient had had three additional children.
4. The earlier trauma was still unresolved, as the patient was forced to relive the depression surrounding her father's death by transferring these fears onto her husband.
5. The child was born almost on the anniversary of the father's death.
6. He was named for the father and became a replacement for the lost father.
7. The patient's entry date into treatment was in part determined by these conflicts, where the therapist stood for the lost father.

With strong, unconscious conflicts of this magnitude, which the passage of time does not heal, one can appreciate how difficult it would be for Ms. R to successfully use weight-reduction programs. In attempting to utilize the value of an anniversary reaction, it is particularly helpful during an initial workup to obtain a careful history of significant figures, births, deaths, and traumatic events. Aspects of death and separation are of special significance because of the vulnerability that psychosomatic patients experience in the face of loss.

For Further Study

Boyer LB: Counter transference with severely regressed patients, in Counter Transference: The Therapist's Contributions to the Therapeutic Situation. Edited by Epstein L, Feiner AH. Northvale, NJ, Jason Aronson, 1979, pp 347–374

Cohen KD: Bulimia, orality, and the Oedipus complex in an adult female, in Psychodynamic Techniques in the Treatment of the Eating Disorder. Edited by Wilson CP, Hogan CC, Mintz IL. Northvale, NJ, Jason Aronson, 1992, pp 211–219

Deutsch F: Symbolization as a formative stage of the conversion process, in On the Mysterious Leap from the Mind to the Body: A Workshop Study on the Theory of Conversion. Edited by Deutsch F. New York, International Universities Press, 1959, pp 75–97

Epstein L, Feiner AH: Counter Transference: The Therapist's Contribution to the Therapeutic Situation. Northvale, NJ, Jason Aronson, 1979

Fenichel O: Organ neuroses, in The Psychoanalytic Theory of the Neuroses. New York, WW Norton, 1945, pp 236–267

Hitchcock J: The importance of aggression in the early development of children with eating disorders, in Psychodynamic Techniques in the Treatment of the Eating Disorder. Edited by Wilson CP, Hogan CC, Mintz IL. Northvale, NJ, Jason Aronson, 1992, pp 223–236

Hogan CC: The adolescent crisis in anorexia nervosa, in Psychodynamic Techniques in the Treatment of the Eating Disorder. Edited by Wilson CP, Hogan CC, Mintz IL. Northvale, NJ, Jason Aronson, 1992, pp 111–127

Karol C: The role of primal scene and masochism in asthma, in Psychosomatic Symptoms: Psychodynamic Treatment of the Underlying Personality Disorder. Edited by Wilson CP, Mintz IL. Northvale, NJ, Jason Aronson, 1989, pp 309–326

Koblenzer C: Psychocutaneous Diseases. Orlando, FL, Grune & Stratton, 1987

Mintz IL: Air symbolism in asthma, in Psychosomatic Symptoms: Psychodynamic Treatment of the Underlying Personality Disorder. Edited by Wilson CP, Mintz IL. Northvale, NJ, Jason Aronson, 1989, pp 211–249

Mintz IL: The fear of being fat in normal, obese, starving, and gorging individuals, in Psychodynamic Techniques in the Treatment of the Eating Disorder. Edited by Wilson CP, Hogan CC, Mintz IL. Northvale, NJ, Jason Aronson, 1992, pp 99–107

Mushatt C: Mind-body environment: toward understanding the impact of loss on psyche and soma. Psychoanal Q 44:81–106, 1975

Mushatt C, Werby I: Grief and anniversary reactions, in Psychosomatic Symptoms: Psychodynamic Treatment of the Underlying Personality Disorder. Edited by Wilson CP, Mintz IL. Northvale, NJ, Jason Aronson, 1989, pp 147–169

Nemiah JC, Sifneos PE: Affect and fantasy in patients with psychosomatic disorders, in Modern Times in Psychosomatic Medicine, Vol 2. Edited by Hill OW. New York, Appleton-Century-Crofts, 1970, pp 26–34

Reiser MF: Toward an integrated psychoanalytic physiological theory of psychosomatic disorders, in Psychoanalysis—A General Psychology. Edited by Lowenstein RM, Newman LM, Schur M, et al. New York, International Universities Press, 1966, pp 570–582

Reiser MF: Changing theoretic concepts in psychosomatic medicine, in American Handbook of Psychiatry, Vol 4. Edited by Reiser MF. New York, Basic Books, 1975, pp 477–510

Savitt RA: Conflict and somatization: psychoanalytic treatment of psycho-physiological responses in the digestive tract. Psychoanal Q 46:605–622, 1977

Schneer H: The Asthmatic Child. New York, Harper & Row, 1963

Schur M: Comments on the metapsychology of somatization, in The Psychoanalytic Study of the Child, Vol 10. New Haven, CT, Yale University Press, 1955, pp 119–164

Schwartz HJ (ed): Bulimia: Psychoanalytic Treatment and Theory. Madison, CT, International Universities Press, 1988

Sperling M: Children's interpretation and reaction to the unconscious of their mothers. Int J Psychoanal 31:1–6, 1950

Sperling M: Psychotherapeutic techniques, in Psychosomatic Medicine. Edited by Bychowski G, Despert J. New York, Basic Books, 1952, pp 297–301

Sperling M: Transference neurosis in patients with psychosomatic disorders. Psychoanal Q 36:342–355, 1967

Sperling M: The clinical effects of parental neurosis on the child, in Parenthood. Edited by Anthony E, Benedek T. Boston, MA, Little, Brown, 1970, pp 539—569

Silverman MA: Power, control and the threat to die in a case of asthma and anorexia, in Psychosomatic Symptoms: Psychodynamic Treatment of the Underlying Personality Disorder. Edited by Wilson CP, Mintz IL. Northvale, NJ, Jason Aronson, 1989, pp 351–364

Wilson CP, Mintz IL: The symptom and the underlying personality disorder, in Psychosomatic Symptoms: Psychodynamic Treatment of the Underlying Personality Disorder. Edited by Wilson CP, Mintz IL. Northvale, NJ, Jason Aronson, 1989, pp 1–9

Wilson CP, Mintz IL: Family psychopathology, in Psychosomatic Symptoms: Psychodynamic Treatment of the Underlying Personality Disorder. Edited by Wilson CP, Mintz IL. Northvale, NJ, Jason Aronson, 1989, pp 63–82

Wilson CP, Mintz IL: Dream interpretation, in Psychosomatic Symptoms: Psychodynamic Treatment of the Underlying Personality Disorder. Edited by Wilson CP, Mintz IL. Northvale, NJ, Jason Aronson, 1989, pp 133–145

References

Alexander F: Psychosomatic Medicine. New York, WW Norton, 1950

Alexander F, French TM, Pollock GH: Psychosomatic Specificity. Chicago, IL, University of Chicago Press, 1968

Boyer LB, Giovacchini PL: Treatment of characterological and schizophrenic disorders, in Tactics and Techniques in Psychoanalytic Therapy, Vol 11. Edited by Giovacchini PL, Farsheim A, Boyer LB. New York, Jason Aronson, 1975, pp 341–373

Boyer LB, Giovacchini PL: Psychoanalytic Treatment of Borderline and Characterological Disorders, New York, Jason Aronson, 1980

Cullinan ER: Ulcerative colitis: clinical aspects. British Medical Journal 2:135, 1938

Daniels GE: Treatment of a case of ulcerative colitis associated with hysterical depression. Psychosom Med 2:276–285, 1940

Deutsch F: The Psychosomatic Concept in Psychoanalysis. New York, International Universities Press, 1953

Deutsch L: Psychosomatic medicine from a psychoanalytic viewpoint. J Am Psychoanal Assoc 28:653–702, 1980

Deutsch L: Reflections on the psychoanalytic treatment of patients with bronchial asthma, in The Psychoanalytic Study of the Child, Vol 42. Edited by Solnit AJ, Neubauer PB. New Haven, CT, Yale University Press, 1987, pp 239–261

Dunbar HF: Psychosomatic Diagnosis. New York, Hoeber, 1943

Engel GL: Psychological aspects of the management of ulcerative colitis. New York State Journal of Medicine 22:2255–2261, 1952

Engel GL: Studies of ulcerative colitis, III: the nature of the psychologic process. JAMA 19:231–256, 1955

Engel GL: Studies of ulcerative colitis, IV: the significance of headaches. Psychosom Med 18:334–346, 1956

French TM, Alexander F: Psychogenic factors in bronchial asthma. American Journal of Psychiatry Monographs, Vols 2 and 4. Washington, DC, National Research Council, 1941

Fromm-Reichmann F: Contribution to the psychogenesis of migraine. Psychoanal Rev 24:26–33, 1937

Gerard MW: Bronchial asthma in children. Nervous Child 5:327–331, 1946

Giovacchini PL: The psychoanalytic treatment of the alienated patient, in New Perspectives in the Psychotherapy of the Borderline Adult. Edited by Masterson J. New York, Brunner/Mazel, 1977, pp 1–39

Grinker RSR: Psychosomatic Research. New York, WW Norton, 1953

Hogan CC: Technical problems in psychoanalytic treatment, in Fear of Being Fat: The Treatment of Anorexia Nervosa and Bulimia, Revised Edition. Edited by Wilson CP, Hogan CC, Mintz IL. Northvale, NJ, Jason Aronson, 1985, pp 197–216

Hogan CC: Inflammatory disease of the colon, in Psychosomatic Symptoms: Psychodynamic Treatment of the Underlying Personality Disorder. Edited by Wilson CP, Mintz IL. Northvale, NJ, Jason Aronson, 1989, pp 367–400

Karush A, Daniels GE: Ulcerative colitis: the psychoanalysis of two cases. Psychosom Med 15:140–167, 1953

Kernberg OF: Internal World and External Reality: Object Relations Theory Applied. New York, Jason Aronson, 1980

Knapp PH: Acute bronchial asthma, II: psychoanalytic observations on fantasy, emotional arousal, and partial discharge. Psychosom Med 22:88–105, 1960

Knapp PH: Psychotherapy for somatizing disorders, in Psychosomatic Medicine, Theory, Physiology, and Practice, Vol 2. Edited by Cheren S. Madison, CT, International Universities Press, 1989, pp 813–839

Knapp PH, Nemetz SJ: Personality variations in bronchial asthma—a study of 40 patients: notes on the relationship to psychosis and the problem of measuring maturity. Psychosom Med 19:443–465, 1957

Knapp PH, Mushatt C, Nemetz SJ: The asthmatic child and the psychosomatic problem of asthma: toward a general theory, in the Asthmatic Child: Psychosomatic Approach to Problems and Treatment. Edited by Schneer H. New York, Harper & Row, 1963, pp 234–255

Knapp PH, Mushatt C, Nemetz SJ: The context of reported asthma during psychoanalysis. Psychosom Med 32:167–188, 1970

Lindemann E: Psychiatric problems in conservative treatment of ulcerative colitis. Archives of Neurology and Psychiatry 53:322, 1945

Mahler MS: On child psychosis and schizophrenia: autistic and symbiotic infantile psychosis, in The Psychoanalytic Study of the Child, Vol 7. New York, International Universities Press, 1952, pp 286–305

Mahler MS: Overview: individuation in perspective, in The Psychological Birth of the Human Infant: Symbiosis and Individuation. Edited by Mahler MS, Pine F, Bergman A. New York, Basic Books, 1975, pp 3–17

Mintz IL: The anniversary reaction: a response to the unconscious sense of time. J Am Psychoanal Assoc 19:720–735, 1971

Mintz IL: Multi-determinism in asthmatic disease. International Journal of Psychodynamic Psychotherapy 8:593–600, 1980–1981

Mintz IL: Treatment of a case of anorexia and severe asthma, in Psychosomatic Symptoms: Psychoanalytic Treatment of the Underlying Personality Disorder. Edited by Wilson CP, Mintz IL. Northvale, NJ, Jason Aronson, 1989a, pp 251–308

Mintz IL: Varieties of somatization, in Psychosomatic Symptoms: Psychodynamic Treatment of the Underlying Personality Disorder. Edited by Wilson CP, Mintz IL. Northvale, NJ, Jason Aronson, 1989b, pp 171–206

Mintz IL: The unconscious role of teeth in anorexia nervosa and bulimia: the lizard phenomenon, in Psychodynamic Technique in the Treatment of the Eating Disorders. Edited by Wilson CP, Hogan CC, Mintz IL. Northvale, NJ, Jason Aronson, 1992, pp 331–352

Mushatt C: Psychological aspects of non-specific ulcerative colitis, in Recent Developments in Psychosomatic Medicine. Edited by Wittkower ED, Cleghorn RA. Philadelphia, PA, JB Lippincott, 1954

Mushatt C: Mind-body-environment: toward understanding the impact of loss on psyche and soma. Psychoanal Q 44:81–106, 1975

Mushatt C: Loss, separation, and psychosomatic illness, in Psychosomatic Symptoms: Psychodynamic Treatment of the Underlying Personality Disorder. Edited by Wilson CP, Mintz IL. Northvale, NJ, Jason Aronson, 1989, pp 33–61

Pollock GH: Anniversary reactions, trauma, and mourning. Psychoanal Q 39:347–371, 1970

Pollock GH: The ghost that will not go away: specificity theory today. J Am Acad Psychoanal 5:421–430, 1977

Pollock GH: Anniversaries and time, in The Mourning-Liberation Process, Vol 1. Madison, CT, International Universities Press, 1989, pp 183–319

Selinsky H: Psychological study of the migraine syndrome. Bulletin of the New York Academy of Medicine 15:757–763, 1939

Sperling M: Psychoanalytic study of ulcerative colitis in children. Psychoanal Q 15:302–329, 1946

Sperling M: Problems in the analysis of children, in Psychosomatic Disorders of Childhood. Edited by Sperling O. New York, Jason Aronson, 1978a, pp 11–16

Sperling M: The role of the mother in psychosomatic disorder in children, in Psychosomatic Disorders of Childhood. Edited by Sperling O. New York, Jason Aronson, 1978b, pp 17–30

Sperling M: Psychoanalytic study of ulcerative colitis, in Psychosomatic Disorders of Childhood. Edited by Sperling O. New York, Jason Aronson, 1978c, pp 61–98

Volkan VD: Primitive Internal Object Relations: A Clinical Study of Schizophrenia, Borderline and Narcissistic Patients. New York, International Universities Press, 1976

Weiss E, English OS: Psychosomatic Medicine. Philadelphia, PA, WB Saunders, 1957

Wilson CP: Psychosomatic asthma and acting out. Int J Psychoanal 49:330–333, 1968

Wilson CP: On the limits of the effectiveness of psychoanalysis: early ego and somatic disturbances. J Am Psychoanal Assoc 19:552–564, 1971

Wilson CP: Ego functioning in psychosomatic disorders, in Psychosomatic Symptoms: Psychodynamic Treatment of the Underlying Personality Disorder. Edited by Wilson CP, Mintz IL. Northvale, NJ, Jason Aronson, 1989, pp 13–31

Chapter 21

The Patient With Bulimia

Harvey J. Schwartz, M.D.,
and Martin Ceaser, M.D.

Current Psychodynamic Perspectives

Eating disorder patients can be confusing, enraging, and frustrating to work with. They seem to be possessed by a concreteness that defies psychological meaning. Their preoccupation with their literal selves—their bodies, their calories, their pounds—can lead therapists to themselves feel possessed, which encourages them toward a complementary form of literalness. This can lead therapists away from the all-important task of understanding what feelings, desires, and fears have led these patients to forsake people for food. Instead therapists often find themselves drawn into their patients' preoccupation with the inanimate world—a preoccupation that all too often only serves to keep hidden the conflicted passions that have led to the creation of the symptom.

The thesis of this chapter is that even though they themselves might be unaware of it, eating disorder patients are in fact struggling with powerful and frightening feelings and fantasies toward people. It is in response to these people-related interests and their associated anxiety and guilt that these patients regress, leading them to *turn to their own bodies,* upon which they then inflict a variety of violent and erotic manipulations. The clinical task is to help these patients recognize that the stimulus for their defensive retreat into themselves is a specific desire—a fantasy—that exists in relation to another person. Furthermore, patients need to come to recognize that the symptomatic narcissistic act itself contains the object-related fantasy in coded form.

In a successful treatment, the primary relationship within which these feelings and their avoidances take place is the one with the therapist—the transference. Before discussing how one invites the transference to blossom or what one then does with it, we would like to detour for a moment to sketch out an overview of the psychology of patients with bulimia.

Overview of Coexisting Symptoms

As will be discussed in the section on differential dynamic diagnosis, bulimia is merely a symptom that can occur in a neurotic, borderline, or psychotic patient. There are nevertheless a number of constituents of this symptom that are common to many patients and that contribute to the other symptoms that regularly coexist with bulimia.

Intolerance of affect. First and foremost, bulimic patients manifest an *intolerance of affect*—that is, when such patients experience anxiety, they attempt to sidestep it by acting. The act may take the form of a food binge, impulsive shopping *(oniomania),* anonymous sex, or an asthma attack. The symptoms themselves are interchangeable (C. P. Wilson 1990), with the form that they take initially being less important than the function they serve to obliterate any delay of action. Pausing, imagining, remembering, and feeling sad are all avoided through the impulsive act. In this process of impulsiveness, one's body is not recognized as a potentially lovely medium for internally derived and tolerable anger, arousal, or grief; instead, it is registered as something foreign—a perception that brings with it an obsessive emphasis on the body's exterior aspects, a decreased registration of enteroceptive signals, and even a diminished sensitivity to pain (Lautenbacher et al. 1991). As part of this defensive state of self-alienation, the body image is either numb or overexcited, with generic sensations that are perceived to be without distinctiveness. The buildup of these anonymous sensations creates the tension state that the patient feels can only be relieved by the monotonous impulsive act. The body image that is the medium for these discharges is without the capacity for gracefulness or love, as it derives from the sense that one's body is not one's own, separate from one's mother.

Maternal enmeshment. It has been commonly recognized that patients with bulimia exist in a state of *enmeshment with their mothers.* Clinically, one sees this even before the initial evaluation, as it is often the mother calling to make the appointment for her 30-year-old daughter. For a variety of motivations that began in early childhood, in adolescence these patients have unconsciously made a pact with their internal image of their mothers. It is as if they live by the credo "Don't worry, Mother. I will not leave you and grow up to be a mature woman with adult concerns of autonomy, sexual desire, and childbearing. Instead, I will remain as if an ill child devoted to preoccupying myself and tormenting you with my eating." Quite commonly and for reasons very much their own, these patients' mothers often have made their own unconscious pact with their internal images of their daughters that reciprocally proclaims "I am distracted from my sadness by your not leaving me. I will agree to remain obsessed about your childlike body in order to protect you (and me) from the terrible dangers that would befall you (and me) if you allowed yourself to care for and be cared about by a man." Through this complementarity, each generation colludes with the other to sidestep the internalization of conflict.

The daughter's failure to establish an essentially tender identification with her mother and her genitality leaves her capable of only a disdainful vision of her femininity. This hateful attachment to the mother limits the daughter's sense of separateness so that the only sexual self she can construct is one that is permeated with aggression. Often, both parties fear that if the daughter is strong enough to separate from her mother, she is strong enough to be her rival.

Imbrication of anxieties over separation and sexuality. It is almost ubiquitous in bulimic patients for there to be an *overlapping of fears of separation and sexuality.* This overlap has contributed to a significant division in the field between those who emphasize one or the other of these components in the etiology of the disorder (see Schwartz 1990a, 1990b; Tabin and Tabin 1990). Although a mixture is quite common, one also finds some patients who engage in nonemotional sexual activity in order to avoid feeling alone and others who act clingy and helpless in order to avoid feeling sexual. As one patient put it, "I'd rather feel sick then feel sexy." With bulimic patients, inorgasmia and avoidance of sexual behavior are more the rule, with counterphobic promiscuity occurring somewhat less often. In both situations, what is being avoided by the patient is the anxiety associated with experiencing herself to be an individuated woman with her own mature genitals who feels aroused and desirous toward a man who is recognized as separate and different from her. For the bulimic patient, this state of object relatedness is assumed to be calamitous and hence is avoided. To her, such a state entails an unforgivable abandonment of mother; an exposure of her own sense of femaleness, which she sees as dirty; a recognition of a man's maleness, which she regressively resents; and the commission of an incestuous transgression.

Dissociation of self. Underlying these gender-related fears and distortions is a *dissociated sense of self* whereby patients view themselves as if they existed in the third person. They live as if their bodies were their own imaginary companions. They measure them, abuse them, and speak of them from an "objective" distance as if they didn't inhabit them. This remoteness leads these patients to a peculiar self-consciousness whereby they know themselves only through how they imagine others see them. In an effort to avoid their angry visions of others, they preoccupy themselves with their own images as seen in the mirror. They obsessively look at their bodies as an outside observer, through the eyes of their imagined mother. Within this regressive state, they feel that they can never be perfect for this mother, so they return to the mirror in an angrily monotonous effort seeking "her" satisfaction. One sees this in the transference in patients' desperate demands that the therapist see them in a fixed way (e.g., as pathetic, fat, arousing). Rather than acknowledge their actual feelings *toward* the therapist, they insistently project their images of themselves onto the therapist and then feel self-consciously watched. As a result, the therapeutic relationship is drained of spontaneity and evokes for these patients the controllingness that they felt as a child—and that they currently inflict on their imagination.

Interchangeable object relatedness. This, then, becomes the bulimic patient's version of relatedness—a version that, in fact, is a caricature of relatedness. As they felt they were related to as a child, these patients reduce others in their life into a controllable extension of themselves. *People are related to as interchangeable inanimate objects.* Clinically, one boyfriend is often interchangeable with another, who is interchangeable with carbohydrates. There have been many different terms applied to such relationships that serve primarily to regulate one's self-esteem. Reich (1953) concluded that they are formed from "narcissistic object choices." Object relations theorists describe these relationships as deriving from "part object" status (Ogden 1986). Jeammet (1988), a French analyst, reported that eating disorder patients use their boyfriends to create a "self-sufficiency *à deux.*" We find it clinically useful to consider that like the patients' own bodies, their boyfriends exist for them as if they were their imaginary companions—indispensable, the containers of their disavowed affects, and the distracters from their sadness. When such boyfriends leave them, these patients, being unable to mourn, instead panic. They then attempt to solve the perceived narcissistic injury of having lost an extension of themselves by dissociating their own body into a frenzied *à deux.* This leads to the binge-purge, in which they simultaneously assume the bisexual roles of the aggressor and aggressee. In place of sadness over a lost lover, bulimic patients turn to regressive expressions of missing someone. In such situations, they use abdominal fullness in lieu of companionship.

Inaccessibility to intimacy. These defensive narcissistic preoccupations lead such patients to be particularly *inaccessible to be open and revealing about their emotional lives.* For some patients, any exploration of their inner world leads to outbursts of complaints about their protruding stomach, their calorie quota, or their self-disgust. When anxious, they return to looking at themselves. They avoid any sense of vulnerability, as it would expose them to their feared childhood feelings of shame, smallness, and hostility. Without realizing it, the more uncomfortable they feel about being intimate with the therapist, the more they demand that the therapist be intimate with them. They project their own inaccessibility onto the therapist and attack him or her for it, all the while keeping everyone in their life at arm's length. This characterological avoidance of the personal is often traceable to childhood defensive responses to their parents' own narcissistic preoccupations.

Negative transformation of positive affects. One common unconscious mechanism by which bulimic patients attempt to avoid experiencing their people-related anxiety is by *turning any opportunity for warmth into bitterness*—that is, by transforming "love-desire into hate-desire" (Kaplan 1984, p. 264). When one bulimic patient called me to cancel a session because she was ill and sounded it, I spontaneously asked what was wrong. She later became, as was characteristic for her, slightly paranoid, accusing me of trying to trick her by my question. In fact, she was deeply moved by my query but was frightened of the flood of loving feelings that she felt in response to it. In an effort to avoid this positive transference, with its history of painful longings as a neglected child, she defensively assumed the position of self-righteous accuser. In fact, in response to any expressions from me that she felt to be caring, she became suspicious or demeaning and declared that she merely had forced them out of me. This is the patient who at the same time continuously railed against me for not being warm toward her. Rather than acknowledge the vulnerabilities and guilt associated with wanting love, the patient instead turned to the ideal of control and the certainty of being able to provoke anger. She, like many bulimic patients, defensively transformed her lifelong and vulnerable wishes to receive into active impulses to take. Similarly, she transformed self-empathy into masochism and impregnation fantasies into vomiting.

Impregnation Fantasies

There is probably no issue in the field of eating disorders more confusing and controversial than that of the *impregnation wish* that is said to underlie bulimic patients' preoccupation with their weight. Many critics declare such ideas to be relics of antiquated and sexist psychoanalytic dogma that "blame the victim" for what are actually familial and cultural obsessions with thinness. Others reject this formulation on the grounds that it fails to acknowledge the centrality of these patients' preoedipal conflicts over separation from the mother.

What is essential to recognize in this controversy is the differing tools of investigation that are utilized to discover the psychological data and the differing levels of abstraction they are each designed to recognize. If one auscultates these patients' thoughts on the topic by surveying them about any thoughts they might have about pregnancy, one may hear an array of manifest responses that—if at all revealing—suggest a "realistic" concern that their "illness" might damage the fetus. On the other hand, to further extend the medical metaphor, if one x-rays such patients to determine the shadows of their deeper psychic structures, one often finds that their aversions to sexuality and their daydreams about their protruding abdomens preconsciously refer to some disguised references to being pregnant. If, however, one performs open-heart surgery with an analytic instrument attuned to the inner experiences of these patients and to recognizing the metaphoric meanings of their associative imagery (Arlow 1979), one is in a position to discover the full breadth of patients' unconscious fantasies about impregnation. It is quite common for patients to express such fantasies in derivative forms—which can include dreams of enlarging enclosed spaces and of new ideas being "conceivable," as well as the creation of metaphoric products of conception (i.e., works of art, growing bank accounts, or successful garden plantings, to name just a few).

> For example, one bulimic patient noticed a pregnant woman sitting outside her therapist's office and concluded that this woman was his wife. That evening she had

an enormous binge and obsessed about her protruding abdomen. With interpretive help, she came to affectively recognize that through her binge, she was attempting to mimic the woman she had seen because she was enraged at her therapist for giving someone else a child while neglecting her. Soon thereafter, this patient became intrigued with the inside spaces of closed refrigerators.

Another bulimic patient, who periodically put on so much weight from bingeing that she had to wear loose-fitting clothes, would be asked by her friends if she were pregnant. Once, although her period was not unusually late, she panicked and, with little evidence, became convinced that she was pregnant. Despite these manifest fears, her preoccupation with being pregnant proved to be not reality but a wish. Reflecting on her need to throw up all her food immediately after eating it, this well-educated patient asserted: *"If I don't throw it up, it will grow."* The childhood image that a baby grows from food in the stomach persists unconsciously throughout life.

For this patient, as for others, the wish to be pregnant represented her trying to make herself more acceptable to her mother in the hope of finally receiving her love and healing her depression. Such scenarios commonly emerge in the transference, which is the arena that allows them to be jointly observable and thereby curative.

The more subtle question that can be raised about this issue is that if impregnation fantasies are a normal and ubiquitous part of a girl's development, why is it that eating disorder patients appear to be so conflicted about them? In and of themselves, these fantasies are neither unusual nor noteworthy and in fact often contribute a pleasurable backdrop to a young woman's realistic desires to become pregnant.

The analytic investigation of patients with bulimia reveals that it is in two ways that they uniquely struggle with impregnation fantasies. First, for these patients, such fantasies are concrete and monotonous obsessions. They have not been endowed with the playfulness and optimism that would characterize them if they were fully symbolized imaginings. Instead, they are only semisymbolic and hence are imbued with an anal-level violence and disgust. Second, for these patients, the impregnation fantasies are filled with an all-or-nothing desperateness. Both these dimensions indicate that what is being expressed does not specifically represent a developmentally advanced oedipal level wish but instead *preoedipal longings disguised as genital wishes.*

It is quite common for these patients to have experienced severe early childhood disappointments that they attributed to their mothers. These disappointments, in turn, led them to develop an intolerable rage at her, which they coped with by projection. One expression of this mechanism is that bulimic patients often fear that food is attacking them. This badness may contaminate their image of their mother, which encourages them to prematurely turn to their idealized "good" father, toward whom they then direct their physical yearnings. In this scenario, the wish to be impregnated and/or the wish not to be female comes to represent a final common solution for an array of paternal and maternal frustrations. Alternately, the father may be the recipient of the maternal badness, which infuses the girl's feminine wish to be impregnated with a terrifying violence. This leads her to a psychology of defensive impenetrability and with it a regressive return to the idealized mother. Both schemata more or less derive from the excessive guilt that surrounds tender sexuality and the ready availability of sadomasochistic aggression to define intimacy.

The success of a toddler girl's development often hinges on her being able to recognize her aggressive wishes toward her mother while maintaining an identification with her. This task differs from that of a boy, who can more easily acknowledge his autonomy and hostility toward his mother by safely identifying with the outside figure of his father. Specifically, the girl's task of both separating from her mother while *at the same time* needing to identify with her as a female sets the stage for her to have transient dissociations of identity to cope with this dilemma. This developmental task, which is unique to females, has been suggested as a cause for the greater incidence in women of both eating disorders (Tabin and Tabin 1990) and imaginary companions (Rucker 1981).

A number of factors contribute to a girl's ability to tolerate her frightening aggressive wishes. Perhaps the most important is her mother's respectful empathy for her separate yet intimate existence. As mentioned, the mothers of bulimic patients often reinforce their children's defensive retreat into narcissistic preoccupation by themselves being excessively self-involved. In the mother's effort to sidestep a loneliness that she fears would be intolerable, she perceives her child as an extension of herself—a process that has been called "appersonation" (O. Sperling 1943–1945). One such mother introduced her 22-year-old bulimic daughter to the therapist by saying "she's my doll"—and she wasn't joking. Through the simultaneous psychoanalysis of a mother and her symptomatic child, M. Sperling found that as the child's symptoms resolved, the mother often became depressed and developed an eating disorder of her own. In a similar vein, analytic treatment of the mother often leads to amelioration of the child's symptoms (M. Sperling 1949, 1978).

The fathers of these patients often have had difficulty in benevolently but firmly extricating their daughters from dyadic enmeshments with the mother and introducing them into a world of tolerable triangularity. In addition, these fathers have been found to frequently have eating peculiarities of their own. More malignantly, however, it is common for these fathers to relate to their daughters by enthralling them while also intensely teasing them. This treatment leads them to be covertly rejecting of their daughters' femininity even as they are being overstimulatingly seductive toward them (Sours 1974; M. Sperling 1983).

Childhood Environmental Conditions

It is not unusual to find a history of actual trauma either in bulimic patients' conscious memories or through the analytic lifting of repressions. Whether eating disorder patients have a significantly higher frequency of childhood abuse than patients with other disorders, however, remains controversial. Recent findings suggest that compared with other female psychiatric patients, those with eating disorders do not have a higher incidence of childhood sexual abuse (Palmer 1991). Nonetheless, it appears that patients who present with multiple impulsive symptoms, especially laxative and substance abuse, frequently have a childhood history of physical and/or sexual abuse (Lacey 1990).

A psychodynamic approach to patients with a history of abuse is described in detail in Chapter 19 of this volume. What is important to appreciate in bulimic patients is that the explosive tension state that precedes and accompanies the binge-purge is a reenactment of the dissociated rage the patients encoded during their abuse. They now do to themselves what was done to them.

> One patient who was brutally abused by her father throughout her childhood developed this state of intense tension whenever she began to experience tender feelings toward her male therapist. She could relieve herself of this tension only by bingeing, cutting herself, having an asthma attack, or provoking her father to beat her. She could not, however, allow herself to leave her father, as this would have exposed her to the profound feelings of neglect she had earlier felt at the hands of her alcoholic mother.

There are two other environmental conditions in the childhoods of bulimic patients that are more common yet less appreciated than that of actual abuse. The first is that of excessive parental nudity. Exhibitionistic parental sexual and toilet behavior is a common phenomena in these families, the significance of which is totally denied by the patient and her parents (C. P. Wilson 1986). Doors in these homes are commonly not locked, with bedroom and bathroom doors often being left open for the curious child. Such overstimulation, often coupled with parental manifest hypermorality, inhibits the child's development of a comfortable and autonomous sexual sense of self.

The other, often minimized, external stimulation is that of surgery during childhood. This experience, especially when accompanied by minimal parental preparation and working through, often leaves an unmetabolized psychic scar in the child. Young girls in these circumstances often take the violence of the surgical intrusion to be both the prototype for sexual intimacy and the mutilating punishment for masturbatory fantasies. This experience of enforced helplessness can lead the child to adopt a stance of absolute anorectic "no" when later faced with situations that she can control (i.e., eating and heterosexuality). It can be valuable to recognize in patients' transference states of passive defiance the reliving of their rage at being surgically intruded upon.

Therapeutic Foci

The technique of working dynamically with bulimic patients entails first and foremost recognizing that these patients are unknowingly hiding their people-related desires in their self-abuse. When they describe their symptoms and loathsome body image, they are in fact speaking to the therapist *about* a patient. These individuals lack a sense of their own inner-derived affects and therefore present to the therapist only the pseudocooperation that is characteristic of their false selves. Hence, *the essential therapeutic task is to make contact with the patient.*

Patients' object disappointments are experienced as narcissistic injuries (e.g., rage at mother is registered as ugliness in the mirror). Similarly, the only way these patients know how to express, for example, their loving feelings for their therapist is to proclaim, "I'm fat." This self-preoccupation simultaneously expresses feelings such as "I miss you when you go away," and "I'm angry at you for changing my appointment time." The therapist needs to recognize that these patients' object longings are for them without distinctiveness and are confusingly condensed in their overexcited narcissistic states.

The task is to direct patients from their defensive self-involvement toward the early awareness of their feelings toward the therapist—that is, to enter their narcissistic *à deux.* When one can accomplish this, one regularly finds that these patients associate any sense of needing or desiring another person with profound fears of shame and ridicule. The vulnerability that is thus awakened in turn mobilizes an intensely conflicted aggression, which leads to a collapse of self-esteem. For higher-functioning patients, this accessibility entails a sense of humiliation and guilt in recognizing their forbidden genital fantasies. More disturbed patients, in contrast, use their monotonous sadomasochistic self-involvements to avoid experiencing an enraging and terrifying aloneness.

One patient described her reaction to hearing that a man she had dated had spurned her for another woman. While thinking of him, she *looked into a mirror* and, seeing her sunken cheeks, bitterly declared "I hope they shrivel into nothing—that would get back at him!" She had transformed her castrating rage at this man into a dissociative (i.e., mirror) self-preoccupation and enacted her violence on her own body. *She was unable to miss him.* This phenomenon is a *sine qua non* of the eating disorders. These patients—and often, their parents—have not been able to elaborate their capacity to mourn—known by some as reaching the depressive position. In its place, they are capable only of somatic outbursts (i.e., depressive equivalents), which in treatment need to be translated into the object longings they were designed to repudiate.

Accordingly, the therapeutic task with bulimic patients is to assist them in recognizing that their symptomatic explosions are a response to feelings they have toward others, especially toward the therapist. This task applies to patients who indifferently deny the therapist's importance to them as well as to those who defend against their more subtle desires by overexcitedly idealizing the therapist. From this consistent interpretive stance, patients can come to recognize that symptoms that initially are experienced as being a function of their "affect intolerance" are in fact an expression of their *intent* to hurt the therapist. Stated differently, the patient's masochism comes to be felt as part of a more fully developed *masochistic attack.*

This is the transition stage at which patients begin to recognize their object desires. Another indication of this period is that patients' symptoms may increasingly emerge in the manifest content of their dreams, leading to the growing recognition that *their bulimic outbreaks are temper tantrums* that are unconsciously designed to engage, provoke, and punish the therapist. This recognition becomes the link to these patients' childhood desires, frustrations, and tragedies, which have for years remained hidden in the monotonous narcissism of their symptoms.

Historical Review

A number of archival surveys of the history of bulimia have been described in the medical literature over the past 300 years (Parry-Jones and Parry-Jones 1991). These reports have documented in impressive descriptive detail the consistency of the symptom picture over the centuries independent of the varying cultural forces that existed during those times. Hypotheses of etiology have varied from worms, head trauma, "nervous atrophy," and cerebral tumor.

For the purposes of this chapter, we will focus on conceptualization of the eating disorders that has evolved since Gull (1874) and Lasègue (1873) first described the syndrome that has come to be recognized as anorexia nervosa. Its history and that of bulimia are intertwined and are fully reviewed in Kaufman and Heiman (1964).

The struggle to understand the eating disorders in the last century parallels the overall evolution in medicine and the greater appreciation of the permeability of the psyche/soma barrier. Lasègue (1873), who first named anorexia, thought that it was caused by the "mental disposition of the patient." He observed, as we do today, the powerful impact both of the family on the patient's symptoms and of the patient's symptoms on the family. However, both he and Gull (1874) were working from a prepsychoanalytic paradigm and thus failed to study the childhood antecedents of the adolescent eating disorders. Their model remained ahistoric.

In the decades since this original work, the recognition of the psychological factors in these illnesses has seesawed with a strictly descriptive/organic approach. During this early period, adherents of both orientations were mired in all-or-none thinking. For example, early id-oriented analytic findings emphasized the exclusive etiological role of oedipal impregnation fantasies. Early phenomenologists insisted that anorexia was schizophrenia, hysteria, and finally, Simmonds' disease.

Although these initial propositions were incorrect, researchers in these two areas have forged ahead and pushed their respective tools of investigation to ever more subtle levels. On the neurochemical side, major advances in measuring and altering brain transmitters have led to recognizing the short-term utility of antidepressants in bulimia. Similarly, advances in ego psychology and object relations theory have allowed the deeper preoedipal layers of psychic functioning to be amenable to analytic treatment. As each field has progressed in this century and deepened its appreciation of its foundations, many feel that a common ground is being discovered. Rather than an either/or perspective, investigators are now studying the impact on brain functioning of early psychic trauma as well as the role of serotonin in mediating the ego capacity to delay discharge (see Soubrie 1986).

In the area of psychoanalysis, there has been one particular development in the last half-century that has played a vital role in advancing our understanding and treatment of eating disorder patients. Specifically, the old concept of countertransference as an unfortunate contamination of the analytic arena has progressed to the point where we now recognize that phenomenon as an inevitable and invaluable data-gathering instrument. It is especially useful in working with the many bulimic patients who use projective mechanisms in an effort to disavow their separateness and aggression. The boredom and overstimulation that these patients evoke in the receptive analyst can be central in appreciating their narcissistic withdrawals and rages, which are initially nonverbal.

Differential Dynamic Diagnosis

Bulimia may be caused by medical conditions (Krahn and Mitchell 1984) and may also be associated with acute posttraumatic stress disorder (Torem and Curdue 1988). Most often, however, it is one symptomatic manifestation of either a neurotic or a borderline character organization. It is the severity of the character disorder and not the severity of the symptoms that is prognostically significant (G. Wilson and Eldredge 1991).

It is not unusual for adolescent girls to have transient periods of mild anorexia nervosa or bulimia. These can occur in girls who are otherwise meaningfully engaged in nonfamilial pursuits and are otherwise more or less adapting to the developmental challenges of adolescence. For them, such episodes represent a defensive regression from and a disguised representation of oedipal conflicts that have been activated by genital maturity and environmental stimulation. These patients are capable of abstract and symbolic thinking, are able to tolerate to some degree ambivalence toward and separation from their mothers, and are able to be sad when they suffer a loss. For them, the "too much" that they experience in relation to their confusing affects serves as a defense against recognizing their specific inner sensations of arousal that are linked to incestuous objects. The repression barrier leads them to hide their object-related sexuality in an oral and narcissistic mode.

Many of these patients do not reach a psychiatrist's office either because the symptoms spontaneously remit or because they respond to supportive counseling from guidance counselors or family doctors. If these symptoms persist over time, intensive psychotherapy or psychoanalysis is indicated.

More often, the patients with bulimia who present to a psychiatrist are those with long-standing global deficits in affect and impulse modulation; multiple symptoms including kleptomania, laxative or substance abuse, and asthma; and infantile object dependency. For these patients, the only sense of pleasure or mastery they experience is through the ability to control themselves and others. One consequence of this character organization is that they use projective identification in order to feel familiar and secure with those with whom they are close. The therapist, accordingly, may find him- or herself possessed by a sense of being intensely enraged, guilty, worthless, or aroused when working closely with such patients.

Generally for the bulimic patient, and occasionally for the therapist, affects are mostly experienced in either the "too much" mode or else its flip side of numbness. For the more disturbed patient, this manner of experiencing self and others usually does not solely derive from a defensive response to forbidden incestuous fantasies; rather, it represents a fixation as a consequence of either pregenital maternal strain trauma or later sexual/physical shock trauma. These patients are unable to register sadness or affectionate sexual arousal. Instead, as a result of the pervasiveness of their aggression, they are only able to experience somatic reactions when exposed to a loss and inorgasmia or genital anesthesia when exposed to sexual stimulation.

Treatment Approaches

The treatment of these patients is extremely difficult. For the most disabled, who initially have almost no capacity for psychological mindedness, cognitive and behavioral approaches are useful in that they bypass the need for introspection. For the higher-functioning individuals in this group, titrated exploratory psychotherapy may enable patients to begin to be aware of the anger that they have for so long been turning upon themselves. Some of these patients will do well in psychoanalysis when it is conducted by experienced analysts.

For some patients, bulimia serves as a "somatic memory" (Kramer 1990) of past abuse. This "memory" encapsulates in nonverbal form the rage, arousal, guilt, and depression that was initially dissociated when experienced with the original object. Working the traumatic relationship through the transference can lead to therapeutic progress.

Male patients with bulimia generally belong to the sicker group (Falstein et al. 1956; Sours 1974). These boys tend to be very tied to their mothers with whom they identify. Gender identity disturbances are pervasive, homosexual compromises are common, and there is a failure of an aggressive emulation of their father. Excessive anxiety over their active phallic strivings leads these boys to regress to a narcissistic preoccupation with their own bodies that is associated with a partial loss of differentiation from their image of their mothers.

There are two additional approaches to treatment that need to be kept in mind, especially for the sicker group of patients. The first concerns the use of antidepressants, which have been demonstrated for some patients to decrease the frequency of bingeing for a temporary period of time. There is no reliable predictor of who will respond to medication, as the presence of depression is not a helpful indicator. What is most useful about these drugs is that they appear to raise the impulse threshold; that is, they decrease the immediacy of the patient's need to relieve him- or herself through action of the affects that are experienced as overwhelming sensations. This can permit the patient the opportunity to pause and recognize a transference-related fantasy before it is impulsively reduced into a binge, theft, or sex act.

The other treatment approach to consider for the adolescent patient living at home is to recommend couple treatment for the parents. It is common for the patient's parents to share their difficulty in recognizing and tolerating fantasies, especially those related to their daughter's autonomy and sexuality. Instead, they overstimulatingly connect themselves to their daughter and use her to modulate their own internal and marital discomforts. If, through her treatment, the daughter begins to develop a meaningful transference to her therapist and thereby becomes able to experience desire and loss, she will remove herself from her impostor intimacy with her parents. Parents, at such times, will frequently interfere with their daughter's treatment in response to their own as well as the daughter's anxiety. It is often crucial to the success of the daughter's treatment for the parents to redirect their defensive possessiveness toward their therapist for analysis rather than toward their daughter for enactment.

Case Examples

Case 1

Ms. S, a bright, 25-year-old art student, was referred for analytic treatment because of a 5-year history of intermittent anorexia nervosa and episodic severe binge vomiting. She presented as a very thin but not cachexic woman who was both seductive and childlike in appearance and behavior. Her family history was significant for its absence of psychiatric disorder including alcoholism, obesity, and affective disorder. Her parents, both accomplished musicians, had divorced when Ms. S was in early adolescence.

The patient was seen in three-times-per-week face-to-face analytic psychotherapy and intermittently consulted with a nutritionist for dietary guidance. In her treatment, Ms. S all too quickly engaged with a readiness for emotional involvement and a pressure to action. Often, at the end of sessions, Ms. S would anxiously stand in front of me (M.C.), asking to be able to remain longer or tearfully pleading for some further response and for something to take with her. In the sessions she sought repeated stimulation and reassurance reminiscent of what she had obtained through cocaine use with older lovers early in college.

The patient's anxious dependence within the sessions—reflective of more pervasive panicky feelings in her outside life—was, of course, not random. Despite her history of instability and proneness to action, Ms. S, from the start, was able to use her mental agility and curiosity to reflect back on her behavior and her *seeming* need for an immediate response from me. She recognized in this the same pressure for response from her parents she had felt as a young child before and after undergoing repeated bladder catheterizations. Not only did Ms. S undergo multiple genitourinary procedures, but she also recalled, during bathing, having experienced highly exciting cleansing of her genitals by her parents, especially her father, presumably to prevent infection. In addition, she recounted periods of being with her father, riding on his shoulders at parades, and feeling guilty over the excitement. In the therapy hours, Ms. S fantasized that her standing and walking about would evoke a feared and welcomed prohibition from me—just as in a screen memory, her father had yelled at her, when she was a child, "Stop moving about" while he watched television or read with her nearby.

In her sessions, Ms. S would, in response to anxiety, erotize the experience by becoming seductive. In one session toward the end of the second year of treatment, and just after talking about her upcoming out-of-town visit to her fiancee, Ms. S stood up, approached me, insisting on the need to be close, and provocatively sat on the ottoman at the foot of my chair. It was possible, then and there, to explore her need for action in response to a disturbing fantasy she was able to verbalize: in going away to be with her fiancee, she imagined that I, like one of her separated parents during childhood, would feel excluded by her and be totally devastated. (Psychodynamically, it seemed that the patient identified with me as the victim of her own aggressive rejection fantasy, and she herself then experienced separation fears.)

Her return of binge vomiting after over a year of abstinence, just prior to the visit with her fiance, was also seen in part as a way of reassuring me that I was still valued and needed by her.

The bulimia condensed other conflicts as well. For example, upon learning that her father had remarried a young "hussy" who may have been pregnant, Ms. S had a resurgence of her binge vomiting. The thought of her father being sexually active was very much on Ms. S's mind. Without apparent conflict, she recalled early adolescent memories of fantasizing herself and her father having intercourse. Most important, these thoughts occurred in the treatment hours as a displacement away from the present, when the patient suddenly developed nausea over disgusting unacceptable, vague sexual thoughts toward her analyst.

A very powerful transference picture reappeared around the patient's seeming object hunger for—and subsequent need to distance herself from—both me and her fiance. Ms. S would focus on my hands, which she saw as natural and thin, suggesting weakness and vulnerability. She equated this image with seeing her fiance waiting at the airport and looking frail and defenseless, reminding her of moments after sex when her partner was depleted and therefore under her power. It was at these times that Ms. S would suddenly become uncomfortable, fearful of closeness, and then seek to disengage.

In her analytic psychotherapy, Ms. S had successfully begun the process of examining this powerful transference fantasy of hurting a perceived weaker partner. Today, she is productively in treatment with an analytic colleague in the city, where she is completing her graduate studies and living with her new husband.

Case 2

Ms. T was a 20-year-old law student referred for evaluation of depression and binge eating. She had been in weekly counseling for several months with another therapist but had left because of a lack of progress. In her initial sessions, Ms. T presented as a very shy, despondent woman who spoke in barely audible tones. She was easily startled and uncomfortable with a male therapist, but recognized that working with a man might help her understand her present mistrust of all men in her life.

Ms. T described having hated her family, and had fled her home by seeking work in a distant city. She recalled having grown up in a household with a cold, despotic father who was physically abusive to his submissive wife, an older sister, and a younger retarded brother. She felt guilty for having been spared the abuse that her father had dealt to the others in the home. Yet she despised her mother, who apologized for the father's behavior and had even lied to the police when Ms. T had called them during a family brawl. The patient had conscious memories of wanting to kill her father with a kitchen knife and of hoping that both her parents would die. While growing up, Ms. T remembered having been told repeatedly by her mother and, later, by her older sister, that her fears of her father's abuse were exaggerated and part of her imagination.

Because of her long history of severe mood swings and vegetative signs of depression, Ms. T was started on an antidepressant and seen in twice-weekly psychotherapy. The patient responded to the medication with a lifting in mood and a decrease in her overeating. However, with each improvement in her mood, she would "forget" her medication therapy, with a resultant gradual return to despondency. As therapy unfolded, Ms. T was clearly struggling with her wish to feel better and her guilt and fear of that wish's consequences.

In her treatment, Ms. T began reexperiencing bizarre physical sensations: pain in one eye, constriction in her throat, and a strong feeling of having something in her right hand. These sensations were accompanied by extreme fright; at the same time, she would describe feeling detached and separated from her body and from her surroundings. Often, within sessions or from one session to the next, Ms. T noticed that her voice sounded different and that her therapist seemed like a stranger.

However, despite experiencing considerable and dramatic upheaval, especially within the therapy sessions, Ms. T was increasingly able to reflect back on her bizarre experiences. For example, she was able to articulate a quasi-belief or conviction that the therapist was tormenting her—that he was an evil person conducting a strange experiment, the nature of which remained unclear. Ms. T described shaking as she sat in the waiting room before her therapy sessions, imagining that she were entering a prison with no chance of escape. In this image, she could recognize a gratifying sense of being punished for a crime, the nature of which eluded her.

As Ms. T related these frightening fantasies during her therapy sessions, she began to experience unclear, frightening childhood images of having been with a dark-haired neighbor, the father of her closest girlfriend. Other pictures, such as a "still frame" of her father's head, also occurred to her. In the therapy hours, the tantalizing quality of these vague images, abetted by the therapist's curiosity, spurred Ms. T to recreate early life memories of herself having felt forced to submit to another person's will.

Ms. T's transference images of the therapy as her punishment alternated with her concern that her indecisiveness and doubts about herself and her treatment were a way of punishing the therapist. She was torturing him, testing his patience and driving him crazy, yet feared that he would become so frustrated that he would become enraged and kick her out.

As the therapy continued, Ms. T was able to look at her shifting views of herself and of the therapist and to relate them to critical junctures in the sessions that aroused anxiety. For example, when the patient allowed herself to look the therapist in the eye, she became fearful and would dissociate. Behind her dread that he would be as untrustworthy as all the men she had known was a greater concern that she might see him as attractive. Whenever Ms. T had fleeting thoughts of being an adult woman with an adult man, she immediately became a little girl.

Ms. T's greatest struggle was about whether or not she was "crazy"; whether the various physical sensations, feeling states, and movielike images that raced before her eyes were just her "imaginings" (as her mother had said) or were actual hints of terrifying past experiences. To accept that abuse had happened in the past was to be "marked forever," and to be a bad person in the present. As she returned again and again to this point, the motive for her regression became clearer: along with her shame was an uncontrolled, murderous rage directed at her therapist. At such moments, Ms. T would retreat, saying, "This is all in my mind. I should be locked up. Everything is fine. I'm just a silly girl."

As this therapy proceeds, the focus remains on helping Ms. T understand the barriers to integrating present experiences, affects, and bodily states. This work in the present, especially in the transference, is facilitating integration with past, split-off memories and fantasies. The patient is increasingly tolerating the benefits of her medication and the productive use of her intellect. Hypnosis or other intrusive interventions have not been necessary.

Case 3

Ms. U, a 28-year-old single professional woman, sought therapy for bulimia and for depression. She presented as a bedraggled, sad individual who felt out of control with her daily binge vomiting. She was quick to attack herself for many perceived failings. Her symptoms had begun during her junior year in high school, when her parents were divorcing and she began to "feel fat." After an unsuccessful attempt at dieting, she began to binge-vomit and to abuse laxatives.

Since high school, Ms. U had had recurrent lows, characterized by overeating, fatigue, and low self-esteem. She had never been suicidal or unable to function in school or professionally. Family history was positive for both depression and eating disorder. Her younger sister was also bulimic, and her mother was overweight and chronically depressed. The patient's father had been depressed—moody and withdrawn—and addicted to barbiturates. Both parents had lost most of their family members during the Holocaust.

Ms. U recalled childhood memories of constant criticism about her looks. Her mother accused her of being either too fat or too thin, and told her she needed a nose job. The patient reported that her mother never prepared her for menarche and informed her about sanitary napkins only after her menses had begun.

After an extended evaluation, Ms. U was diagnosed as having recurrent atypical depression, bulimia, and a masochistic personality disorder (with borderline features). Individual insight-oriented twice-weekly psychotherapy was recommended and begun. The patient was adamant, however, about not wanting to take any antidepressant medications. She agreed to see an internist to monitor the physical effects of her eating disorder.

In psychotherapy, Ms. U was able to clarify the conditions under which she binged and vomited. She would overeat on sweets both to compensate for loneliness and to block out intense feelings she feared would be uncontrollable. She fantasized that if she expressed her feelings, she would go insane and never be able to stop them. By contrast, when she binge vomited, she felt that she was in charge of whether or not she went out of control and of when to stop. (Later, during her analytic treatment, she recognized that she preferred masturbation over intercourse for the same reason.)

Ms. U also described fearing that the world would overwhelm her by "getting too big" and would "enter her and wash her away." She also feared that if she allowed her own feelings to emerge, they would overwhelm and flood others. (There was no conscious memory expressed of incest; however, during analysis the patient recalled vague memories of frequent enemas by her mother.) Ms. U saw herself as a "cannon about to explode." She could allow in only feelings of failure, not those of success.

Ms. U was uncomfortable competing with either men or women and chose male lovers who were domineering and abusive. She was consciously aware of finding strength when feeling pain. In her relationships, the patient had to deny that she did, in fact, take initiative, because that would mean that she manipulated others and used them to meet her own needs. Instead, she felt safer feeling that others were forcing and controlling her.

After 2 years of therapy, Ms. U's symptoms and mood changes had at least stabilized. Her episodes binge vomiting had decreased from daily to a few times per week, and she had become interested in working analytically on the psychological origins of her bulimia. During therapy, Ms. U had formed a working alliance, was curious about herself, and seemed to have sufficient ego strength to have at least a trial at psychoanalysis.

Ms. U remained in four-times-weekly classical psychoanalysis for 3 years, leaving prematurely at the time of her marriage. At times during the analysis, she had difficulties recognizing the "as if" nature of the transference. Her potential for regression was great and her fear of it set limits on what could be accomplished analytically. Nevertheless, Ms. U did have symptomatic improvement and was able to partially analyze some core transference conflicts. Her bulimia had virtually stopped by the second year of analysis. Although her chronic depressive symptoms improved, the underlying psychobiological basis for her mood disturbance remained: during treatment for an ear problem, Ms. U took moderate doses of steroids and became markedly depressed until the medication was tapered.

Nonspecific factors associated with therapy of all kinds can and do lead to symptomatic improvement. In this case, the transition from psychotherapy to psychoanalysis with the same psychiatrist offered a window into the different effects of one treatment as compared with the other. Ms. U's relinquishment of her bulimia during the second year of analysis and her improvement in object relations coincided with and seemed the consequence of progressive analysis in the transference of her experiencing herself as a victim—of her bulimia, of professional pressures, and of her lovers. Most powerfully, these issues were experienced in her treatment around brief periods of silence, at times of separation, and over the issue of payment.

The following excerpt illustrates how Ms. U responded to anxiety over sadistic fantasies toward the analyst by retreating to safe, masochistic self-images:

In one session during the first year of analysis, Ms. U described how uncomfortable she felt around weak men. The previous evening, she had been with a man whose "softness" reminded her of a dream of a childhood pet rodent who appeared trapped and was unable to escape. Ms. U felt that she could easily damage the new man in her life if she were to "cut him off cleanly." With disgust, she remembered squashing a bug in her room the previous night. She then pictured her analyst as soft, weak, and depressed like her father, into whom she had to pour everything in order to be the "spark that electrifies." Instantly, Ms. U felt unable to sustain the thought of herself as a "prodder," instead experiencing herself subservient to her more powerful analyst.

Another example demonstrates how Ms. U's protective turning of "active into passive" was understood analytically. During the second year of analysis, the patient was planning a 2-week trip out of the country:

Within the session, Ms. U felt that the analyst was trying to take advantage of her by charging her for missed appointments that might not be filled during her absence. She felt panicky thinking of oppressive financial details, and felt as though somebody were forcing something inside her chest.

The next session followed a 3-day holiday weekend, during which time Ms. U reported having felt abandoned by her analyst. She became upset, noticing that the couch was "hot" from the previous patient. As her thoughts of being hurt and abandoned were explored, Ms. U began to have conscious fears about people she would leave behind, picturing the analyst in a wasteland where a bomb had exploded and feeling guilty that a sick aunt would die in her absence. She laughed nervously as she described feeling "like Atlas, holding up the world," as if everything would crumble without her. Following a brief pause, Ms. U turned her attention to a memory of the previous evening, when she had felt desperate, alone, and compelled to place a long-distance call to an old boyfriend.

Patient and analyst were able to observe that at the point of feeling responsible and guilty for leaving the analyst and others, it was *Ms. U* who then experienced being cut off and alone. In this way, the defensive guilt-reducing function of her masochism was understood analytically.

During the third year of analytic treatment, Ms. U's intermixing of guilt, punishment, and abandonment continued to be analyzed, especially as it related to her decision to marry a man she had been seeing for the past year. Again, she felt abused and enraged at the thought of being charged for time away during her honeymoon, threatening that she would have to quit. By this time, Ms. U could better appreciate how these feelings of being *forced* to leave the analyst coincided with her guilty thoughts of betrayal and fears of retaliation.

Ms. U imagined the analyst watching enviously as she and her fiance had sex, then thought of people seated at tables with low-back chairs who were "stabbed in the back." She became more and more worried about having something of value taken from her. During another session, Ms. U thought about binge vomiting after talking about her fiance, whom she had "plucked from a limited supply."

She described taking care not to flaunt what she had, fearing that it would hurt and pain others, as she had been pained in the past. At that instant in the hour, Ms. U wondered if the analyst were still present. The analyst observed that perhaps she had to picture him gone because he would be envious and hurt, and might angrily take away from her what she had taken from the "limited supply." The origins of this transference fantasy were in part related to the guilty feelings Ms. U had had as a child when leaving her depressed mother to be with others, such as her father, whom she felt had a sexual interest in her.

In the months before her marriage, Ms. U was also able to appreciate how her feeling of being forced to leave the analyst was, in part, due to her fear of being closer to him. She was increasingly aware that to allow herself to think of the analyst in a positive way meant to allow very uncomfortable sexual feelings, as she had had for her father and believed he had had for her. Her overwhelming fear of being too close and of then losing control of sexual sadomasochistic feelings had been a powerful unconscious motive in her bingeing and vomiting.

Ms. U left analysis following her marriage. Within the limits of her personality organization, she had benefited from her treatment. A greater tolerance in her conscious awareness of her sadism and defensive omnipotence, and a perception that she protected herself by being a victim and a martyr, enabled her to replace her "need" for a self-destructive, maladaptive behavior—her bulimia—with a feeling of choice and greater voluntary control. She was also able to tolerate and to accept being close with a man who was neither abusive nor openly inviting of abuse. The competitive sexual and aggressive issues of the oedipal phase of development, although ever present, were too threatening for the patient to analyze within the time she remained in treatment.

Summary

Bulimia represents the final common pathway for a variety of pregenital and oedipal conflicts. Patients struggle with intense difficulties over recognizing themselves as autonomous beings who are therefore capable of aggressive and erotic affects toward others in their lives. Keeping these desires dissociated and indistinct and turning them on themselves are two commonly employed defenses that are unconsciously designed to create a regressive pseudointimacy that denies their past and their memory.

A major challenge in working with patients with bulimia is the syntonic indifference with which they treat the doctor. Instead of relatedness, the physician encounters the patient's numbing and provocative self-involvement with their own caricatured image of their bodies. The therapeutic task is to avoid as much as possible enacting the common countertransference temptation to sadistically intrude, which can include manipulating a patient's diet. Analyzing one's own provoked inclinations to act enables one to begin to bring to the patient's attention the defensive role that their self-preoccupations play in distracting them from their object directed fantasies and affects. Such a treatment can help the patient recognize that within the defensive certainty of her enacted sadomasochism lies a vulnerable sadness from which her capacity for love can grow.

For Further Study

Bach S: On sadomasochistic object relations, in Perversions and Near-Perversions in Clinical Practice. Edited by Fogel G, Myers W. New Haven, CT, Yale University Press, 1991, pp 75–92

Bruch H: The Golden Cage. Cambridge, MA, Harvard University Press, 1978

Ceaser M: The role of maternal identification in four cases of anorexia nervosa. Bull Menninger Clinic 41:475–486, 1977

Coriat I: Sex and hunger. Psychoanal Rev 8:375–381, 1921

Friedman L: Defensive aspects of orality. Int J Psychoanal 34:304–312, 1953

Geleerd E: The analysis of a case of compulsive masturbation in a child. Psychoanal Q 12:520–540, 1943

Gero G: An equivalent of depression: anorexia, in Affective Disorders. Edited by Greenacre P. New York, International Universities Press, 1953, pp 117–139

Goldberg P: The role of distractions in the maintenance of dissociative mental states. Int J Psychoanal 68:511–524, 1987

Hamburger W: The occurrence and meaning of dreams of food and eating. Psychosom Med 20:1–16, 1958

Jeammet P: The anorexic stance. Journal of Adolescence 4:113–129, 1981

Kaplan LJ: Anorexia nervosa—a feminine pursuit of perfection, in Adolescence: The Farewell to Childhood. New York, Simon & Schuster, 1984, pp 249–283

Kaufman RM, Heiman M (eds): Evolution of Psychosomatic Concepts: Anorexia Nervosa—A Paradigm. New York, International Universities Press, 1964

Oliner M: The anal phase, in Early Female Development. Edited by Mendell D. New York, SP Medical & Scientific, 1982, pp 25–60
Risen SE: The psychoanalytic treatment of an adolescent with anorexia nervosa. Psychoanal Study Child 37:433–459, 1982
Ritvo S: The image and uses of the body in psychic conflict—with special reference to eating disorders in adolescence. Psychoanal Study Child 39:449–469, 1984
Rizzuto A: Transference, language, and affect in the treatment of bulimarexia. Int J Psychoanal 69:369–387, 1988
Sackin HD: The parents of children with psychosomatic diseases: a critical review of the literature, in Parental Influences in Health and Disease. Edited by Anthony EJ, Pollock G. Boston, MA, Little, Brown, 1985, pp 403–423
Sarnoff CA: Derivatives of latency in the psychopathology of anorexia nervosa, in Psychotherapeutic Strategies in Late Latency Through Early Adolescence. New York, Jason Aronson, 1987, pp 69–82
Schwartz HJ: Bulimia: Psychoanalytic Treatment and Theory. Madison, CT, International Universities Press, 1990
Schwartz HJ: Bulimia: encountering the sadomasochistic temptation. Neuropsychiatrie de l'Enfance 41:5–6,364–368, 1993
Sours JA: The anorexia nervosa syndrome. Int J Psychoanal 55:567–576, 1974
Sours JA: Starving to Death in a Sea of Objects. New York, Jason Aronson, 1980
Sperling M: Trichotillomania, trichophagy, and cyclic vomiting: a contribution to the psychopathology of female sexuality. Int J Psychoanal 49:682–690, 1968
Thomä H: Anorexia Nervosa. New York, International Universities Press, 1967
Wilson CP (ed): Fear of Being Fat: The Treatment of Anorexia Nervosa and Bulimia. New York, Jason Aronson, 1983
Wilson CP, Hogan C, Mintz I: Psychodynamic Technique in the Treatment of Eating Disorders. New York, Jason Aronson, 1992

References

Arlow J: Metaphor and the psychoanalytic situation. Psychoanal Q 48:363–385, 1979
Falstein E, Feinstein S, Judas I: Anorexia nervosa in the male child. Am J Orthopsychiatry 26:751–772, 1956
Gull W: Anorexia nervosa. Transactions of the Clinical Society of London 7:22–28, 1874
Jeammet P: Discussion of Regina Casper's presentation: psychodynamic psychotherapy in acute anorexia nervosa. International Journal of Adolescent Psychiatry 1:225–237, 1988
Kaplan LJ: Adolescence: The Farewell to Childhood. New York, Simon & Schuster, 1984
Kaufman RM, Heiman M (eds): Evolution of Psychosomatic Concepts: Anorexia Nervosa—A Paradigm. New York, International Universities Press, 1964

Krahn D, Mitchell J: Case report of bulimia associated with increased intracranial pressure. Am J Psychiatry 14:1099–2000, 1984

Kramer S: Residues of incest, in Adult Analysis and Childhood Sexual Abuse. Edited by Levine HB. Hillsdale, NJ, Analytic Press, 1990, pp 149–170

Lacey H: Incest, incestuous fantasy and indecency. Br J Psychiatry 157:399–403, 1990

Lasègue E: De l'anorexie hystérique. Archives Générales de Médecine 1:385–403, 1873

Lautenbacher S, Pauls A, Strain F, et al: Pain sensitivity in anorexia nervosa and bulimia nervosa. Biol Psychiatry 29:1073–1078, 1991

Ogden T: The Matrix Of The Mind. New York, Jason Aronson, 1986

Palmer M: Childhood sexual experience with adults and later eating disorders. Paper presented at the International Symposium on Eating Disorders, Paris, France, April 17, 1991

Parry-Jones B, Parry-Jones W: Bulimia: an archival review of its history in psychosomatic medicine. International Journal of Eating Disorders 10:129–143, 1991

Reich A: Narcissistic object choice in women. J Am Psychoanal Assoc 1:22–44, 1953

Rucker NG: Capacities for integration, oedipal ambivalence and imaginary companions. Am J Psychoanal 41:129–137, 1981

Schwartz HJ: Introduction, in Bulimia: Psychoanalytic Treatment and Theory. Edited by Schwartz HJ. Madison, CT, International Universities Press, 1990a, pp 1–29

Schwartz HJ: Bulimia: psychoanalytic perspectives, in Bulimia: Psychoanalytic Treatment and Theory. Edited by Schwartz HJ. Madison, CT, International Universities Press, 1990b, pp 31–53

Soubrie B: Reconciling the role of central serotonin neurosis in human and animal behavior. Behavioral and Brain Sciences 9:319–364, 1986

Sours JA: The anorexia nervosa syndrome. Int J Psychoanal 55:567–576, 1974

Sperling M: The role of the mother in psychosomatic disorders in children. Psychosom Med 11:377–385, 1949

Sperling M: Case histories of anorexia nervosa, in Psychosomatic Disorders in Childhood. Edited by Sperling O. New York, Jason Aronson, 1978, pp 139–173

Sperling M: A reevaluation of classification, concepts and treatment, in Fear of Being Fat. Edited by Wilson CP. New York, Jason Aronson, 1983, pp 51–82

Sperling O: On appersonation. Int J Psychoanal 24–26:128–132, 1943–1945

Tabin CJ, Tabin JK: Bulimia and anorexia: understanding their gender specificity and their complex of symptoms, in Bulimia: Psychoanalytic Treatment and Theory. Edited by Schwartz HJ. Madison, CT, International Universities Press, 1990, pp 489–522

Torem M, Curdue K: PTSD presenting as an eating disorder. Stress Med 4:139–142, 1988

Wilson CP: The psychoanalytic psychotherapy of bulimic anorexia nervosa, in Adolescent Psychiatry. Edited by Feinstein S. Chicago, IL, University of Chicago Press, 1986, pp 274–314

Wilson CP: Bulimic equivalents, in Bulimia: Psychoanalytic Treatment and Theory. Edited by Schwartz HJ. Madison, CT, International Universities Press, 1990, pp 489–522

Wilson G, Eldredge K: Frequent binge eating in bulimic patients: diagnostic validity. International Journal of Eating Disorders 10:557–561, 1991

Chapter 22

The Bereaved Patient

Richard S. Blacher, M.D.

Current Psychodynamic Perspectives

A chapter on mourning and bereavement might at first glance seem out of place in a textbook on psychodynamic psychiatry. After all, isn't mourning an expectable and "normal" response to loss? What possible interest would this phenomenon hold for an understanding of the inner life of our patients? Clinical experience teaches us otherwise. Reactions to loss can have a major effect on our functioning and our daily lives; a major loss, such as the death of a loved one, may play a profound, long-standing, and even dominant role in our psychic functioning.

Loss and separation are background themes in all human development, and the child's ability to tolerate them are marks of its growing maturation. When the child is able to maintain an internal image of a comforting parent, it is easier to accept a separation. The toddler can explore the world as long as it notes the presence of its mother in the background; *it* can leave mother, but if *mother* leaves, then the child becomes anxious. What we often mean when we talk of "separation anxiety" is really anxiety in reaction to being left. The comings and goings of parents—in combination with the time sense of children, which makes short periods seem long and long periods interminable—often result in an intolerance to being left. Thus, in adulthood we encounter a cliche—"You can't fire me; I quit!"—that reflects the persistent need to attempt to control separations—separations over which children have no control.

Until the 20th century, loss and bereavement were matters dealt with by the clergy. In his rich clinical and theoretical paper, "Mourning and Melancholia" (1917/1957), Freud noted that mourning and depression share many of the same symptoms, such as a sense of loss and emptiness, painful sadness, guilt, shame, hopelessness, helplessness, anorexia, sleep difficulties, and loss of interest in the world—social, personal, and work. Vegetative symptoms are often prominent as well. However, people are usually able to differentiate the two states if they are asked, and depressed people are not usually able to shed tears. "If only I could cry, I know I would feel better," a depressed patient may say. Above all, in the differential diagnosis, as Freud pointed out, is the sense of self-regard lost in depression. Frequently, the theme of the depressed person is that "The world is all right, but I am worthless." The mourner, in contrast, feels that "The world is terrible without the person I've lost; I'm all right and would feel good if I could just recover that person."

The phenomenological similarities between mourning and depression may make it difficult at times to determine which problem we are dealing with, especially since the two conditions are rarely seen in pure form. Not infrequently, there may be depressive elements intermixed with the grief of the mourner. But it is important to make a diagnosis because the two conditions may require very different treatments. It would be quite inappropriate to interpret a patient's productions in pure mourning, not to mention how wrong it would be to give such a person antidepressants. On the other hand, an overly concerned and sympathetic ear may not be at all helpful to a depressed patient. Here a careful history and examination are essential. If one knows the patient from previous treatment, one can of course understand the symptoms more easily—for example, by observing how these symptoms fit the patient's usual coping style. Often though, the consultee is a stranger, and here it is most important to attempt to evaluate the individual's self-regard.

Definitions

What is mourning and what is its natural history? In its uncomplicated form, mourning is a characteristic response to loss. Although we think of mourning usually in relation to the loss of a loved person, it can also reflect our feelings about someone we didn't know, but admired, such as a political leader or entertainer. Mourning is also a reaction to the loss of one's valued possessions, status, ideals, or home or homeland as a result of conquest or immigration. Grief may often follow divorce or the ending of a long-term relationship between two people. Last, but frequently overlooked, mourning is the response to the loss of a body part or function; such mourning is often described as a "postoperative depression" although it may not be a depression at all.

On learning of loss, the usual reaction is one of shock and an attempt to deny reality. Gradually, the person allows him- or herself to accept the loss and develops the symptoms described above. This phase diminishes in intensity over weeks and months and a longer period of recovery ensues, during which there is a gradual withdrawal of emotional investment in the memory of the lost person and an accompanying freeing of libido as well as increasing interest in other people and activities. This last phase often takes about a year, going through holidays and seasons without the other person.

Historical Review

It was natural for the early psychoanalysts to study loss, especially in relation to depression. Here, after all, was a situation that led to mourning in some people and to depression in others. Freud and Abraham were much later followed by Melanie Klein, and in 1944 by Lindemann, who investigated mourning reactions after a major public disaster—the Coconut Grove fire. Lindemann described the feelings of the bereaved and the various forms that grief could take, including both underreaction and overreaction to the loss. He discussed how the psychiatrist may help to move the grief into adaptive channels by listening and sharing the grief work with the patient. Morbid grief reactions were seen, and here, too, the psychological work could transform the distortions into resolvable issues. Lindemann's classification of these reactions included the following:

1. Postponement of grief—for days, weeks, or even years (in these cases, there may be little mourning at the time but a later dramatic reaction to a lesser loss)
2. Overactivity
3. Identification with the deceased via developing symptoms that the latter had in his or her last illness
4. A medical illness
5. Marked hostility to the deceased's doctors
6. Loss of feelings
7. Change in social patterns
8. Self-destructive behavior
9. Agitated depression (seen especially in those with obsessive-compulsive personalities)

This spectrum of reactions is familiar to those who work with grief and loss.

In 1961, Engel raised an interesting question in his paper entitled "Is Grief a Disease?" (Engel 1961). He pointed out that although we look on grief as a normal response to bereavement, it shares characteristics with many diseases, with its own morbidity and mortality. As such, it is a legitimate subject for research. Indeed, in 1977, Bartrop et al. demonstrated how the immune system changed in bereavement. Later work by Schleifer et al. (1985) showed in more detail the variations in T-cell levels in the face of loss. Engel and Schmale (1967) had previously demonstrated how reactions to loss could serve as a backdrop for the onset of all sorts of illnesses. In the early 1960s, Bowlby began a series of volumes on mourning and the results of this process on children's subsequent development. He described several varieties of pathological mourning in which anxiety, depression, anger, and denial are prominent, along with the excessive need in some patients to care for others who are bereaved (Bowlby 1969).

At the end of the 1960s, increasing interest in grief led to the formation of an organization focused on thanatology—the study of death and dying—but with a special interest in mourning. A series of books have followed symposia on related subjects sponsored by the Foundation of Thanatology. *Loss and Grief* (Schoenberg et al. 1970) was the first major contribution of this organization; it discussed the medical management of all types of losses.

This sampling of the history of our concerns about mourning indicates an increased interest in the subject on the part of our profession, but hardly reflects a lack of interest on the part of the ancients in the subject. Rather, it indicates our ability to understand more fully now, from a dynamic point of view, what the bereaved person goes through.

Differential Dynamic Diagnosis

What is the role of the psychiatrist in dealing with the bereaved patient? In order to make rational sense of our role, we must first understand some factors that influence the mourner's reactions. The first of these factors is our society's view of death. Whatever the therapist's personal outlook, he or she must be aware that no society looks upon death as the end of life. Rather, all societies picture death in terms of immortality—in the West, we posit Heaven and Hell; the East talks of reincarnation. Death becomes an altered state of consciousness with the dead eternally asleep in the grave, either pleasantly so or uncomfortable and id-deprived. Freud (1915/1957) stated, "It is indeed impossible to image our own death; and whenever we attempt to do so we can perceive that we are in fact still present as spectators . . . in the unconscious, every one of us is convinced of his own immortality" (p. 289). Freud suggested that the idea of immortality is related to the need to retain love objects lost to death. "Man could no longer keep death at a distance . . . but he was nevertheless unwilling to acknowledge it, for he could not conceive of himself as dead. So he devised a compromise. He conceded the fact of his own death as well but denied the significance of annihilation. . . . It was beside the dead body of someone he loved that he invented spirits" (Freud 1915/1957, p. 294).

These concepts of death are bound to determine to some degree how the bereaved person responds, given our definition of grief work as the decathecting of the representation of the lost love object. If the object is not really lost, the task is further complicated. Most religions provide landmarks concerning death. Those people without strong beliefs picture death in a number of ways—as a pleasant release from the pain of a terminal illness or as a fearful entry into an unknown domain. Shakespeare suggested this in Hamlet's speech:

> To die, to sleep—To sleep, perchance to dream—Ay, there's the rub; For in that sleep of death what dreams may come, when we have shuffl'd off this mortal coil, must give us pause . . . . (Shakespeare, *Hamlet, Prince of Denmark,* act 3, scene 1)

This "fear of the unknown" has nothing to do with the truly unknown. It is the fear of a future already prematurely peopled by monsters, dragons, and assorted horrors projected by us onto our expectations, rather than from the future itself.

Factors in Bereavement

Among the factors that determine the form and even the outcome of bereavement, we can include the following:

1. **The type of dying.** A sudden death resulting from trauma or an unexpected cardiac event requires a different adaptation than does a loss following a long illness. The shock of an "acute" dying will usually be greater, the denial will be more sustained, and the image of the lost person will be different from the one retained by someone watching the slow, often painful deterioration of a loved one from a chronic illness. In the latter situation, a task often confronting the survivors is dealing with their natural tendency to begin the mourning process prematurely. The gradual withdrawal of their emotional investment in the patient may ease their response when he actually dies, and may even result in the commonly seen reaction of relief at the end. "He is out of his pain and misery now," may be a true statement but could be seen as including the mourners' relief as well. The danger of this prophylactic mourning can be experienced by the dying patient as an emotional withdrawal at a time when he might like people to be closer to him. For the survivors, the image they retain afterward is frequently that of the cachectic, listless patient in his last days rather than that of the vibrant, energetic person they had known for years.
2. **The relationship to the dead person.** One expects that, in general, the relationship of the survivor to the deceased will affect the experience of loss. The death of aging parents may be expected; the death of a child is rarely anticipated. Such an event feels out of the natural order of things and may never be fully mourned by the parents (Pollock 1989). Siblings play varying roles in people's lives, and the meaning of losing a brother or sister can be influenced by when the loss occurs (in childhood or in adulthood) and the emotional relationship between the survivor and the dead sibling. An allied problem is the complicated situation in which a child is conceived in order to replace a dead sibling and this expectation is constantly present in its subsequent growth and development (Cain and Cain 1964, as discussed by Pollock 1989). A child's reaction to the death of a sibling or to the loss of other relatives can be strongly affected by the upheaval in the household and by whether or not attention is paid to the child's emotional needs at the time.

It goes without saying that it is the emotional relationship and not the familial tie with the dead person that determines the reaction to the death. An estranged sibling may experience the loss as a revival of early positive feelings from before the separation from the brother or sister, and of course there may well be the addition of guilt feelings centering on the conflict that led to the alienation.

It should be noted that the mourner may be the dying patient him- or herself (Aldrich 1963). Often unappreciated is how patients who know they are terminally ill may grieve for the loss of all those they are leaving behind. Dying patients often want to talk about such issues and may find their medical attendants too uncomfortable to help them (Blacher and Fitzgerald 1992). It is often the psychiatrist who spends time with these patients, allowing them to explore their feelings. Usually there is an alternation of acceptance/mourning and denial, and the sensitive therapist gives patients room to place themselves where they want to be on this spectrum at any one time.

Case Example

An 83-year-old man dying of cancer noted that he knew he had only a few weeks to live (this was true) and talked of his full and productive life. He then sighed and said, "I'm 83. If I live to be 90, it will be amazing." The discrepancy between the two statements was striking, but not commented on by the psychiatrist, who allowed the patient to deny his impending death without challenge.

The role of denial is often unappreciated. When this mechanism does not interfere with obtaining good care, it may serve a useful, adaptive role.

The physician listening to a dying patient's thoughts may find him- or herself in an anxiety-provoking situation. Not only does death challenge our own immortality, we know that the patient may implicitly resent the fact that he or she is dying and we are going to live. The temptation may be to protect ourselves at times by a casual demeanor. One colleague in such a situation had a patient complain, "Dying may be something you're used to every day; to me it's a unique experience."

Treatment of Pathological Grief

It is evident that those who either seek help or are referred to the psychiatrist are those who suffer excessively or else have symptoms that they might not connect with the bereavement itself. Many people whose grief is markedly prolonged and whose symptoms may merge into depression can rationalize their distress and avoid therapy. Although they correctly point out that treatment cannot restore their loss, they miss the point that the suffering they are experiencing results not only from the loss but, more important, from the inability to decathect the dead loved one.

At times, the psychiatrist may have the opportunity to see a recently bereaved person—either someone currently in treatment or someone whose loss occurs during a hospitalization for some medical condition. In the latter situation, the psychiatrist may well be called in by the attending physician. The consultant's role then is usually to listen in a supportive and empathic way and to determine whether the bereaved person's responses are reasonable. Although the consultant may feel that his or her proper role in such a situation is to step back from the case, he or she should also offer the bereaved patient the opportunity for further contact if the patient feels this is needed. The offer to be there for the patient can be felt as very helpful.

Some of the typical problems of a difficult bereavement were presented by the following patient:

Ms. V, a 43-year-old researcher, was referred by her physician after a workup for severe angina pectoris revealed no cardiac or chest pathology. For the past year, she had been experiencing substernal pains that awakened her in the early morning. These pains were often disabling enough to keep her from her work as head of a medical research laboratory. Usually, Ms. V managed to drag herself to her office, but she found that her work—which had formerly been exciting and challenging—now gave her little pleasure, and she went through the day rather mechanically. Her internist, a sensitive and experienced woman, noted a marked change in the her usually animated and outgoing patient and convinced her to seek help.

On interview, Ms. V was somewhat subdued, but not overly depressed. She was preoccupied with her concerns about her heart but also felt regretful that she had been ignoring the needs of her two teenage children, a 15-year-old son and a 12-year-old daughter. Formerly, she had been attentive and enjoyed family activities; lately, she just hadn't had the energy to get involved much in their lives.

It all began about a year and a half before, when her husband, a successful businessman of 50 years of age, had died of injuries sustained when his automobile was struck by a drunken driver. Despite the shock, Ms. V had maintained a calmness that was admired by her friends. She had directed most of the funeral arrangements herself and emotionally supported her children and her husband's aging mother, who was at the point of collapse. She had cried some in the privacy of her bedroom but returned to work after a few weeks. Ms. V was herself amazed by how well she had managed, noting that her marriage was a close and loving one, marred only by a sense from the beginning that she could never please her husband enough. Whether this feeling emanated from him or from her she could not tell, and had at one time thought of seeing a psychiatrist to explore this, but now of course that question was purely academic.

Ms. V was raised in an upper-middle-class family in a medium-sized midwestern city. A sister 4 years older than the patient was the local beauty who compensated for her poor grades in school with her social graces. After barely finishing high school, this sister had upset the family by marrying the ne'er-do-well son of the local bank president. Ms. V was the academic star of the family and it was clear early on that her father had high aspirations for her. He himself had come from a poor family and had struggled through law school. A brilliant career in practice had led to a state judgeship. Now socially and financially secure, he pictured great things in the future for his bright daughter and hoped she would follow in his legal footsteps. Her mother supported the father in his ambitions for the patient.

To her dismay, in college, Ms. V realized that she had no interest in things pertaining to the law, but was instead drawn to biological and biochemical studies. When she shared this with her parents, her father erupted in an emotional storm. All his ambitions for her were going up in smoke; all the connections he could use to smooth her professional path would be wasted. And all for an enterprise he could neither appreciate nor understand. Why anyone would want to devote a life to fiddling with test tubes was beyond him. For Ms. V, this was the worst confrontation in her life and in retelling it in my office, she suddenly realized that it was the culmination of a childhood spent trying to please her father and never feeling able to do so. For a while she had even contemplated trying law school to earn back his regard, but found the thought too distasteful. Her next visit home from college was during Christmas vacation, and following another minor contretemps with her father, he complained of chest pain but refused to call the doctor. He died in his sleep that night. What had struck Ms. V at the time was how surprisingly unmoved she was by his death, and how little she grieved. After all, she had loved him deeply and had suffered so much in not satisfying his ambitions for her.

Ms. V returned to college and went on to gain her doctorate from a prestigious program, obtained a faculty position, and rose fairly rapidly through the tenured ranks on the basis of her elegant research. She met and married a bright and loving entrepreneur, a man who owned a thriving business. She enjoyed her children and regretted that her busy schedule kept her away from them too much. She maintained a cordial tie with her mother and sister, but always felt a bit depressed when visiting them.

In an early session, Ms. V noted that although she was considered quite successful in her work, in reality she was dissatisfied, for she could have gone much further in one line of investigation, even becoming world-class had she pushed a little bit more. In other words, she felt that something in herself had kept her from really succeeding. She also rather reluctantly revealed that the picture she presented to the world of vivacity and joyousness hid a long-standing sense of depression and gloom. Her facade had been quite successful throughout most of her adulthood but she had felt it crumbling over the past year.

Her husband had died in August and she had carried on well until the end of December of that year, when on Christmas Eve she had awakened in the middle of the night with a terrible pressing pain in her chest. Her doctor was out of town and unreachable so she suffered an hour, and then the pain passed, only to recur the next night. When the psychiatrist pointed out the double connection of her father's death at Christmas and of his chest pain, Ms. V gasped in astonishment and immediately broke down in tears and sobbing. She reported the next hour that she had spent most of her time since the last session crying and thinking both of her father *and* her husband. Oddly, she noted, she hadn't had any chest pain in 3 days, since our last session.

What became clear as treatment progressed was that Ms. V had been unable to grieve her father's death because of her ambivalence and guilt. Her husband's death had revived the loss of her father, but again she could not grieve because of the unconscious equation she had made, centering on the feeling that she could not please either of them. Bringing these connections to consciousness had freed Ms. V enough to begin the mourning process for both, although it goes without saying that much therapeutic work was necessary to sort out her complicated feelings from her earlier years.

This case illustrates a number of issues in bereavement. First, losses seem to be connected with each other—that is, new losses revive old ones—and the survivor does not become immune to repeated separations. Rather, one tends to become "anaphylactic" and may call into play emergency defenses in order to cope with the overwhelming anxiety. This woman was unable to mourn her father; the loss of her husband revived her father's death and the chest symptoms represented an identification with her father and his illness, which she felt her behavior had brought on. The nagging feeling that she could never please her husband was clear evidence of her equating him with the father she really didn't please.

Her inability to mourn led to a form of subclinical depression manifested both by an inability to achieve as much as she had felt herself capable of in the profession her father had opposed and by a sense of gloom and depression despite the facade of happiness she presented to the outside world.

Although major losses occur at some time for most people, there is no set formula for bereavement. Some symptoms are usually present—sadness, a sense of loss, tearfulness, a loss of interest in the world. However, each person brings to the situation a different personal history and past experiences of response to separation and loss. There is a revival of past losses, both from early childhood and from later years.

Because a major reaction to frustration and loss is anger, one would expect this affect to be involved in mourning. Anger as a response to loss is most clearly seen in children, but it does play an important role for adults as well. Adults may have a more difficult struggle with such a response—"How can I be angry at someone for dying?!" Indeed, the need to speak only good about the dead *(de mortuis nil nisi bonum)* may indicate a reaction formation concerning our resentment that they have deserted us, as well as an attempt to appease powerful spirits who can affect us from the grave.

Anger is indeed important in the mourning process for many people, and the inability to tolerate anger, with the guilt this affect evokes, may lead to depression, as in the case of Ms. V. Survivors often struggle with resentments about the behavior of the deceased: "He smoked a lot" and "He was reckless with his health and never took care of himself" are frequently heard statements. The therapist should realize that those complaints may be attempts on the part of the mourner to deal with his or her own past resentments about the dead person. The theme becomes "It wasn't my angry feelings that killed him—he brought it on himself." In our case, Ms. V's comment about her father's refusal to call the doctor for his chest pain on the night of his death fit this theme. The ability to tolerate anger may determine the ease of mourning for many patients.

The fact that Ms. V's physical symptoms appeared on Christmas was significant, both for the timing as an anniversary reaction (Pollock 1989) and for the content of the symptoms—that is, the patient's identification with the father. Emotional reactions to anniversaries are common. As a society, we tend to mark the dates of death of significant figures as well as their birthdays. Individually, we note these dates for people important to us, and we do this either consciously or unconsciously. A religious person may go to a house of worship to say a special prayer on those dates, but a survivor may also describe feeling sad from the time of awakening "for no reason," until realizing that the day marked the anniversary of the death of a significant person.

Ms. V was able to start the grief work only with psychotherapeutic help. Most people do not need such an intervention. On the other hand, those mourners with severe characterological difficulties may present to their physicians with a variety of complaints, and later find their way to the psychiatrist when the primary doctor becomes overwhelmed by the difficulties of treating them. The issues of loss may evoke in these patients markedly exaggerated exacerbations of their underlying characterological styles—for example, a compulsive individual may show an accession of obsessive ruminations, and a person with hysterical traits may become markedly histrionic. The psychiatrist's approach must be individualized to the needs of the specific patient, with the emphasis on encouraging such patients to talk about their suffering. It is only rarely that these patients require hospitalization.

Summary

Mourning is a universal phenomenon and one looked upon by society as a simple response to a loss. The thoughtful clinician recognizes it as a complicated matter involving the person's armamentarium of defenses and indeed his or her entire past history, especially that portion of the history involving separations and losses. Usually, people are able to mourn—to decathect the memory of the deceased loved one. At times, however, the psychiatrist is called upon to help a derailed process get back on track.

The role of the therapist in a case of pathological mourning is the same as in any psychotherapy; however, even in evaluating patients that may not be extremely pathological, it is important for the therapist to listen to the patient's productions with an understanding of the dynamic issues. The realization that symptoms always have a meaning and are not random enables the listener to appreciate that the patient's struggle makes some internal sense in coming to terms with the loss.

For Further Study

Bowlby J: Attachment and Loss, Vol 3. New York, Basic Books, 1980

Engel GL: The death of a twin. Int J Psychoanal 56:23–40, 1975

Freud S: Mourning and melancholia (1917), in The Standard Edition of the Complete Psychological Works of Sigmund Freud, Vol 14. Translated and edited by Strachey J. London, Hogarth Press, 1957, pp 243–260

Kutscher A, Carr A, Kutscher L (eds): Principles of Thanatology. New York, Columbia University Press, 1987

Lindemann E: Symptomatology and management of acute grief. Am J Psychiatry 101:141–148, 1944

Parkes CM: The effects of bereavement on physical and mental health. BMJ 2:274–279, 1964

Pollock GH: The Mourning-Liberation Process. New York, International Universities Press, 1989

Schoenberg B, Carr AC, Peretz D, et al. (eds): Loss and Grief. New York, Columbia University Press, 1970

Weisman AD: Dying and Denying: A Psychiatric Study of Terminality. New York, Behavioral Publications, 1972

References

Aldrich CK: The dying patient's grief. JAMA 184:329–331, 1963

Bartrop RW, Luckhurst E, Lazarus L, et al: Depressed lymphocyte function after bereavement. Lancet 1:834–836, 1977

Blacher RS, Fitzgerald SM: Teaching in thanatology: stimuli and resistances, in Medical Student Education: Meeting the Challenges of Life-Threatening Illness, Death and Bereavement (proceedings of Conference on Death, Bereavement and Medical Student Education, held December 1991 at Columbia University, New York). Edited by Bulkin W, Kutscher AH, Brown WW. New York, Foundation of Thanatology, 1992

Bowlby J: Attachment and Loss, Vol 1. New York, Basic Books, 1969

Cain AC, Cain BS: On replacing a child. Journal of the American Academy of Child Psychiatry 3:443–456, 1964

Engel GL: Is grief a disease? Psychosom Med 23:18–22, 1961

Engel GL, Schmale AH: Psychoanalytic theory of somatic disorder. J Am Psychoanal Assoc 15:344–365, 1967

Freud S: Thoughts for the times on war and death (1915), in The Standard Edition of the Complete Psychological Works of Sigmund Freud, Vol 14. Translated and edited by Strachey J. London, Hogarth Press, 1957, pp 273–302

Freud S: Mourning and melancholia (1917), in The Standard Edition of the Complete Psychological Works of Sigmund Freud, Vol 14. Translated and edited by Strachey J. London, Hogarth Press, 1957, pp 243–260

Lindemann E: Symptomatology and management of acute grief. Am J Psychiatry 101:141–148, 1944

Pollock GH: The Mourning-Liberation Process. New York, International Universities Press, 1989

Schleifer SJ, Keller SE, Siris SG, et al: Depression and immunity. Arch Gen Psychiatry 42:129–133, 1985

Schoenberg B, Carr AC, Peretz D, et al. (eds): Loss and Grief. New York, Columbia University Press, 1970

CHAPTER 23

The Suicidal Adolescent

Aaron H. Esman, M.D.

Suicidal acts are alarmingly frequent among American adolescents. A recent survey (Gallup Organization 1991) reported that 6% of persons between 13 and 19 years of age acknowledged attempting such an act, and 15% said that they had come close to succeeding. This frequency represents a significant public health issue and confronts the practicing psychiatrist with a major clinical problem. Suicide remains the third leading cause of death among Americans between the ages of 15 and 25; despite at least three decades of social concern, this figure shows no signs of abating. Indeed, in the years between 1964 and 1984, the rate of suicide among white males aged 15–24 years tripled; that among females grew by about one-third. Clearly, there are important factors within both the culture and the developmental experience of adolescence that continue to generate such despair and hopelessness as to precipitate self-destructive feelings, wishes, and actions among those who have been called the hope of our society.

Current Psychodynamic Perspectives

Although some recent work suggests the possibility of a biological contribution to suicidal behavior (for a review of this literature, see Mann et al. 1989), the preponderance of the literature has addressed these developmental and sociocultural factors. The psychiatric literature (Kandel et al. 1991; Petzel and Kline 1978; Petzel and Riddle 1981; Shaffer et al. 1988) has delineated a profile of the adolescent who is most likely to commit suicide: the individual is apt to be male, white, and from an unstable family in which another member has attempted or committed suicide. He is likely to have made at least one previous attempt, and to have a long history of emotional difficulty. Most frequently, there has been a recent experience of loss or major disappointment in a love relationship or an important life activity, such as school or work. He may be, or imagine himself to be, in some sort of trouble with authority. It is important to remember that although adolescent girls are three times as likely as boys to attempt suicide, three times as many males will succeed, primarily because they are likely to use more violent and/or lethal means (e.g., guns, hanging, jumping). Like Shaffer, Carlson and Cantwell (1982) found that the great majority of suicidal adolescents were clinically depressed, but in their series, up to one-third were not so diagnosed; many appeared to have been schizophrenic and to have killed themselves in response to command hallucinations or delusional ideas.

Far more than suicidal acts, suicidal ideation is widespread among adolescents. Harkavy-Friedman et al. (1987) found that as many as 60% of "normal" adolescents surveyed admitted that they experienced such thoughts; although, in most cases, such thoughts were ephemeral, in one-third they were persistent. Consideration of this fact necessitates a review of the developmental issues specific to adolescence that predispose many young people to the depressive moods that may generate such thoughts and actions.

Fragility of Self-Esteem

For many adolescents, the normative transformations of body image and body sensations generate a preoccupation with the self that is highly susceptible to the effects of intercurrent events. Especially in the absence of strong parental support, many adolescents will experience deviations from peer group norms in any aspect of pubertal maturation (e.g., breast development, penis size, timing of growth spurt, acne) as an abnormality and a mark of inferiority. Adolescents are acutely dependent on others for self-esteem regulation, and any perceived deficiency or failure can easily evoke feelings of self-loathing, self-depreciation and, in the extreme, hopelessness. This is particularly true—as the case cited later in this chapter will demonstrate—in adolescents who have internalized lofty parental expectations for social or academic performance or who are rivalrous with parents or siblings who are "high achievers." Such adolescents may experience any lapse from these now-self-imposed standards as a failure of major proportions. For others, social rejection or a general feeling of social inacceptance may similarly evoke feelings of self-loathing and despair. In short, a profound sense of failure to live up to an idealized (and often unattainable) self-image may, in an otherwise predisposed adolescent, precipitate a suicidal action.

Fragility of Object Relations

A central aspect of normal adolescent development is the process defined by Katan (1937) as "object removal"—the loosening of the primary affective attachment to the parent(s) and the shift toward the expected adult investment in a nonfamilial object. In Western cultures, at least, this process is normally characterized by extensive experimentation, with back-and-forth movements between autonomy and dependence, often marred by disappointments and enhanced by transitory triumphs, until a more or less definitive attachment is formed. During the course of this transition (called by Blos [1967] the "second individuation process"), the adolescent may experience episodes of objectlessness, of a sense of isolation and abandonment, or of the absence or withdrawal of supportive attachment; these episodes will engender feelings of depression that in normal circumstances will be warded off by activity, hectic object seeking, or the use of chemical pacifiers (e.g., alcohol, drugs). In those adolescents predisposed by early experiences of loss of parents or other major figures, or by emotional or material neglect or deprivation, however, the combination of felt abandonment and rage at the abandoning object may lead to violent destructive wishes which, defensively turned on the self, may eventuate in suicide.

A special variant of this situation can be seen in families in which, for one reason or another, the adolescent is the target of parental hostility or is seen as an interference or a burden by one or both parents. In such families, the young person may be the target of explicit or implicit communications that he or she should die; this adolescent becomes what Sabbath (1969) has called "the expendable child." Many of the "accidental" deaths of adolescents, incurred in the course of injudicious risk-taking behaviors (e.g., automobile crashes, drug overdoses, Russian roulette) have been seen as the consequence of unconscious compliance with such parental wishes. A recent report by Prowda and colleagues (K. Prowda, P. Marzuk, R. Gallagher, and A. Leon, "Risk-Taking Behavior and Suicidality: A Case-Control Study," [unpublished manuscript], May 1991), however, casts doubt on this correlation between suicide and risk-taking behaviors, at least in adults.

Suicide in adolescents can be seen, then, as a final common pathway for a number of dynamic and developmental determinants. Impaired self-regard, exaggerated self-criticism, feelings of loss and/or disappointment in personal relationships, a sense of parental rejection or hostility, and a deficiency in internal self-soothing mechanisms can, in combination, so intensify the normatively transitory dysphoric affects as to generate suicidal wishes and behaviors. Underlying these acts are often fantasies of reunion with lost objects and/or of vengeance against the now-hated abandoner ("They'll be sorry when they find me dead!"). Behaviors such as increased social isolation, deterioration in school performance, or increased drug or alcohol intake are frequent manifestations of the depression that often goes unnoticed by parents and other adults in the adolescent's world.

Historical Review

In his classic two-volume tome, the first systematic treatise on adolescence as a defined stage of development, Hall (1904) devoted 11 pages to the topic of suicide in adolescence. Allowing for his inveterate moralism, his text contains flashes of modernity: he speaks of hostility and revenge, and disillusionment and disappointment in love as primary motives and, like many contemporary "authorities," considers the role of imitation and contagion in stimulating adolescent suicide. Hall cited a "committee of Swiss physicians [who] lately petitioned for a law to prohibit the printing of suicides to avoid suggestion" (1904, p. 385).

Later, more specifically psychiatric and psychoanalytic contributions play variations on many of these themes. Bender and Schilder (1937) concluded their study of child and adolescent suicides thus:

> The child reacts to an unbearable situation with an attempt to escape. Mostly these unbearable situations consist of the deprivation of love or are at least based upon such an assumption. The deprivation provokes aggressive tendencies which are primarily directed against those who deny love. Under the influence of feelings of guilt, these aggressive tendencies are turned against oneself. The aggressive tendencies may be increased by constitutional factors and identification with an aggressive parent or other aggressive members of the family and all the other factors which may increase aggressiveness. The suicidal attempt constitutes also a punishment against the surroundings and a method to get a greater amount of love. The suicidal death represents also a reunion with the love object in love and peace. There may be also an identification with a dead love object. Suicides which follow disappointments in love in children are again attempts to regain the love object which in the deeper sense is always one of the parents. (p. 233)

Toolan (1962) similarly cited the following "causes" for adolescent suicide attempts:

> 1) Anger at another which is internalized in the form of guilt and depression. Usually parents or parent surrogates are the original objects . . . 2) Attempts to manipulate another, to gain love and affection, to punish another . . . 3) A signal of distress . . . 4) Reactions to feelings of inner disintegration, as a response to hallucinatory commands, as a desire for peace and a nirvana-like existence . . . 5) A desire to join a dead relative . . . (p. 722)

Both Bender and Schilder (1937) and Toolan (1962) refer to the notion of "turning aggression against the self." Derived from Freud's (1917/1957) views on melancholia, this concept delineates a complex defensive process, through which 1) a lost object is retained in fantasy by being assimilated into the self-representation, which then 2) becomes the target of the aggressive or hateful wishes directed against that object. In a somewhat simpler formulation, the rage against the object (not necessarily lost) is defensively diverted from object to self in order to achieve a compromise between the rage and the protection of the object from destruction (i.e., both drive and superego aims are achieved).

Schneer and Kay (1961) considered adolescent suicide to be "omnipotent, regressively infantile behavior in coping with an explosive oedipal conflict involving loss (destruction) of the sadomasochistic . . . object . . . mainly a phallic narcissistic mother image" (pp. 180, 200). Sabbath (1969), as noted earlier, described cases in which an adolescent responded to overt or covert communications from one or both parents that he or she was unwanted, hated, or in the way by committing a suicidal act. "This appeared to occur at the time when the adolescent's ego, already compromised by previous developmental faults and/or current narcissistic injuries and losses, succumbed to the felt parental wish for them to die" (p. 285).

Erlich (1978) suggested that both affective and cognitive developmental issues in adolescence played a role:

> I propose that adolescence, conceived of as a developmental disturbance, contributes to suicide by precipitating and exacerbating affects and wishes connected with the loss of the maternal object; and second, that in the adolescent in whom such stirred up longings for maternal union are coupled with the operation of a specific cognitive factor [i.e., cognitive rigidity and increased egocentricity], we encounter a heightened potential for suicide. (p. 276)

Asch (1971), Doctors (1981), and others have described a pattern of parasuicidal behavior seen most frequently in adolescent girls—the syndrome of "delicate wrist scratching." According to Asch, such behavior occurs most often in girls who have suffered significant maternal neglect and/or abuse, who have failed to achieve object constancy, and who have no capacity to experience genuine affect. Frustration or object loss "stimulate massive rage reactions, which result in depersonalization both as a defense and as a result of a fragile self-representation. . . . Wrist scratching is a specific technique for dealing with both the rage and depersonalization. . . . The induced bleeding in the cutting is an attempt to undo the current separation by identifying with the bleeding woman (mother), symbolic of the mother-infant unity in the past" (Asch 1971, p. 617).

Laufer and Laufer (1984) viewed the suicidal act in an adolescent as a sign of an acute psychotic breakdown—a temporary loss of the ability to maintain the link to external reality. From their particular perspective, they argued that "at the time of the decision to kill himself, the adolescent's body is no longer part of him but instead becomes the object that can express all his feelings and fantasies. . . . The body has become totally identified with the fantasied attacker who must now be silenced" (pp. 112–113).

Although not psychodynamically oriented, the recent epidemiological study of adolescent suicide by Shaffer et al. (1988) offered some important clues to dynamic issues. Contrary to common assumption, for example, these authors found that "youngsters who commit suicide are not more likely to come from a 'broken' home than are other youngsters of the same ethnic group. However, suicide attempters probably do come from more disturbed families" (p. 2). Furthermore, "a high proportion of youth suicide victims or suicide attempters have had a close family member or friend who attempted or committed suicide"

(p. 2). Implied in these findings are two corollaries: 1) successful suicide is more likely to be the outcome of serious mental illness which, in the authors' view, is predominantly biologically based, and 2) either genetic affinity or identification with a suicidal relative or friend may play a significant role in suicidal acts. On the other hand, Miller (1981) and Esman (1990) have proposed that the documented increase in the incidence of depression among American adolescents in recent decades (Klerman 1988) can be accounted for and is coincident with the steady rise in the divorce rate, such that at present about "40% of U.S. children will witness the breakup of their parents' marriages before they reach 18" (Cherlin et al. 1991, p. 1386). Indeed, in many cases this breakup will occur during the child's adolescence, especially when the parents have held on to a shaky marriage "for the sake of the children." This family disorganization and the all-too-frequent chaos, violence, and turmoil that both precede and follow it have appeared both to clinicians and to epidemiologists to contribute in major ways to the impotent rage, feelings of hopelessness and disappointment, guilt, and poor self-esteem (Wallerstein 1991) that predispose many adolescents to clinical depression and suicidal acts.

Finally, the question of media influence has been widely discussed. Just as with Hall's Swiss physicians nearly a century ago, many contemporary observers have been concerned about the role of imitation and "contagion" in response to newspaper, radio, television, and cinematic accounts of youth suicide, actual or fictitious. Anecdotal accounts of such influence abound, but empirical studies have resulted in somewhat ambiguous findings. Phillips et al. (1989) found a significant increase in adolescent suicides following news stories about such events; indeed, the greater the publicity, the sharper the increase. Kessler et al. (1988), however, discovered that, over a longer time span, this increase did not hold up. Nonetheless, Brent et al. (1989) described an outbreak of suicidal behavior in a high school following the suicides of two students in a 4-day period. Students who were vulnerable because of previous psychiatric disorders were most likely to develop suicidal behaviors; whether they might have done so at a later date in any case could not be determined. Strikingly, having a close relationship to the initial victim did not seem to play an important role.

In short, although the data are unclear, it seems as though imitation and/or identification with suicides, both in the immediate life situation and through media exposure, may have some influence on the suicidal behavior of otherwise predisposed adolescents. It is striking that such influence does not appear to occur in adult groups; adolescents seem to possess a special vulnerability in this respect (Shaffer et al. 1988).

Differential Dynamic Diagnosis

In descriptive psychiatry (e.g., DSM-IV [American Psychiatric Association 1994]), the differential diagnosis of suicide and attempted suicide ranges among the various levels of affective disorder (e.g., dysthymia, adjustment disorder with depressed mood, major depressive disorder, bipolar disorder) and schizophrenia. From the psychodynamic standpoint, however, the differential diagnostic questions are directed less toward the formal syndrome than toward the presumed conflicts and/or developmental issues that serve to motivate the suicidal act. The aim of such a diagnostic process is to formulate, at least provisionally, the meaning—or, more likely, the meanings—of the act so as to better focus the therapeutic effort and to anticipate the kinds of transference/countertransference issues that may arise in the course of treatment. In the actual clinical experience, such as in the case example presented below, there are likely to be multiple and overlapping levels of conflict at work, making the dynamic formulation more complex but no less important (Shapiro 1990). Some of the principal differential possibilities include the following:

1. **Loss of reality testing with acting out of grandiose/omnipotent fantasies.** This factor is often involved in so-called accidental suicides, such as those resulting from risk-taking behaviors. Illustrative is the case (described in detail in Esman et al. 1983) of a 15-year-old manic boy who had refused treatment (including lithium) because "it would ruin my creativity." This boy's body was found in the courtyard of his apartment building, where he had apparently fallen from the roof. It was believed that he had fallen while walking along the edge of the roof in a death-defying gesture.
2. **Object loss with disappointment, rage, and revenge fantasies turned against the self.** This factor is perhaps the most frequent precipitant of suicidal acts in adolescence, resulting, as it often does, from a failed love relationship in which the loss is experienced as an injury to one's self-esteem ("narcissistic rage"). For example, a 17-year-old boy was hospitalized because of intractable rage reactions following his rejection by a female schoolmate with whom he had had an intense sexual relationship. These rages were so violent that he was expelled from his boarding school; he blamed the girl for this indignity. In the hospital, his rage reactions subsided and he appeared reasonable and euthymic, denying any suicidal ideation or intent. He expressed both an interest in learning to control his rages and a wish to return to school and get on with life. On the day of his discharge, he went home to his father's twelfth-story apartment, wrote a suicide note, and jumped from the terrace to his death.
3. **Ego fragility, with shame, self-loathing, and self-punishment.** Shapiro and Freedman (1987) described a borderline adolescent girl with a history of sexual abuse, family conflict, drug use, and impulsive promiscuity. In response to the impending breakdown in her parents' marriage, she spent a night seeking solace in serial intercourse with two boyfriends. The next morning, filled with shame, guilt, self-denigration, and despair, she tried to throw herself off a bridge and was barely prevented from doing so.
4. **Fantasies of reunion with lost objects.** As the case example provided below will illustrate, suicide may appear to some adolescents as a means for achieving reunion with dead parents or other important nurturing figures. In such

cases, the normal mourning process has failed to occur; the lost object has not been given up, replaced, or internalized. In times of stress, lowered self-esteem, or disappointment, self–object boundaries are loosened and the fantasy of rejoining the lost "selfobject" ("One's subjective experience of another person who provides a sustaining function to the self within a relationship . . . one's experience of images needed for the sustenance of the self" [Moore and Fine 1990, p. 178]) through death becomes irresistible.

Case Example

The patient, Mr. W, was a young man seen first at age 20 after he had dropped out of his second year of college because of unmanageable depression. He could not concentrate on his work, became increasingly isolated, and felt helpless and incapable of functioning. Of note were the facts that his mother had died about 1 year earlier, and that his father had, after a divorce when the patient was 11, committed suicide when the patient was 13.

In fact, this episode was the second depression Mr. W had experienced. Two years earlier, he had similarly withdrawn from another university shortly after beginning his freshman year in the context of his mother's illness, which had both physical and psychiatric components. At that time, he returned to her home, gradually recovering sufficiently to transfer to his current school the following year. Exceptionally bright and intensely intellectual, this young man was profoundly self-depreciatory and totally lacking in self-confidence. Gradually it became clear that his self-criticism and poor self-esteem were the reverse of a set of overweening grandiose expectations and unachievable ideals; inevitably, his failure to live up to them left him feeling incompetent and degraded. He could not settle for the good; only the best would do, and if that was not attainable he would abdicate.

Mr. W entered eagerly into a twice-a-week therapy program, confidently expecting that he would return to his out-of-town college. The early phase of the treatment was dominated by his self-denigration and his inability to mobilize himself socially or intellectually. After a few months of this, I introduced antidepressant medication. He responded quickly to imipramine, and after 2 months he was activated, optimistic, and perhaps even a bit hypomanic. Against my advice, he terminated treatment in mid-June, planning to resume therapy in the fall with someone in his college town.

I did not hear from Mr. W again for 18 months. Then I received a call from him letting me know that he was in the hospital recovering from a serious and almost lethal suicide attempt. I found him in bed fully alert but still being monitored after an overdose of his asthma medication. He had again become depressed, ostensibly because of academic difficulties, concluding that he could not go on because he could not complete a crucial term paper, and decided to end it all. His academic performance was in fact excellent otherwise—good enough, in fact, to engage the respectful attention of a number of prominent faculty members who took on the role of parent-surrogates for him. Characteristically, however, his work did not meet his own lofty self-expectations. On returning to school, Mr. W had consulted with an analyst, but when told it would have to be analysis or nothing, he undertook instead a course of cognitive therapy with no benefit and had avoided resuming either psychodynamic therapy or medication during the 18-month interval.

Over the next 3 years Mr. W resumed both. It became apparent that the major psychological determinant of his chronic dysphoria and its acute exacerbations was the traumatic loss of both parents, his profound sense of aloneness, and the desperate, unconscious fantasy that ideal intellectual performance would somehow restore to him his lost objects. Aggravating his situation was an intensely dependent and masochistic relationship with a girl who had on two separate occasions abruptly abandoned him, reactivating his earlier losses and plunging him each time into self-abasing ruminations and desperate attempts—ultimately fruitless—to restore the connection. Paralyzed by his self-depreciations (i.e., by his inability either to live up to or relinquish his grandiose self-expectations), Mr. W withdrew from an attempt to return to school locally, avoided finding work because nothing challenging enough seemed available and nothing available was challenging enough, and spent most of his time listening to music and more or less aimlessly reading in his chosen field, always with the feeling that he did not understand enough.

In therapy, Mr. W urgently sought direction and "explanations," his attitude alternating between pleading dependence and caustic sarcastic provocation. The rage against those who had abandoned him was primarily self-directed, although it emerged in the transference in the form of passive-aggressive negativism, deprecatory comments, and the pervasive sense that he was not getting enough. Although suicidal thoughts were persistent and recurrent, no further suicidal acts were carried out or even contemplated. He had taken a private oath that, having failed once, he would never repeat the attempt. Trials of various antidepressants provided only marginal benefit at best, and finally were abandoned. Ultimately, as the painful feelings about his losses and his restitutive efforts were in part worked through, Mr. W began to elaborate plans for once more returning to graduate school, this time in another city. Although it was clear that much further therapeutic work needed to be done, we agreed that his plans seemed realistic and appropriate to his career objectives, and, since he had succeeded in gaining admission to a highly competitive and prestigious school, we agreed to terminate his treatment and to refer him to a colleague in his new location.

This patient exemplifies many of the phenomena common to suicidal adolescents. His genetic loading for depression was massive; one parent had committed suicide and the other had suffered from depressive episodes for years before her death. He had always been socially awkward, and after his parents' death felt abandoned, acutely dependent on parent-surrogates, and suffused with unconscious rage in response to any feeling of rejection or desertion. His ego ideal was grandiose and implacable—all the more so because his father's suicide had deprived him of the opportunity to test the reality of his early idealization against the more realistic perception that comes with adolescence. Underlying his depression was a stubborn, inflexible, and obsessional personality whose unconscious primitive rage was barely controlled by his fragile defenses of intellectualization, isolation, and reaction formation. Of particular importance was the absence in this young man of internalized self-soothing, self-esteem regulatory structures. He was in continuous need of external supporting figures—"selfobjects," in the language of self psychology—to sustain even minimal levels of self-regard; without them, his archaic, tyrannical superego exacted a debilitating toll.

Summary

As suggested earlier, suicidal behavior in adolescence emerges from the confluence of many dynamic and developmental streams; there is no universal pattern. The normative maturational and developmental events of adolescence—the bodily changes of puberty, the shifts in patterns of personal relationships, the (explicit or implicit) demand for giving up dependence and assuming greater self-reliance, and the need to adjust to the de-idealization of parent figures—leave many adolescents vulnerable to depressive moods, painful self-consciousness, and feelings of isolation and loneliness. Losses, disappointments, personal failures actual or self-perceived—or, in some cases, delusional breaks with reality—may precipitate a suicidal act that the adolescent sees either as a way out of a hopeless situation and/or as a communication to those he deems responsible for that situation.

For Further Study

French A, Berlin I (eds): Depression in Children and Adolescents. New York, Human Sciences Press, 1979

Kaplan LJ: Adolescence: The Farewell to Childhood. New York, Simon & Schuster, 1984

Mack J, Hickler H: Vivienne: The Life and Suicide of an Adolescent Girl. Boston, MA, Little, Brown, 1981

McLean G (ed): Suicide in Children and Adolescents. Toronto, Canada, Hogrefe & Huber, 1990

Pfeffer C: The Suicidal Child. New York, Guilford, 1986

Sudak H, Ford A, Rushworth N (eds): Suicide in the Young. Boston, MA, Wright, 1984

References

American Psychiatric Association: Diagnostic and Statistical Manual of Mental Disorders, 4th Edition. Washington, DC, American Psychiatric Association, 1994

Asch S: Wrist-scratching as a symptom of anhedonia: a predepressive state. Psychoanal Q 40:603–617, 1971

Bender L, Schilder P: Suicidal preoccupations and attempts in children. Am J Orthopsychiatry 7:225–234, 1937

Blos P: The second individuation process of adolescence. Psychoanal Study Child 22:162–186, 1967

Brent D, Kerr M, Goldstein C, et al: An outbreak of suicide and suicidal behavior in a high school. J Am Acad Child Adolesc Psychiatry 28:918–924, 1989

Carlson G, Cantwell D: Suicidal behavior and depression in children and adolescents. Journal of the American Academy of Child Psychiatry 21:361–368, 1982

Cherlin A, Furstenberg F, Chase-Lansdale PC, et al: Longitudinal studies of effects of divorce on children in Great Britain and the United States. Science 252:1386–1389, 1991

Doctors S: The symptom of delicate self-cutting in adolescent females: a developmental view. Adolesc Psychiatry 9:443–460, 1981

Erlich HS: Adolescent suicide: maternal longing and cognitive development. Psychoanal Study Child 33:261–278, 1978

Esman A: Les troubles de l'humeur a l'adolescence (Mood disorders in adolescence). Psychiatrie de l'enfant 33:93–111, 1990

Esman A, Hertzig M, Aarons S: Juvenile manic-depressive illness: a longitudinal perspective. Journal of the American Academy of Child Psychiatry 22:302–304, 1983

Freud S: Mourning and melancholia (1917), in The Standard Edition of the Complete Psychological Works of Sigmund Freud, Vol 14. Translated and edited by Strachey J. London, Hogarth Press, 1957, pp 243–260

Gallup Organization: Teenage Suicide Study: Executive Summary. Princeton, NJ, The Gallup Organization, 1991

Hall GS: Adolescence, Vol 1. New York, Appleton, 1904

Harkavy-Friedman J, Asnis G, Boeck M, et al: Prevalence of specific suicidal behaviors in a high school sample. Am J Psychiatry 144:1203–1207, 1987

Kandel D, Raveis V, Davies M: Suicidal ideation in adolescence: depression, substance use and other risk factors. Journal of Youth and Adolescence 20:289–308, 1991

Katan A: The role of displacement in agoraphobia. Int J Psychoanal 32:41–50, 1937

Kessler R, Downey G, Milavsky J, et al: Clustering of teenage suicides after television news stories about suicides: a reconsideration. Am J Psychiatry 145:1379–1383, 1988

Klerman G: The current age of youthful melancholia: evidence for increased depression among adolescents and young adults. Br J Psychiatry 152:4–14, 1988

Laufer M, Laufer E: Developmental Breakdown and Psychoanalytic Treatment in Adolescence. New Haven, CT, Yale University Press, 1984

Mann J, De Meo M, Keilp J, et al: Biological correlates of suicidal behavior in youth, in Suicide Among Youth: Perspectives on Risk and Prevention. Edited by Pfeffer C. Washington, DC, American Psychiatric Press, 1989, pp 185–202

Miller D: Adolescent suicide: etiology and treatment. Adolesc Psychiatry 9:327–342, 1981

Moore B, Fine B: Psychoanalytic Terms and Concepts. New Haven, CT, Yale University Press, 1990

Petzel S, Kline D: Adolescent suicide: epidemiological and biological aspects. Adolesc Psychiatry 6:239–266, 1978

Petzel S, Riddle M: Adolescent suicide: psychosocial and cognitive aspects. Adolesc Psychiatry 9:343–398, 1981

Phillips D, Carstensen L, Paight D: Effects of mass media news stories on suicide, with new evidence on the role of story content, in Suicide Among Youth: Perspectives on Risk and Prevention. Edited by Pfeffer C. Washington, DC, American Psychiatric Press, 1989, pp 101–116

Sabbath J: The suicidal adolescent: the expendable child. Journal of the American Academy of Child Psychiatry 5:272–289, 1969

Schneer H, Kay P: The suicidal adolescent, in Adolescents: Psychoanalytic Approaches to Problems and Therapy. Edited by Schneer H, Lorand S. New York, Hoeber, 1961, pp 180–201

Shaffer D, Gould M, Fisher R, et al: Suicide and Depression in Children and Adolescents. New York, Columbia University College of Physicians and Surgeons, 1988

Shapiro E, Freedman J: Family dynamics of adolescent suicide. Adolesc Psychiatry 14:191–207, 1987

Shapiro T: The psychodynamic formulation in child and adolescent psychiatry. J Am Acad Child Adolesc Psychiatry 28:675–680, 1990

Toolan J: Suicide and suicide attempts in children and adolescents. Am J Psychiatry 118:719–724, 1962

Wallerstein J: The long-term effects of divorce on children: a review. J Am Acad Child Adolesc Psychiatry 30:349–360, 1991

Chapter 24

The Depressed Geriatric Patient

Wayne A. Myers, M.D.

Psychodynamic Perspectives on Depression, Past and Present

In his earliest psychoanalytic conceptualization of depression, Freud (1893/1966) saw the condition as being a variant of the anxiety neurosis. At that time, his ideas were based on his work with patients who developed anxiety symptoms after engaging in sexual practices that did not lead to orgiastic gratification, such as coitus interruptus. In such people, he perceived the undischarged sexual (libidinal) energy as being directly transformed into anxiety. Depression was seen by him as a long-lasting type of anxiety state caused by the chronic damming up of libido secondary to such sexual practices. This state was to be differentiated from the more severe melancholic ones, which Freud imagined to be caused by an actual loss or depletion of libidinal energy.

A quarter of a century later, in his classic monograph on depression, "Mourning and Melancholia" (Freud 1917/1957), Freud noted that in mourning, there was an actual loss of a person and that the process involved an unconscious detachment of feelings from the lost person over a period of time without any significant disturbance in self-esteem. In melancholia, on the other hand, the loss was experienced as if it had occurred to the self and was accompanied by a marked diminution in self-regard. Thus, mourning was seen as a normal state and melancholia as a pathological one.

Freud's close observations of melancholic individuals suggested to him that the reproaches directed against the ego (or self) were really meant for someone else—specifically, the lost person (lost love object). For example, the loyal wife who, depressed after the death of her husband, berates herself for being unfaithful may actually be referring to her husband's tendencies to cheat with other women and to his ultimate infidelity in having abandoned her by dying.

Freud additionally noted that melancholic persons tend to choose people with whom to be involved on a narcissistic basis. By this, he meant that they chose their love objects on the basis of those objects' similarity to themselves. Thus, a loss of a loved one, for such individuals, carried a concomitant threat of a loss of a highly valued aspect of the self and had to be defended against by an unconscious process of internalization or identification with parts of the personality of the lost person (love object). Depending on the degree of angry (ambivalent) feelings felt toward the lost person, this process of identification might lead to self-reproaches and melancholia or to mourning and a subsequent working through of the feelings for the lost object and a consequent shift of interest to others. From their observations, Freud (1917/1957) and Abraham (1916/1927) theorized that inadequate oral gratification provided by the mother for the infant in the earliest libidinal stage of life (roughly seen as spanning the first year) and excessive anger toward the object led to a potential in that child to develop melancholia in later life. Abraham (1916/1927) was the first analyst to postulate a state of primal depression in early infancy that occurred following blows to the child's infantile feelings of narcissistic omnipotence and control over objects, particularly the mother.

At this point, Freud (1923/1961) revamped his earlier topographic model of the mind, in which the psyche was divided into conscious, preconscious, and unconscious realms and substituted for it a tripartite theory of the psychic apparatus known as the *structural theory.* In this model, the sexual and aggressive drives were ascribed to the id, the conscience and ego ideal to the superego, and the representations of the self to the ego. The ego and superego were seen as being formed, in part, by internalizations of and identifications with various aspects of the important objects in the individual's life, such as the parents. "Normal" individuals—that is, those who had experienced a moderate (optimal) amount of frustration at the hands of the important love objects in their lives and thus had a relatively small amount of ambivalence toward those selfsame love objects (because they only had a modest quantity of aggression that was unneutralized by libido)—were able to develop a perception of themselves as being separate from the objects and were less susceptible to becoming depressed in later life. Individuals who had experienced more intense frustration from objects very early in life felt a greater degree of ambivalence toward them and were therefore both less able to separate from these objects and more susceptible to later-life depression.

Put another way, in this model of depression, orally fixated individuals were seen as attempting to defend against the potential arousal of depressive affect following the loss of an object or a narcissistic slight by internalizing and merging the unconscious representations of the ambivalently invested love object with those of the self and then by directing their reproaches against this merged representation. To state this in terms of the structural theory, the melancholic individual's ego can be seen as being made to masochistically suffer at the hands of the sadistic superego because of intolerable feelings of guilt (and an unconscious need to be punished) caused by excessive anger toward the love object.

Melanie Klein (1932), from her work with children, postulated a normal developmental phase—*the depressive position*—that occurred early in the first year of life. She believed that the child feared that its own anger, secondary to its recognition of the mother as an object separate from itself, could lead to the destruction of the object and to a state of primal depression. To Klein, as to Abraham earlier, the depressions of later life are merely revivals of these early experiences of object loss or separateness.

In a study of 170 institutionalized infants, Spitz and Wolf (1946) observed that those infants deprived of mothering care underwent a marked behavioral change in the second 6 months of life. They became weepy, withdrawn, apathetic, and retarded and some even died after 3 months of separation from their mothers. Spitz and Wolf termed these reactions *anaclitic depressions* and saw these early separation experiences as predisposing the infants to later adult depressive states. Similar findings were later reported on separation reactions in infants (Bowlby 1960). Another worker who saw depression as a universal concomitta of childhood was Benedek (1956). She viewed premature experiences of separation as leading both to a heightened feeling of aggression toward the mother and to what she referred to as *the depressive constellation.*

Mahler (1966) also saw depression as a basic affective component of the separation-individuation phase of childhood. She related the feeling to a depletion of confident expectation in the mother following experiences of separation in childhood and to a concomitant diminution in self-esteem because one cannot presumably control the erratically appearing and disappearing love object. Mahler's work can be seen to be similar to much recent psychiatric work connecting panic disorders with depression.

Jacobson (1946), in her extensive work with depressed patients, came to believe that adult depressions were the result of the presence of an overabundance of primitive aggression directed against the libidinal investment of the ego (self) as a consequence of excessive experiences of frustration in childhood. Episodes of loss or frustration in adult life were thus seen by her as being the triggers leading to a devaluation of the ego by the ego ideal and to a profound diminution in self-esteem.

In 1953, Edward Bibring placed an even greater emphasis on the concept of self-esteem in his psychodynamic description of depression. In his model, the depressive affect is seen as resulting from a state of perceived helplessness and powerlessness of the ego, with a concomitant diminution in self-esteem, rather than as being solely determined by a reaction to object loss. He hypothesized that all individuals desire to be deemed worthy, strong, secure, and lovable, and that their awareness of their inability to achieve these narcissistic aspirations leads to a state of depression and to a depletion in self-esteem. For Bibring, early infantile states of helplessness were more significant than states of primal depression in laying the foundation for adult states of depression. Dorpat (1977) followed Bibring's thinking in believing that depressive affects arose from early traumatic states of infantile helplessness. In Dorpat's view, however, true depressive feelings do not develop until the child has learned to make the distinction between temporary and permanent losses of the object.

Beck (1976), in his work with depressed patients, has offered a combination of a behavioral and a psychodynamic model of depression. He postulated that depression results from a series of learned experiences or cognitions of a negative nature. These then lead the individual to develop a pessimistic perception of him- or herself that becomes intensified over a period of time as it is reinforced by life experiences. Such negative cognitive sets lead to feelings of sadness and depression and to a perception that the individual is lacking in the elements essential for happiness and success in life. Beck and his followers utilize behavioral treatments that attempt to modify these negative cognitive sets.

In summation, one might say that most of the psychodynamic theories of depression currently view the state as a response to the loss of a significant and ambivalently invested object—one that has never been experienced as being fully separated from the self. In an attempt to retain it, the representation of the lost love object is psychically merged even more closely with the representation of the self. The resulting depression is an expression of the conflict between these two representations. In addition, the degree to which an individual feels unable to match up with the dictates of his or her ego ideal determines the degree of self-esteem difficulty seen. Although these views emphasize the unconscious psychodynamics of depression, they are not to be interpreted as being in any way at variance with the biochemical factors leading to depressive states.

Historical Review

Use of the psychoanalytic method with older patients was delayed for many years because Freud (1898/1962, 1904/1953, 1905/1953) felt that individuals in this age range would have too much material to deal with and would be ineducable because of the presumed inelasticity of their mental processes. It was only after Abraham (1919/1953) wrote of his successful analytic treatment of patients in their 40s and 50s—an age considered old for that time period—that psychoanalysis began to be used more often with even older people.[1]

[1] A number of the articles that followed (Alexander 1944; Grotjahn 1940, 1951, 1955; Kaufman 1937; Meerloo 1953, 1955) dealt more with the use of analytically oriented therapies with such patients than with analyses per se, but the thrust of their theses was to the effect that such insight-oriented treatments were both practical and desirable in the older age group. One issue of importance noted by Grotjahn (1951) and Meerloo (1953) was that the defensive structure of the individual may become more malleable with advancing age, thus making it easier to treat such people than their younger counterparts. Grotjahn (1955) further observed that older people were also capable of forming intense transference feelings toward their analysts and that analysts quite readily experienced strong countertransference feelings toward their older patients. Meerloo's (1953, 1955) observations about the difficulties older people encounter in self-esteem regulation and their prominent fears of death were also quite cogent.

A number of other relevant observations about grief and loss in older patients can be found in a volume published by the Boston Society for Gerontological Psychiatry (Berezin and Cath 1965). The first actual case report to cite clinical material in any depth from the analysis of an older depressed patient, however, was presented by Segal in 1958. Other, briefer reports of such treatments followed some years later (Hurn 1969; Wolff 1971), as did a detailed study of the treatment of an older narcissistic man with depression (Sandler 1978).

King (1980) presented brief clinical vignettes from the analyses of three older individuals. In her paper, she noted the sense of enhanced urgency and motivation lent to the patients' treatments by their awareness that their life expectancies were limited—a cognizance on their part of the fact that this was probably their "last chance" to change. Kernberg (1980) noted that older narcissistic patients who became depressed were easier to treat than younger ones because of the inroads made by reality on their grandiose selves.

Two important collections of articles on older people (Colarusso and Nemiroff 1990; Nemiroff and Colarusso 1985) present a variety of case studies and theoretical papers, some of which deal with the issue of older depressed patients. The most important new point introduced in these works is that psychological development does not stop in either childhood or adolescence, but continues throughout the life cycle. This insight is important with respect to the issue of therapy with older, depressed individuals in that it recognizes that these patients are capable of forming new concepts and relationships and of investing in their treatments in as meaningful a manner as many younger people do. This idea is crucial in terms of combating the attitude of therapeutic nihilism with which many younger therapists regard the older patients they see.

In my own studies in this area (Myers 1984, 1985, 1986, 1987a, 1987b, 1988, 1990a, 1990b, 1990c, 1991), I have described my use of psychoanalysis and psychoanalytically oriented psychotherapy with more than a dozen individuals in their 50s, 60s, and 70s. Most of the aging patients whom I have seen initially presented with symptoms of depression. This frequently led to my using antidepressant medications early in their treatments. The impact of this parameter or "deviation" from the "classical" psychoanalytic model—in which intrapsychic change is supposed to be mediated solely through interpretive efforts on the part of the analyst—on the subsequent treatment course had to be analyzed during a later phase of the analysis. In working with these older patients, I, too, have noted that their defenses were frequently more malleable than those seen in younger individuals and that intense transference and countertransference situations were often encountered. In addition, I have observed that dreams whose manifest content deals with the death of, or separation from, loved ones are also considerably more common in older people than in younger ones (Myers 1987b), a phenomenon that I have related to the frequency of object losses experienced by older people and to their need to come to terms with the issues surrounding their own impending death. The most important finding to evolve, from my own work as well as from that of the earlier studies cited, is that analysis is both a viable and a meaningful treatment modality for many older people.

Differential Dynamic Diagnosis

When first meeting with an older depressed patient, it is important for the therapist to obtain as complete and careful a history as possible. It is also frequently necessary to obtain the results of a recent physical examination in order to rule out any possible organic causes of late-life depression. Among the more obvious of such causes are a panoply of physical illnesses with mental features, such as diseases of the thyroid, pituitary, or adrenal glands; collagen disorders; metabolic problems; deficiency diseases; and primary or metastatic tumors involving the brain itself.

In addition, depression is quite commonly seen in patients with Alzheimer's disease and other organic mental disorders as well as in elderly individuals who abuse substances such as alcohol. In an important recent study (Rubin et al. 1991), it was found to be quite difficult to distinguish depressed subjects without concurrent dementia from nondepressed subjects with very mild dementia (Clinical Dementia Ratings of less than 1 on the dementia rating scale of Hughes et al. [1982]). Both groups of patients demonstrated global psychometric impairment of memory, speech, visuospatial abilities, and motor performance. One possible way to distinguish between the two groups involves tests of incidental recall (Hart et al. 1987), although this assertion has been debated. It may be necessary to offer patients with uncertain diagnoses an empirical trial with antidepressant medication in order to differentiate the two groups, inasmuch as the psychometric impairments will disappear in the group suffering solely from depression after the medication has had a salutary effect.

Case Example

At the time that I began to see Ms. X, a 71-year-old widow, I was in my late 40s. As a consequence of having had two mild cerebrovascular accidents within the 6 months prior to her referral to me, she was suffering from moderate feelings of sadness but had no clear-cut vegetative symptoms of a major depression. The strokes had also caused a now barely discernible paresis on one side that left her with a minimal limp when she walked.

I was immediately struck by her evident self-consciousness in attempting to "hide" her difficulty in walking when she entered my office and by her failure to make eye contact with me in her initial visits. I felt quite certain that her physical disability must pose a considerable difficulty for her in the sphere of self-esteem, but the reasons for this problem were not readily apparent.

In taking a detailed history about her background, I learned that Ms. X had been an active, athletic person all her life. Horseback riding had been a passion of hers as a child, and when she married, she and her husband had spent many idyllic moments riding together on ranches and black sand beaches around the world. Although she had mourned him at his death, the difficulty that her current infirmity posed for her in mounting a horse and the pains that she incurred in her leg when she was seated astride a saddle seemed to further reinforce the idea of his loss by robbing her of the means of reliving the motoric memories of their intimate rides together.

Despite her feelings of sadness and her recent history of cerebrovascular accidents secondary to a moderate degree of hypertension, it was clear that Ms. X's sensorium was intact and that her overall physical condition was good. It was also quite apparent that she was determined to regain as much as possible of her former athletic skills. In this sense, she seemed similar to many younger patients who place a strong priority on maintaining certain high levels of physical performance.

Although she maintained a number of friendships with people her own age, Ms. X's primary social interactions were with her two daughters. Both of them were middle aged women with children of their own who lived in communities nearby their mother in Connecticut. As I came to learn more about her interplay with her daughters, I was struck by the fact that my patient seemed to take their attentions for granted, as if their catering to her physical well-being and to her narcissistic need for attention and admiration was something to be expected. Ms. X was, however, quite bothered by her perceptions that her present life seemed "empty" and "without meaning" to her, and she wondered if this had not been a long-standing problem that had somehow been masked by the myriad activities that had occupied her attention throughout her life.

In her interactions with me, Ms. X seemed quite outgoing. She frequently commented on the photographs from different trips that adorned the walls of my office and mentioned having been to many of the same places with her husband. After her initial self-consciousness began to wear off, she started to pay attention to her dress before each visit and seemed almost flirtatious in her manner with me. Despite her age and her modest infirmity, she was still a slender, attractive woman with a considerable sense of style that obviously set her apart from many of her peers.

In addition, Ms. X found it fairly easy to freely associate in sessions and was rather well attuned to her own unconscious processes, as evidenced by the number of dreams she spontaneously reported. As a result of this, we agreed to undertake an analysis in an attempt to address and modify her longstanding characterological (narcissistic) issues and, after a few sessions of sitting up, she began to use the couch.

On the couch, Ms. X began to speak in greater depth about her parents. Both of them had been accomplished athletes. Her mother had been an excellent swimmer who had fantasies of gaining fame from swimming the English Channel, and her father had been a mountain climber and skier. It quickly became apparent to me that Ms. X's first love was skiing, surpassing even her passion for horseback riding. In her associations, sexual pleasures with her husband in the past or in her occasional masturbatory episodes in the present seemed to rank second to the thrill of schussing wildly through the deep powder of a distant mountainscape. I could readily appreciate her feelings for the sport, inasmuch as I shared her passion for skiing and indulged it at every possible opportunity.

After Ms. X had been in treatment for a number of months, I went on a spring skiing trip. During the trip, I sustained a serious injury to my left knee that led to my wearing a soft cast on part of my leg for some time. Needless to say, I felt somewhat dispirited upon my return, as my vacation had been anything but what I had hoped it would be and I was worried about whether I would ever be able to ski again.

As soon as Ms. X saw me hobbling about on my crutches as I greeted her upon my return, she responded as if my injury had been one inflicted on her and not me. The color appeared to drain from her face and her flirtatious manner seemed to have been aborted in midstream. It was as if she had experienced my injury as a slap across her face. When she made a brief gasping sound and tears welled up in her eyes, I felt quite irritated with her. In my own state of anxiety about my physical well-being, a countertransference reaction of needing some sort of maternal comforting had arisen in me. Ms. X's antithetical response had angered me, as if she were not giving me the warmth and mothering I felt I deserved at that moment. When she framed the one-word question "Skiing?," I nodded in the affirmative without even bothering to attempt to analyze her query. I did not respond to her further inquiries about whether I would be able to ski again, but the expression on my face and the slumping of my shoulders obviously spoke volumes about the nature of my fears.

When I saw Ms. X the next day, she seemed as depressed as she had been at any time since she had begun her treatment. The limp in her left leg, which had barely been discernible in recent weeks, appeared quite accentuated. "I've been very upset since our last visit," she announced. "Your accident has sent me into a tailspin."

Ms. X's words made me feel vaguely guilty. I recognized this as a response to the irritation I had felt with her during the previous session. I had the impression that my injury had somehow emasculated me in her eyes, as if I had been rendered impotent to help her deal with her own physical difficulties.

As I began to associate to myself about the feelings she had engendered in me, I realized that they were related to specific early life interactions with my own mother. With this nascent awareness of the roots of my countertransference feelings, which I increasingly worked on in the next few days in my ongoing process of self-analysis, I was able to once more assume a therapeutic stance with my patient and to begin working with her negative feelings toward me. The process of monitoring one's countertransference feelings is of importance in psychodynamic treatments with patients of any age, but is especially important in situations involving younger therapists and older patients (Myers 1986, 1987c).

The following day, Ms. X brought in a dream. It was short and the meaning seemed obvious enough. "Someone close to me had just died and I was at the cemetery. It was a cold day and there was snow on the ground. I felt very, very sad."

When I asked her about her associations to the dream, she seemed stopped up and told me that she was feeling "blank" and "empty." She had no thoughts about who it was who might have died or why there was snow on the ground. When I suggested that the dream might be connected with my skiing accident, she agreed and began to cry again and spoke of feeling quite depressed.

Over the next several weeks, Ms. X's condition began to worsen and she soon manifested clear-cut vegetative signs of a major depression. Her ability to free-associate in sessions became markedly inhibited and she began to reproach herself quite sternly and quite often for being selfish and ungiving. In this setting, I had to institute treatment with a tricyclic antidepressant.

Her positive therapeutic response to the medication I had prescribed seemed to be synchronous in time with my own positive response to the treatment that I had been receiving for my knee. It was as if both our moods had brightened, hers by being on the medication and mine by being able to shed my cast and crutches and to walk freely about again.

She commented one day on how glad she was that my leg was getting better and then her associations drifted back to the dream about the death of someone close to her that had preceded her falling into the depths of depression. "I have some other thoughts about that dream now," she said.

"What are they?" I asked.

"I'm not really sure, but it's as if I need you to be totally intact physically in order to offer the possibility of helping me to overcome my own physical problems. You're supposed to be young, so that I can count on you to keep me alive. If you fall apart, what's going to happen to me? I know there's more to it than that, though."

The two of us remained silent for a while and then Ms. X continued: "It's strange, since you're probably young enough to be my son. But I think I've looked on you as something of a father substitute since the day I first came in here to see you. I was very close to my father when I was growing up. He was the one who first taught me how to ski. We were on a vacation in Zermatt. I can remember it as if it were yesterday. It was so beautiful there, looking up at the Matterhorn. I miss him so, especially now that I can't ski anymore. It's as if I can never relive those moments with the sun and snow and wind in my face again, and my father's voice and arms around me when he put me on his own skis with him that first time, so I wouldn't feel lonely or afraid by myself."

"You really begin to lose people, when you lose the basic ties that bind you. Funny, the expression that I just used. It sounds as if I'm talking about ski bindings. Even with the very words I'm using, I'm trying to hold on to him. And when I came here, I think I put all of that onto you. You were supposed to take over where Daddy and Phillip (her deceased husband) left off. But when you hurt your knee and looked as if you might never ski again, all my hopes to get close to them again felt shattered. You lost all value for me then. I know that must sound like a terrible thing to say, but it's what I felt."

In this speech, Ms. X verbalized her fantasy that my relative youth and athletic vigor would be able to keep her alive forever. In addition, my knee injury interfered with her transference wish for me to reduplicate the earlier relationships with her husband and father. The interference with these fantasies and the attendant intensification of her feelings both of prior object loss and of loss of self-esteem led to the onset of the depression. With the depression, she felt her life drain out of her, as if she were dead. By giving her the medication and by recovering from my knee injury, I was "magically" able to restore her to life and thereby to help resurrect the fantasy that I could keep her alive forever.

In the next few sessions, Ms. X expressed considerable concern that I would dislike her for having verbalized the idea that I had lost all value for her when my knee was injured. She was certain that I would think of her as a "terrible" person for having such feelings, similar to the way she believed her husband, Phillip, had felt about her when she responded negatively to his impotency after he had had prostate surgery for the cancer that ultimately ended his life.

In the months that followed, Ms. X began to recognize that she had always expected those who were close to her to cater to her wishes rather than responding to their own. There had been very little sense of give-and-take in her life. Because of her beauty, wit, and athletic ability, her husband had always been willing to gratify her narcissistic needs, as had her daughters. But when she responded so poorly to his impotency near the end of his life, his angry turning away from her had both wounded her and made her question the values which had theretofore governed her life.

At this juncture in the treatment, the problem of dealing with her lifelong self-esteem issues felt as if it were too difficult a task for Ms. X. She attempted to defend herself against the negative feelings aroused by the contemplation of her long-standing interpersonal inadequacies by projecting these difficulties onto me. I was seen as the "empty," "inadequate" person because I was often silent and had no "pithy insights" to offer her when she wished me to speak. Although she knew objectively that this stance was part of my analytic technique, emotionally she felt deprived and angry if I did not make comments for her on demand, and she began to characterize me as being cold and ungiving.

Her irritation with me grew quite strong and she verbalized ideas of stopping the treatment, as she felt that it was no longer doing anything "positive" for her. In one session her frustration became so great that she even got up off the couch and left early. The following day she seemed quite contrite in her manner. "I had a dream last night," she announced. "I was a little girl in it, no more than 5 or 6. My mother was there and she looked very beautiful, all dressed up in an evening gown. I went over to touch the gown and she got mad at me and told me that I would mess it up, and she went out with my father without kissing me good night."

In her associations to the dream, Ms. X began to convey a different impression of her mother than the one she had previously painted for me. In the new version, her mother had been a rather narcissistic woman who was more interested in being complimented by others and in being adorned in pretty clothes to wear to gala social events than in spending time with her only child or in even gratifying many of her husband's needs for companionship. From this new portrait of the mother, it was a fairly easy step for the patient to see that her transference perceptions of me as cold and ungiving were based on her earlier feelings about her mother, the "blank" and "empty" woman against whose representation within her ego she had directed reproaches during her depressive state. She also recognized that she had unconsciously identified with many of her mother's mannerisms and means of interaction with others in an attempt to maintain some sort of object tie with the woman, particularly after the mother's death during Ms. X's late adolescence. The patient came to see that she had often been vain and selfish herself, especially in her handling of her husband during his terminal illness and in her expectations of obeisance and homage from her two daughters.

In the remaining 2½ years of the treatment, most of the work of the analysis dealt with the freeing up of Ms. X's ability to be a more substantial mothering presence to her children and grandchildren than her own mother had ever been to her. Whereas her anger toward her mother initially surfaced toward me in the transference, as the treatment progressed she was able to allow more of it to be directly perceived. In doing so, Ms. X also began to acknowledge to herself that she had been cheated of maternal warmth in her own life and had shortchanged her children of this quality in theirs. The self-revelations were difficult for her inasmuch as they made her feel quite badly about herself, as if she were not a very "nice" person. Despite these blows to her self-esteem, she did not slip back again into a major depression. Our understanding of this was that she felt a close tie to me in the transference relationship, in that she believed that I perceived her to be a "worthwhile" individual because I had "stuck with her" throughout all her travails and her self-revelations.

When the time came to terminate the analysis, shortly before her 75th birthday, Ms. X became fearful that she would die or become depressed if she lost her tie with me. Although she understood the fact that her fantasy that I could keep her alive by my relative youth was simply that, a fantasy, it was very difficult for her to surrender the idea. She asked if I would mind if she maintained occasional contact with me, either by means of the telephone or by in-person visits, and I said that would be fine. This particular request for an incomplete termination is something I have encountered with a number of older patients. With all of the patients in question, the request appears to be connected both with the fantasy that my relative youth will enable them to remain alive and with the fact that for many older individuals, the therapist has become an important real-life object in addition to being a transference one.

Summary

In looking closely at Ms. X's case, one can see the relevance of many of the psychodynamic conceptualizations of depression suggested by the authors whose works were detailed in the opening section of this chapter. For example, the idea that the reproaches directed against the self are clearly meant for an ambivalently perceived love object whose representation has been merged with aspects of the self-representation in the ego is quite apparent in this case. Even though she can justifiably think of herself as "blank" and "empty" in a number of ways, Ms. X's diatribes against herself were recognized as being more relevant to her narcissistic mother than to herself.

The lack of optimal maternal largesse during her childhood led to early experiences of deprivation (perceived of as object loss) and to the development of a heightened degree of ambivalence toward her mother. Because of an incomplete degree of separation from the ambivalently perceived love object (mother), Ms. X tended to internalize aspects of the mother's personality and to choose or create love objects in her own life (her husband and daughters) who would gratify her needs to be admired and to feel lovable, in order to overcome her feelings of deficit and unlovability.

The self-esteem issues that numerous authors have mentioned as being of importance in patients with depression were also clearly a part of Ms. X's personality. She was, interestingly enough, troubled by her narcissistic issues at the start of the treatment, and dealing with them became the central issue of the analysis. In this regard, the success of the treatment illustrates the point noted in the review of the literature that older patients—especially older narcissistic patients who are able to experience feelings of depression about their lives—are often more amenable to treatment than younger ones.

A few final comments on Ms. X's case seem in order. She was clearly capable of modifying long-standing personality issues, as noted above. Her ability to form an intense and analyzable transference response to me was also beyond question. Finally, she was obviously able to engender a clear-cut negative countertransference response in me during a particular phase in the treatment—a response that I had to analyze for myself in order to allow the treatment to continue in a salutary manner.

For Further Study

Colarusso CA, Nemiroff RA (eds): Frontiers of Adult Development. New York, Basic Books, 1990

Freud S: Mourning and melancholia (1917), in The Standard Edition of the Complete Psychological Works of Sigmund Freud, Vol 14. Translated and edited by Strachey J. London, Hogarth Press, 1957, pp 237–258

King P: The life cycle as indicated by the nature of the transference in the psychoanalysis of the middle-aged and the elderly. Int J Psychoanal 61:153–160, 1980

Myers WA: Dynamic Therapy of the Older Patient. New York, Jason Aronson, 1984

Myers WA: Transference and countertransference issues in treatments involving older patients and younger therapists. J Geriatr Psychiatry 19:221–239, 1986

Myers WA: Dreams of mourning and separation in older individuals, in The Interpretations of Dreams in Clinical Work (American Psychoanalytic Association Workshop Series, Monograph 3). Edited by Rothstein A. Madison, CT, International Universities Press, 1987, pp 125–143

Myers WA: On beginning with an elderly patient, in On Beginning an Analysis. Edited by Jacobs T, Rothstein A. Madison, CT, International Universities Press, 1990, pp 259–269

Myers WA: Psychoanalytic psychotherapy and psychoanalysis with older patients, in New Techniques in the Psychotherapy of Older Patients. Edited by Myers WA, Washington, DC, American Psychiatric Press, 1991, pp 265–279

Nemiroff RA, Colarusso CA (eds): The Race Against Time: Psychoanalysis and Psychotherapy in the Second Half of Life. New York, Plenum, 1985

References

Abraham K: The first pregenital stage of the libido (1916), in Selected Papers. London, Hogarth Press, 1927, pp 248–279

Abraham K: The applicability of psychoanalytic treatment to patients at an advanced age (1919), in Selected Papers. New York, Basic Books, 1953, pp 312–317

Alexander F: The indications for psychoanalytic therapy. Bulletin of the New York Academy of Medicine, Second Series 20:319–332, 1944

Beck A: Cognitive Therapy and the Emotional Disorders. New York, International Universities Press, 1976

Benedek T: Toward the biology of the depressive constellation. J Am Psychoanal Assoc 4:389–427, 1956

Berezin MA, Cath SH (eds): Geriatric Psychiatry: Grief, Loss and Emotional Disorders in the Aging Process. New York, International Universities Press, 1965

Bibring E: The mechanism of depression, in Affective Disorders. Edited by Greenacre P. New York, International Universities Press, 1953, pp 13–48

Bowlby J: Grief and mourning in infancy and early childhood. Psychoanal Study Child 15:9–52, 1960

Colarusso CA, Nemiroff RA (eds): Frontiers of Adult Development. New York, Basic Books, 1990

Dorpat TL: Depressive affect. Psychoanal Study Child 32:3–28, 1977

Freud S: Draft B: the aetiology of the neuroses (1893), in The Standard Edition of the Complete Psychological Works of Sigmund Freud, Vol 1. Translated and edited by Strachey J. London, Hogarth Press, 1966, pp 179–184

Freud S: Sexuality in the aetiology of the neuroses (1898), in The Standard Edition of the Complete Psychological Works of Sigmund Freud, Vol 3. Translated and edited by Strachey J. London, Hogarth Press, 1962, pp 261–285

Freud S: Freud's psycho-analytic procedure (1904), in The Standard Edition of the Complete Psychological Works of Sigmund Freud, Vol 7. Translated and edited by Strachey J. London, Hogarth Press, 1953, pp 249–254

Freud S: On psycho-therapy (1905), in The Standard Edition of the Complete Psychological Works of Sigmund Freud, Vol 7. Translated and edited by Strachey J. London, Hogarth Press, 1953, pp 257–268

Freud S: Mourning and melancholia (1917), in The Standard Edition of the Complete Psychological Works of Sigmund Freud, Vol 14. Translated and edited by Strachey J. London, Hogarth Press, 1957, pp 237–258

Freud S: The ego and the id (1923), in The Standard Edition of the Complete Psychological Works of Sigmund Freud, Vol 19. Translated and edited by Strachey J. London, Hogarth Press, 1961, pp 3–66

Grotjahn M: Psychoanalytic investigation of a seventy-one year old man with senile dementia. Psychoanal Q 9:80–97, 1940

Grotjahn M: Some analytic observations about the process of aging. Psychoanalysis and Social Sciences 3:301–312, 1951

Grotjahn M: Analytic psychotherapy with the elderly. Psychoanal Rev 42:419–427, 1955

Hart RP, Kwentus JA, Wade JB, et al: Digit symbol performance in mild dementia and depression. J Consult Clin Psychol 55:236–238, 1987

Hughes CP, Berg L, Danzinger WL, et al: A new clinical scale for the staging of dementia. Br J Psychiatry 140:566–572, 1982

Hurn HT: Synergic relations between the processes of fatherhood and psychoanalysis. J Am Psychoanal Assoc 17:437–451, 1969

Jacobson E: The effect of disappointment on ego and superego formation in normal and depressive development. Psychoanal Rev 33:129–147, 1946

Kaufman MR: Psychoanalysis in late-life depression. Psychoanal Q 6:308–335, 1937

Kernberg OF: Internal World and External Reality: Object Relations Theory Applied. New York, Jason Aronson, 1980

King P: The life cycle as indicated by the nature of the transference in the psychoanalysis of the middle-aged and the elderly. Int J Psychoanal 61:153–160, 1980

Klein M: The Psychoanalysis of Children. London, Hogarth Press, 1932

Mahler MS: Notes on the development of basic moods, in Psychoanalysis: A General Psychology. Edited by Loewenstein RM. New York, International Universities Press, 1966, pp 152–168

Meerloo JAM: Contribution of psychoanalysis to the problem of the aged, in Psychoanalysis and Social Work. Edited by Heiman M. New York, International Universities Press, 1953, pp 30–35

Meerloo JAM: Transference and resistance in geriatric psychotherapy. Psychoanal Rev 42:72–82, 1955

Myers WA: Dynamic Therapy of the Older Patient. New York, Jason Aronson, 1984

Myers WA: Sexuality in the older individual. J Am Acad Psychoanal 13:88–94, 1985

Myers WA: Transference and countertransference issues in treatments involving older patients and younger therapists. J Geriatr Psychiatry 19:221–239, 1986

Myers WA: Age, rage and the fear of AIDS. J Geriatr Psychiatry 20:127–142, 1987a

Myers WA: Dreams of mourning and separation in older individuals, in The Interpretations of Dreams in Clinical Work (American Psychoanalytic Association Workshop Series, Monograph 3). Edited by Rothstein A. Madison, CT, International Universities Press, 1987b, pp 125–143

Myers WA: Work on countertransference facilitated by self analysis of the analyst's dreams, in The Interpretations of Dreams in Clinical Work (American Psychoanalytic Association Workshop Series, Monograph 3). Edited by Rothstein A. Madison, CT, International Universities Press, 1987c, pp 37–46

Myers WA: I can't play ball anymore. J Geriatr Psychiatry 21:121–139, 1988

Myers WA: Modifications in the frequency of altered ego states throughout the life cycle, in Frontiers of Adult Development. Edited by Colarusso CA, Nemiroff RA. New York, Basic Books, 1990a, pp 488–497

Myers WA: On beginning with an elderly patient, in On Beginning an Analysis. Edited by Jacobs T, Rothstein A. Madison, CT, International Universities Press, 1990b, pp 259–269

Myers WA: Psychotherapy of the elderly, in American Psychiatric Press Review of Psychiatry, Vol 9. Edited by Tasman A, Goldfinger SM, Kaufmann CA. Washington, DC, American Psychiatric Press, 1990c, pp 263–278

Myers WA: Psychoanalytic psychotherapy and psychoanalysis with older patients, in New Techniques in the Psychotherapy of Older Patients. Edited by Myers WA. Washington, DC, American Psychiatric Press, 1991, pp 265–279

Nemiroff RA, Colarusso CA (eds): The Race Against Time: Psychotherapy and Psychoanalysis in the Second Half of Life. New York, Plenum, 1985

Rubin EH, Kinscherf DA, Grant EA, et al: The influence of major depression on clinical and psychometric assessment of senile dementia of the Alzheimer type. Am J Psychiatry 148:1164–1171, 1991

Sandler AM: Psychoanalysis in later life: problems in the psychoanalysis of an aging narcissistic patient. J Geriatr Psychiatry 11:5–36, 1978

Segal H: Fear of death: notes on the analysis of an old man. Int J Psychoanal 39:178–181, 1958

Spitz R, Wolf KM: Anaclitic depression: an inquiry into the genesis of psychiatric conditions in early childhood. Psychoanal Study Child 2:313–342, 1946

Wolff K: Individual psychotherapy with geriatric patients. Psychosomatics 12:89–93, 1971

Section IV

Special Topics

Efrain Bleiberg, M.D.,
Section Editor

Chapter 25

The Psychology of Prescribing and Taking Medication

Fredric N. Busch, M.D.,
and Elizabeth L. Auchincloss, M.D.

In this chapter we review various controversies and clinical issues related to the use of combined psychodynamic psychotherapy and psychotropic medications. We also discuss issues pertaining to the meaning of medications for patients, exploring how the use of the psychodynamic model can lead to both 1) the incorporation of the meaning of medication into the psychotherapeutic process and 2) increased compliance. Finally, we discuss how attention to countertransference issues can aid clinicians in understanding their patterns of prescribing and their interactions with patients around medication. A number of case examples are presented to demonstrate the various meanings that medications can have for patients and to illustrate some approaches to medication management.

In 1938, in the "Outline of Psychoanalysis," Freud wrote of his expectation that "the future may teach us how to exert a direct influence, by means of particular chemical substances, upon the amounts of energy and their distribution in the mind" (Freud 1938/1964, p. 182). It may be, he suggested, "that there are . . . undreamt-of possibilities of therapy" (p. 182). Earlier, in 1933, in "The New Introductory Lectures on Psychoanalysis," Freud stated that "analysis as a psycho-therapeutic procedure does not stand in opposition to other methods used in this specialized branch of medicine; it does not diminish their value nor exclude them. There is no theoretical inconsistency in a doctor who likes to call himself a psychotherapist using analysis on his patients alongside of any other method of treatment" (Freud 1933/1964, p. 152).

Despite the open-minded eclecticism of the father of psychoanalysis, there has been, until recently, a "curiously persistent tendency among psychiatrists to limit their knowledge either to the area of psychotherapy or to that of so-called somatotherapy" (Linn 1964, p. 138). Linn observed that "psychoanalysts often pride themselves on their ignorance of drugs, and their somatically oriented colleagues take no less pride in their ignorance of psychodynamics" (Linn 1964, p. 138). In an editorial on "Pharmacotherapy and Psychotherapy" (1982), Shader and Greenblatt complained that "eclectic or integrated teaching is hard to come by even in the more contemporary programs. There is still an 'either-or approach' to treatment" (p. 1).

At one extreme, psychotherapists have argued that drugs are little more than placebo and could be detrimental to patients in psychotherapy by increasing dependency, blunting the capacity or motivation to seek insight, supporting a tendency to look for quick solutions to complex problems, or lowering self-esteem. Even those analytic pioneers who have written about and studied the combined use of psychoanalysis and drug therapy (Ostow 1962; Sarwer-Foner 1983) have viewed medication as useful only in the treatment of symptoms or in the enhancement of the patient's capacity to engage in analysis, where the "real treatment" would take place. The work of these analysts reflects a theoretical hierarchy in which psychological treatment is considered more deeply curative than medication therapy and best left undisturbed whenever possible.

At the other extreme, psychobiologists have often viewed psychotherapy, at worst, as malpractice, and at best, as unnecessary, irrelevant, or neutral. Some pharmacotherapists have hypothesized that psychotherapy might be deleterious to treatment because symptoms may be aggravated by uncovering defenses. Even those pharmacologists who have seen psychotherapy as useful have considered it helpful only in facilitating compliance with medication or for the improvement of some vaguely defined "psychological problems" left over after the "real" biological treatment had achieved the desired results.

Whatever its origins, it is clear that this polarization between biological and psychodynamic viewpoints in American psychiatry has long inhibited—and, at times, paralyzed—any efforts to describe and make use of the psychology of medication. However, as is sometimes the case, clinical practice is clearly at odds with standard ideologies. Beitman et al. (1984) estimate that as many as 210,000 patients per month are seen in shared arrangements between psychopharmacologists and nonmedical therapists. According to Kahn (1990), "combined treatment undoubtedly is growing as more residents graduate from well-rounded programs and enter practice" (p. 197). At the same time, a second generation of biologically oriented clinical research has begun to produce convincing evidence that treatment approaches combining psychotherapy and medication may be preferable to monotherapy methods in the treatment of depression, schizophrenia, and anxiety states. The research literature may also support a combined approach to other disorders, including anorexia nervosa, drug abuse and alcoholism, obsessive-compulsive disorder, and borderline personality disorder (Beitman and Klerman 1991).

In 1981, the Boston–New Haven Collaborative Study of Depression directly addressed and refuted the claims—made by psychoanalysts and biological psychiatrists alike—that opposite treatments in combination could harm patients (Rounsaville et al. 1981). Kahn (1991) summarized this study as follows:

> The researchers tested the hierarchical view that therapy is superior to drugs and that drugs interfere with therapy. They distilled four traditional hypotheses of negative interaction: 1) drugs could be a negative placebo, increasing dependency and prolonging some kinds of psychopathology; 2) drug relief of symptoms could reduce motivation for further therapy; 3) drugs could eliminate one symptom but create others by symptom substitution if underlying conflicts remained intact; 4) drugs could decrease self-esteem by leading the patient to believe he or she was not interesting enough for insight-oriented work. They also examined the reverse position, that psychotherapy could be harmful in patients sick enough to need medication, either by promoting regression or by encouraging the patient inappropriately not to use drugs. Careful statistical evaluation of outcomes in large samples receiving different treatment combinations revealed no negative interactions. On the contrary, their work supported the theory that the two treatments are additive, not conflicting. (p. 87)

Thus, a combination of practical experience and the latest research findings has contributed to a renewed and revitalized exploration of the interface between psychological and biological treatment in both the psychiatric and the psychoanalytic literature and has set the stage for the development of a sophisticated psychology of medication. It is our opinion that medication and psychotherapy are not mutually exclusive treatments, but in fact may be mutually enhancing in at least three ways. *First,* medication effects may increase the patient's ability to participate in psychotherapy. The patient may become more able to tolerate painful affects, allowing exploration into distressing material that previously needed to be repressed. Relief from symptoms can lead to a more positive sense of the self and an increase in self-esteem. In addition, medication can enhance "verbal skills, cognitive functions, attention, and concentration, and it may also facilitate abreaction by modifying defenses, permitting repressed emotions and memories to emerge" (Marmor 1981, p. 313). *Second,* the exploration of the intrapsychic meaning of taking medication may highlight unconscious conflicts, particularly as experienced in the transference, and lead to greater insight and therapeutic change. *Third,* exploration of the meaning of taking medication may increase compliance with the medication regimen. In the opinion of the authors, the clinician should adopt an attitude that accepts and tolerates our present lack of definitive knowledge about etiology and cure of psychopathology and that sets the tone for maximal exploration of the patient's fantasies about diagnosis, etiology, and treatment strategies. It is crucial in most cases not to adopt an authoritarian attitude that makes compliance the highest goal in the treatment. In a thoughtful paper that addressed issues of noncompliance, Gutheil (1978) stressed the concept of "participant prescribing." In his view, "pharmacotherapy is as much a collaboration as the psychotherapy, involving shared inquiry, shared goals, and mutual participation in both experiencing and observing the process" (p. 219). For Gutheil, "drug prescribing is a legitimate subject for the same therapeutic exploration and sensitivity applied to more abstract and verbal interchanges. The subject is as rich in potentially useful affects, fantasies, and associations as any other aspect of the therapeutic process; indeed, such willingness to discuss and explore will increase the patient's compliance with the medication regimen" (p. 225). Therapeutic exploration of these aspects will also allow patients on medication to learn a great deal from their psychotherapy, particularly in the critical area of conflicts around autonomy and dependence, or blame and responsibility, as these conflicts emerge in the transference.

For example, Mr. Y was a 50-year-old man who presented with symptoms of major depression that had thus far not responded to medication treatment. The history revealed that the patient had intense fears of medication, such as fears of dying in his sleep, and had been able to take only small doses. Realizing his sensitivity to medications, the therapist started Mr. Y on a very low dose of antidepressant (sertraline 25 mg/day). At the next visit, Mr. Y revealed that he had taken only 12.5 mg and had experienced multiple side effects. The therapist gently suggested that perhaps Mr. Y was having such side effects in part secondary to anxiety about the medication. Mr. Y became quite resentful about these comments and at that point discontinued the medication and canceled a follow-up appointment.

At the next visit, Mr. Y discussed his feelings and agreed to restart the medications, with an apparent resolution of his anger at the therapist. Over the next few sessions, the patient slowly increased the dose of the sertraline. The therapist, however, continued to note some guardedness in the patient's approach to the therapist. When the therapist shared this with him, Mr. Y revealed that he still was upset about the therapist's initial response to his reported side effects, and felt as though the therapist still did not believe him when he reported side effects. The therapist stated that because he and Mr. Y should be allied in their wish to help Mr. Y with his depression, it was important to understand why Mr. Y felt they might be at odds. Mr. Y responded by discussing a prior doctor who failed to diagnose his thyroid disease even though he complained of the typical symptoms. Ultimately, a connection could be made between his perception of the therapist and his experience of his father, whom he saw as critical and abusive, often responding negatively to his difficulties.

Thus, Mr. Y gradually revealed an ongoing transference fantasy in which he felt that the therapist was demeaning his intense fears of medications and pressuring him to take medications that he found frightening. If the therapist had not been sensitive to this ongoing disruption in rapport, the treatment could have continued with the patient's being quietly angry and suspicious with the therapist. The therapist's attitude of "participant prescribing" helped the patient to reveal his fantasy and to develop a new view of how the therapist was working with him. In this case, nonjudgmental exploration of the patient's experience of taking the medication led not only to increased compliance but also to increased self-knowledge.

In a second case, the therapist felt that taking medication was a choice that only the patient could make, as the indications for it were not clear. Including the patient in the decision led to profound discoveries in the transference that had a direct bearing on the patient's chief complaints.

> Ms. Z was a 45-year-old executive who, 2 years earlier, had started two-times-per-week psychotherapy for painful episodic feelings of anxiety and depression. Although a prominent businesswoman, Ms. Z had not had successful relationships with men, who she felt were always pushing her around. She had angrily left her previous therapy when the therapist had suggested a trial of fluoxetine. Exploration of her angry feelings toward her parents and of her fears of separating from her mother had improved her interpersonal relationships so that she was now engaged to be married.
>
> Six weeks before her wedding, Ms. Z developed profound, generalized anxiety and became angry with her therapist that she still had this symptom. She began to feel that her boyfriend was forcing her to get married. She asked the therapist if she should take medication. The therapist did not decide right away, but asked Ms. Z what her feelings would be if she were to take medication. Ms. Z revealed that her feelings were mixed and that she wanted the therapist to decide what she should do. The therapist told Ms. Z that although anxiolytic medication might help with her symptoms, so might continued psychological exploration, and that the decision should be hers. The therapist offered to support either choice.
>
> What emerged in the ensuing weeks was an exploration of Ms. Z's anxiety about experiencing the opportunity for autonomous choice. She was initially furious that her therapist would not make the decision for her; and she insisted that her symptoms and her indecisiveness were intolerable. At the same time, she gradually revealed that in the past, she had often gone to doctors with complaints and had "submitted" to a variety of recommended procedures, including surgery, later feeling that these procedures had been forced on her.
>
> Ms. Z began to see that she was inviting the therapist to force medication on her, and she realized that although she would resent such an action, she was terrified by the experience of autonomy. Her associations led to renewed exploration of her fears of separating from her mother and "living her own life"—represented by the experience of autonomy in the choice of whether or not to take medications or to marry. Ms. Z's mother had suffered from multiple phobias during the patient's childhood and had responded to all separations from Ms. Z with intense anxiety and hovering behavior. Ms. Z began to see that her marriage represented a further separation from her mother and that she had identified with her mother's anxious state. At the same time, she had unconsciously invited her therapist to become anxious about her symptoms and to respond fretfully with a prescription like a hovering mother.
>
> Ultimately, although Ms. Z opted not to take medications, exploration of her choice resulted in greater insight into her own experiences. Her masochistic fantasy about feeling "forced into marriage" as she had been forced to undergo various medical procedures had many other sources, but the exploration of her choice about the medication highlighted some crucial psychodynamic themes.

The Meaning of Medications

An understanding of psychodynamics can help the clinician to explore with the patient the meaning of taking medications. The fact that taking medication is full of meanings with profound psychological effects is well known. That these meanings can be psychoactive lies behind the fact that placebo control groups have been part of all medication research studies since the early 1970s. In 1955, in an article discussing the placebo effect, the noted pharmacologist Louis Lasagne described some of the properties of therapeutically successful placebos:

> Some authorities consider the color of the preparation very important. Colorless capsules are presumed to be unimpressive. One writer advises yellow, orange, or brown; another prefers pink, blue, or a mottled design. Similarly, tasteless placebos are considered inferior to bitter or highly flavored ones. It is believed that an extraordinarily large pill impresses by its size, an exceptionally small one by "potency." An injection is thought to be more effective than something taken by mouth: presumably the presence of the nurse or physician necessary for the injection is an important component of the psychological effect. I hasten to point out that most of these "principles" of the art of the placebo are based not on any systematic investigation of the facts but on impressions. Almost no controlled studies of them have been made. (Lasagne 1955, p. 68)

Whereas drug researchers control for the meaning of taking pills and placebo prescribers seek to exploit them, ideally, the clinician psychiatrist should seek to explore these meanings.

To begin with, many patients have strong responses to the idea that the prescription of medication implies a "biological" diagnosis. Some patients welcome such a diagnosis because it gives them the opportunity to blame themselves less for their symptoms. Other patients are happy to find a justification for not trying to get better because they are no longer "responsible."

Just as often, patients may see the medication as a symbol of their having an illness—a fact that represents a narcissistic injury and thus is painful for them to recognize. Not taking the medication may be a way of struggling with or denying the illness.

> For example, Mr. A was a 75-year-old man who presented with panic disorder. He had a long history of good health and prided himself on having never needed medications. He was unwilling to take an antidepressant even though he was told of the potential rapid reduction of his panic symptoms. Clearly, Mr. A's sense of injury had to be addressed in order to help him deal with the presence of illness and the need for medication.

How the patient views medication use in moral terms will also have an important impact on the patient's feelings about the prescription of medication.

Many people, including therapists, feel that it is wrong or weak to rely on medications. The patient's attitude will be influenced by the media, other doctors, religious groups, and of course, family members.

A careful history of family members who have psychiatric diagnoses or who have taken psychotropic or other drugs will often shed light on a patient's feelings about taking medications. Book (1987) describes a case of noncompliance secondary to identification with a relative who had not responded to the same medication in the past. A history of drug abuse in a family member is a common cause of a patient's fearing medication. The following case example (from Busch and Gould 1993) illustrates how productive psychodynamic psychotherapeutic work can help in a situation in which a patient's identification with a family member's experience with medication interfered with the treatment.

> Ms. B, a 39-year-old woman with borderline personality disorder who was in psychodynamic psychotherapy with an analytically trained social worker, developed symptoms of major depression in the context of a breakup with her boyfriend and difficulties in her career. She was referred for a medication consultation with a psychiatrist, after which this consultant recommended an antidepressant trial and further medical evaluation to rule out any organic source for the depression. Ms. B became extremely alarmed at the prospect of a medical evaluation, fearing that she would be found to have a serious disease. Additionally, she was terrified of the medication and unwilling to increase the dose to a therapeutic level. Ms. B's intense anxiety about the medical examination and the medication was explored in psychotherapy. She revealed the intense distress that she had experienced with the doctors who were treating her mother at the time of her mother's death. Ms. B blamed the doctors for the death, which occurred following complications from a medication her mother had been taking. This issue, in addition to the patient's compelling identification with her sick mother, was explored. Projection of Ms. B's destructive wishes toward her mother onto the figure of the doctor was also worked through to the point where she was able to undergo the physical examination. Both her therapist and the psychiatrist worked on these issues with her. Exploratory work on Ms. B's reactions eventually made it possible for her to take adequate doses of her medication, to which her depressive symptoms responded well.

The experience of side effects is also important. Most psychiatrists quickly learn that side effects are an important cause of noncompliance with medication plans. Clinicians may be less aware, however, that emotional responses to side effects are often subtle and frequently defy common sense. For example, Gutheil (1982) described the case of a young man with schizoaffective disorder who preferred Mellaril (thioridazine) to other antipsychotic medications because it caused him to develop retrograde ejaculation. The patient had obsessive-compulsive personality features, and he was gratified by the absence of "mess" secondary to this side effect.

The psychiatrist must also be alert to how the patient experiences any improvements brought about by medications. As with side effects, these experiences may be idiosyncratic. Many patients feel that improvements made on medications are not "real" or cannot be trusted. In other cases, noncompliance occurs in situations in which the patient's symptoms have served some important intrapsychic function. A patient of Linn's (1964) "forgot" to take his medication in the context of new conflicts about his sexual interests, which increased as his depression was treated. This patient developed nightmares that the analyst was an angry father who would destroy him if he acted on these sexual wishes. In the case presented below, a variation of this reaction occurred that became valuable to explore in the setting of ongoing psychodynamic psychotherapy.

> Mr. C was a 32-year-old man who presented in a major depressive episode following a breakup with his girlfriend. He began in two-sessions-per-week psychotherapy and was placed on fluoxetine, to which he had a good response at 40 mg/day. In his sessions, a number of conflicts became apparent, particularly fears of passivity and a feeling that his success would endanger others. After a 9-month period on the medication, Mr. C was successfully tapered off. He had been wondering whether it was him or the medication that led to his newfound assertiveness, and came to realize that he could indeed function in this manner without medication. At that point, Mr. C reported a dream in which he was looking for his therapist in a hospital. In the dream, Mr. C was dressed in a suit and tie and was with his family. He was embarrassed about revealing his name to the secretary. Mr. C met his therapist, who told him he looked good but not "medicationed."
>
> Previous associations to being dressed in a suit and tie indicated that Mr. C viewed these as symbols of success. Dressing this way was an indication of his increased assertiveness at work. Mr. C had also expressed fears of his assertiveness being revealed to his family, in part because he felt that his mother needed to have him dependent. These associations led to the view that the medication provided a means by which he could avoid the conflict and anxiety involved in his being assertive, since he could attribute his assertiveness to the medication. That he looked good but not "medicationed" led to the fear that his newfound assertiveness would be revealed to himself and others.

As the case examples presented above demonstrate, meanings of medication typically become intertwined with the transference to the therapist. In fact, many of the most powerful meanings of taking medications are related to feelings in the transference. For example, pills may represent something positive from the therapist, such as a gift or food, or something highly negative, such as a dangerous intrusion or manipulation. They can be seen as a dependency gratification, a "crutch," a good or bad object, or a sexualized penetration. Medications can be accepted or rejected on the basis of any of these meanings.

Hausner (1985–1986) discussed the concept of medications as transitional phenomena. For example, he noted the soothing function of medication, as in circumstances in which medication is available "just in case" (p. 377) but does not necessarily need to be taken to be effective in reducing anxiety. This soothing function may well be related to the high rate of placebo response found in many studies. Medication can at times be used to "provide a sense of safety in the therapist's absence" (p. 378), as does a child's transitional object. A patient's fear of changing the dose of a medication may represent the need to have a constant object "in a sea of seemingly changing objects" (p. 379). A decrease in medication can be interpreted as withdrawal by the therapist or as the therapist's demand for the patient to improve. Discontinuation of medication may be perceived as a precursor to termination; therefore, when a medication is discontinued, feelings of loss of or separation from the medication must be differentiated from symptoms resulting from relapse of the illness.

Often, medication use interacts with the transference to produce noncompliance. Most obviously, patients with paranoid tendencies or intense needs to control themselves or others may see taking medication as the ingestion of a potentially harmful or dangerous substance that could control or hurt them from within. Hausner (1985–1986), in his discussion of the transitional object functions of medication, referred to situations in which the medication is not felt to have a soothing function but rather is experienced as a "foreign object" (p. 386).

As noted by Gutheil (1982), medications can take on "object" attributes in an extraordinarily concrete way. He described an example of a paranoid schizophrenic patient who was concerned about his homosexual feelings toward the therapist. The patient reported somatic sensations that he attributed to the medication. He asked the therapist "Why is it that medications are always named after people, like Stella, Thor, and Mo?" (p. 326). The patient felt that the medication he was taking, Moban (molindone), was a "male medication" and thus likely to hurt him from inside his body. He wanted his medication changed to "Stella-zine" (i.e., Stelazine [trifluoperazine]).

In another example, described by Book (1987), a patient refused medication in order to defend against wishes to be taken care of by therapist. Other patients may wish to defeat the therapist by not taking a medication that would be helpful, even though such patients can experience significant pain secondary to their refusal. Dangerous acting out and suicide attempts using medication represent potentially lethal negative transference responses to medication that must be carefully monitored and explored.

Roose (1990) has made the important point that a recommendation to take medication at the beginning of treatment will have a very different meaning than a similar recommendation made in the middle of an ongoing therapy. Such a recommendation in the middle of treatment often arises in the midst of a crisis or a therapeutic stalemate. During both such periods, transference and countertransference feelings run high. If the therapist suggests medication, it might mean that he or she feels unskillful and hopeless or is bored by or weary of the patient's unchanging feelings. Patients may variously experience the therapist as giving up on them, as seducing or coercing them, or as exerting him- or herself to do everything possible to help them. The prescription of medication in the middle of treatment may involve related changes in the therapist's behavior, to which the patient will react. The patient's reactions will be particularly marked if the therapist's previous stance was one of nonintervention. Such changes in therapists' behavior include the writing of prescriptions, the inquiring after side effects, and the answering of questions about possible responses. If the medication is helpful, the patient might be angry that it was not suggested earlier.

If the suggestion for medication originates with the patient, it will have many meanings, depending on the state of the transference at the time. The request may represent a desire for love or nourishment or a fear that the therapist is tired of the patient's problems. It may represent an invitation to incest or to sexual closeness. One patient who requested medication was unconsciously testing the therapist to see if he was corrupt, as her father had been, by asking for a prescription for sleeping pills that she could share with her friends. The same patient was also testing to see if the therapist would be careless about a possible pregnancy that might be damaged by medication.

It is our opinion that the precise moment in the treatment when medication is suggested, particularly if that moment is in the middle of an ongoing treatment, almost always reflects a transference-countertransference enactment that should be explored whenever possible. The presence of this enactment does not imply that medication might not be indicated; rather, it highlights the need to investigate the context in which the possibility of medication arises.

In the following case example, a difficult and dangerous sadomasochistic transference was displaced onto the medication, where it was ultimately explored and resolved. This case illustrates many of the issues previously raised regarding the multiple meanings of taking medication.

Ms. D, a 31-year-old woman, entered treatment reporting that she became depressed and dysfunctional whenever she tried to leave home and live on her own. She had a history of suicide gestures following painful separations. She was involved in a relationship with a married man in which she felt used and abused. Ms. D described her childhood as idyllic until the death of a teenage sister from brain trauma sustained in a car accident when Ms. D was 8 years old. The family reacted to the event with silence. During adolescence, Ms. D became more "spaced out" and accident prone.

The therapist was not initially impressed with the extent of the patient's depression. Ms. D began in psychotherapy two times per week, which was later changed to psychoanalysis four times per week. In the initial phase, her sense of weakness as well as her fury and disappointment at her parents for her sister's death were explored. She made progress in understanding her suicide attempts as a wish to join her sister and her identification with her sister as a vulnerable waif. After 3 years of treatment, however, Ms. D still showed persistent low-grade depression, social withdrawal, "spaciness," poor concentration, poor academic functioning, and mildly paranoid ideation. The analyst made the decision to begin her on medication for these persistent symptoms.

The analyst chose phenelzine because tricyclic antidepressants had not been helpful in the past, and because Ms. D's depression was characterized by overeating, oversleeping, and rejection sensitivity. Although Ms. D professed an interest in medication, acting out with the medication began several days after starting the phenelzine. She recurrently ate things that were not safe with monoamine oxidase inhibitors (MAOIs) and reported fantasies of being rushed to the emergency room with her "brains exploded." The analyst told Ms. D to stop the medication until the basis of her using phenelzine in a dangerous way could be explored.

Ms. D became angry, stating that the therapist was too "authoritarian and controlling" and at the same time too casual in giving her the medication. She revealed that she had suicidal ideation and a collection of pills, which the analyst asked her to bring in. She began to be aware of a wish to cause the analyst pain and anxiety. The analyst pointed out Ms. D's wish to enact a drama in which the analyst carelessly or maliciously fed her a dangerous poison. She revealed a wish to provoke a response from the analyst, whom she saw as impassive. This led to memories of impassivity and neglect by her parents in which her older siblings experimented with drugs, mysticism, and truancy, causing Ms. D to experience fear and anger. As the transference evolved, she revealed that she would sometimes bang her head against a wall, often imagining the analyst banging her head. Gradually, she began to sometimes imagine herself as the perpetrator in the violent scenario as opposed to only the victim. Ms. D's acting out using phenelzine as a weapon brought to light a complex, multidetermined sadomasochistic transference that became an important focus of the treatment. Her sadomasochistic fantasies and behavior had previously been hidden behind a veil of depression and withdrawal.

In discussing the phenelzine, Ms. D also revealed that she could not allow herself to get better because that would mean abandoning her sister. She felt intensely guilty about using the phenelzine as a chance to live. About 1 month after insisting that she stop the medication, the analyst told Ms. D that she could restart it. No dangerous acting out or dietary indiscretions recurred. She was now able to discuss rather than act out fantasies that the analyst was careless and uncaring and that it would be the analyst's fault if something dangerous occurred. Ms. D waited a month before restarting the medication.

After restarting the medication, there was a significant increase in dreams of a sexual nature. This and other material provided strong evidence that the patient had experienced taking the drug as sexually stimulating. Fantasies of impregnation were associated with ingesting the medication. After about 3 weeks, Ms. D began to note improvement on the medication. After about 2 months, she reported that her depression had resolved and she appeared more affectively alive and dramatically more talkative in sessions. She became involved in her first serious relationship with an available caring man, whom she later married. Although her symptoms improved significantly, her analysis continued to be difficult but with significantly less acting out.

Clearly, medications were valuable in this case in helping the patient to become more available for analysis. Attention to the meaning of medications appeared to enhance the possibility of analytic exploration rather than interfere with it. For example, analysis of the acting out with phenelzine and the patient's experiences of the analyst's strong response helped open the way to a new understanding of Ms. D's family and of her complex relationship and identification with her older sister who had died. Multiple meanings of the medication became evident as the patient acted out a sadomasochistic transference, struggled with her guilt over surviving her sister, and explored sexual fantasies associated with medication taking. The meaning of the medication evolved during the course of the treatment. In the end, the medication seemed to take part in a competitive triangular/oedipal transference fantasy, as Ms. D imagined that the therapist would be jealous of her love for phenelzine. Each of these meanings could be used in the analysis in a productive fashion.

Therapeutic Triangles

Whereas in the case of Ms. D, the psychiatrist provided both medication and psychotherapy, it is becoming increasingly common for psychiatrists to provide medication consultation to nonphysician psychotherapists. The growing number of nonmedical psychotherapists conducting psychotherapy and the advent of more effective psychotropic medications with fewer side effects have contributed to this increase. Typically, the primary therapist refers the patient for medical consultation as the result of recognizing a pattern of symptoms that is felt to be medication responsive and/or symptoms that have not responded to psychotherapeutic intervention. Such a collaborative effort can lead to the effective treatment of symptoms with increased availability of the patient for psychotherapy. However, the alliance can also be conflictual, with the potential for splitting on the patient's part and problematic countertransference responses on the part of the practitioners (Busch and Gould 1993).

For example, the effective amelioration of symptoms by the medication and the more directive, involved stance of the pharmacotherapist may lead to idealization of the psychopharmacologist and a devaluation of the therapist. If the consultation occurs in the middle of treatment, the patient may wonder why the therapist had not recommended medications sooner. The patient may also wish to discontinue treatment with the therapist and to continue with the psychopharmacologist alone. This decision could represent a resistance to frightening issues that had arisen in the psychotherapy. Such splitting tendencies can be particularly prominent in borderline patients. Being alert to potential splitting and maintaining optimal communication between the practitioners can help to resolve these problems when they arise.

A number of potential countertransference problems can arise between the two practitioners. For example, there may be a sense of having competing ideologies, with each practitioner trying to prove that his or her viewpoint is the correct one. A pharmacologist who is critical toward a psychotherapeutic approach would be susceptible to such a conflict. The pharmacologist could potentially collude with the patient's negative reaction to the therapist, not recognizing that this reaction can represent a resistance to issues in the psychotherapy. Roose (1990) mentions another special case of countertransference issues in which an older analyst refers a patient to a younger psychiatrist for medication treatment. Here, competitive feelings may lead to an oedipal struggle. Communication between the two practitioners about the patient's medications and current psychotherapeutic issues, as well as attention to countertransference, can help to avert such problems. The psychopharmacologist can serve a useful role in educating the therapist about medications and psychiatric illness and should be aware of ongoing psychodynamic aspects of the case.

Countertransference Issues

Although the decision to treat a patient with medication may typically seem to the therapist a rational decision based purely on medical grounds or DSM-IV (American Psychiatric Association 1994) criteria, countertransference issues, as mentioned above, may also play a role in such a decision and should be kept in mind. Goldhamer (1983) and Hausner (1985–1986) suggested several possible sources of countertransference involved in the decision to give medication. For example, the therapist may have difficulty enduring the slow pace of psychotherapy or the patient's intense affects in situations of therapeutic regression. The therapist might also have difficulty tolerating therapeutic passivity and may need to prescribe medications to be more active. Additionally, the therapist may wish to assert authority over the patient or to demonstrate his or her omnipotence.

Gutheil (1982) noted how therapists might take a particular attitude toward prescribing medications that can end up being countertherapeutic: "The same physicians who adopt a receptive, open posture toward their patients' verbal productions may take a rigid, prescriptive stance in relation to drugs, offering direct and specific suggestions, even commands, which they would energetically eschew in the psychotherapeutic interaction" (p. 322). Of course, a more directive stance may be more necessary with regard to medications than with psychodynamic psychotherapeutic approaches, but the tendency to be more authoritative and rigid does create potential problems.

Book (1987) outlined particular forms of countertransference that he feels are likely to occur when the therapist becomes angry at patients for not complying. One such scenario is for the therapist to collude with patients' noncompliance out of a vindictive wish to have them become ill for defying him or her and to show them how much they need the medication. A second form of countertransference is telling patients to go elsewhere for treatment, rejecting patients for noncompliance, or threatening patients with abandonment. A third is for the therapist to behave with reproaches, which can give patients the feeling that they are harming the therapist by not taking their medications. Patients may at that point become compliant out of a sense of guilty obligation.

Psychiatrists may also fail to recommend medications on the basis of countertransference bias. Perry (1985) suggested that physicians may inadequately prescribe pain medication for complex countertransference reasons. Another bias against medication can be seen as stemming from an undue adherence to a caricature of the analytic model. Cooper (1985) noted that analysts who have not medicated patients "may . . . have been coconspirators with these patients in their need to construct a rational-seeming world in which they hold themselves unconsciously responsible for events" (p. 1399).

Roose (1988) described therapists who view the turning to medications as a defeat, feeling that "real analysis" is not being done. He directly confronted the notion that either psychoanalysts or psychopharmacologists could claim to be offering the more profound, deeply curative, or definitive treatment with regard to etiology:

> Just as the dynamically oriented therapist must appreciate that understanding the dynamic meaning attached to behavior is not equivalent to uncovering the etiology of the behavior, that the relationship of dynamic meaning to etiology is at best unclear, so too must the pharmacologist realize that treatment with a medication implies nothing about the etiology of the illness, and though the patient may respond to a medication, this response should not be taken as proof that he has a "biological" illness. (Roose 1990, p. 4)

By calling into question much of the certainty behind our various claims to the truth about the complex issues of etiology and cure, these authors and others have allowed us to make the history of our attitudes regarding medication versus psychotherapy part of the study of the psychology of medication and medication giving. Indeed, our own attitudes toward medication and psychotherapy, which reflect our own experiences of the history of polarization in our field, will be an important aspect of the psychology of medication as it emerges in the clinical setting. As clinicians, we must ask ourselves to understand rather than to act out our attitudes and biases with regard to biological as opposed to psychological approaches to mental phenomena so that we may be able to help our patients understand, evaluate, and work through their prejudices about taking medication and about approaching their problems psychologically.

Conclusion

Although there has been a great deal of controversy about the use of medication with patients in psychotherapy, there is now strong evidence that medications can and should be used for treatable psychiatric illnesses in this setting. Medications can both improve the availability of the patient for psychodynamic psychotherapy and provide a fertile ground for psychodynamic exploration. Attending to the psychodynamic meanings of medication can be clinically valuable and can help the clinician to think about a patient from several perspectives.

For Further Study

Beitman BD, Klerman GL (eds): Integrating Pharmacotherapy and Psychotherapy. Washington, DC, American Psychiatric Press, 1991

Combined psychotherapy and medication. Psychiatr Clin North Am 13:197–376, 1990

Panel of the New York Psychoanalytic Society: The use of medication with patients in analysis: Journal of Clinical Psychoanalysis 1:9–55, 1992

References

American Psychiatric Association: Diagnostic and Statistical Manual of Mental Disorders, 4th Edition. Washington, DC, American Psychiatric Association, 1994

Beitman BD, Chiles J, Carlin A: The pharmacotherapy-psychotherapy triangle: psychiatrist, nonmedical psychotherapist, and patient. J Clin Psychiatry 45:458–459, 1984

Beitman BD, Klerman GL (eds): Integrating Pharmacotherapy and Psychotherapy. Washington, DC, American Psychiatric Press, 1991

Book HE: Some psychodynamics of non-compliance. Can J Psychiatry 32:115–117, 1987

Busch FN, Gould E: Treatment by a psychotherapist and a psychopharmacologist: transference and countertransference issues. Hosp Community Psychiatry 44:772–774, 1993

Cooper AM: Will neurobiology influence psychoanalysis? Am J Psychiatry 142:1395–1402, 1985

Freud S: New introductory lectures on psycho-analysis (1933), in The Standard Edition of the Complete Psychological Works of Sigmund Freud, Vol 22. Translated and edited by Strachey J. London, Hogarth Press, 1964, pp 1–182

Freud S: An outline of psycho-analysis (1938), in The Standard Edition of the Complete Psychological Works of Sigmund Freud, Vol 23. Translated and edited by Strachey J. London, Hogarth Press, 1964, pp 139–207

Goldhamer PM: Psychotherapy and pharmacotherapy: the challenge of integration. Can J Psychiatry 28:173–177, 1983

Gutheil TG: Drug therapy: alliance and compliance. Psychosomatics 19:219–225, 1978

Gutheil TG: The psychology of psychopharmacology. Bull Menninger Clin 46:321–330, 1982

Kahn D: The dichotomy of drugs and psychotherapy, in The Psychiatric Clinics of North America. Edited by Marcus ER. Philadelphia, PA, WB Saunders, 1990, pp 197–208

Kahn D: Medication consultation and split treatment during psychotherapy. J Am Acad Psychoanal 19:84–98, 1991

Hausner RS: Medication and transitional phenomena. International Journal of Psychoanalytic Psychotherapy 11:375–400, 1985–1986

Lasagne L: Placebos. Sci Am 193:68–71, 1955

Linn L: The use of drugs in psychotherapy. Psychiatr Q 38:138–148, 1964

Marmor J: The adjunctive use of drugs in psychotherapy. J Clin Psychopharmacol 1:312–315, 1981

Ostow M: Drugs in Psychoanalysis and Psychotherapy. New York, Basic Books, 1962

Perry SW: Irrational attitudes toward addicts and narcotics. Bulletin of the New York Academy of Medicine 61:706–729, 1985

Roose SP: Psychoanalysis and medication. Bulletin of the Association for Psychoanalytic Medicine 28:89–92, 1988

Roose SP: The use of medication in combination with psychoanalytic psychotherapy or psychoanalysis, in Psychiatry. Edited by Michels R. New York, JB Lippincott, 1990, pp 1–8

Rounsaville BJ, Klerman GL, Weissman MM: Do psychotherapy and pharmacotherapy of depression conflict? Arch Gen Psychiatry 38:24–29, 1981

Sarwer-Foner GJ: An overview of combined psychopharmacology and psychotherapy, in Psychopharmacology and Psychotherapy. Edited by Greenhill MH, Gralnick A. New York, Macmillan, 1983, pp 165–180

Shader RI, Greenblatt DJ: Pharmacotherapy and psychotherapy (editorial). J Clin Psychopharmacol 2:1, 1982

Chapter 26

Interruptions of Treatment

Eugene L. Goldberg, M.D.

Time present and time past
Are both perhaps present in time future,
And time future contained in time past.

T. S. Eliot, *Four Quartets [Burnt Norton]* (1935)

In the course of training, with the progression from one level to another, or in natural rotations of services, the psychiatric trainee is faced with a recurrent series of interruptions in the treatment of patients. These interruptions can be seen as a series of terminations of both brief and longer treatment. According to Mann (1973), "In any dynamic psychotherapy, the restless guardians of time are aroused. . . . We have tended to pay little attention to it until the issue of the termination of treatment arises" (p. 11). This issue is particularly powerful for neophyte therapists at the conclusion of their own training who are relinquishing their protected roles to enter the "outside world." Issues of separation are universal and have often played a role in the therapist's choice of profession. The therapist attempts to master his or her previous helpless role of child by actively ministering to others who are currently overwhelmed by those same painful affects; by identifying with these patients, the therapist is also working through more of his or her own early trauma. Therefore, therapists overidentify with their patients in these parallel situations, which are most acute in these endings. In most programs, residents are encouraged to treat a few long-term

I wish to thank Dr. Bruce Levine, Dr. Lyle Rosnick, and Dr. Steven Silverman for so generously sharing with me their rich experience in working with inpatients.

cases. In all of these transitions, particularly in the work with the highly invested long-term cases, these identificational issues intensify the mutual anxiety and doubt and often lead to potential enactments in both patient and therapist. Recognition of these problems has been a recent development on the part of supervisors. It has also led to a strong recommendation for specific seminars or workshops on the issue of termination to be introduced at times of transition, and particularly at the end of residencies (Pumpian-Mindlin 1958).

As the opening quotation, from Eliot, expresses the existential timelessness of the unconscious, so the idea of a finite ending represents a confrontation with reality. Only when children have learned to tell clock time, according to Schecter et al. (1955), are they forced to gradually relinquish an omnipotent union of past, present, and future.

It is understandable that immortality is exemplified in our imagination as a woman, whereas Father Time, with his scythe, is the Herald of Death, the ultimate castration. In an early paper on "Time and the Unconscious," Marie Bonaparte (1940) focused on the fantasy of the "paradise" of childhood, from which we must depart. Only in adolescence does the reality of time become an obsession and a source of developmental conflict. "We destroy time from the moment we begin to use it . . . for in living out time we die of it" (Bonaparte 1940, p. 431). It is also during this period that the emerging adult first confronts the idea of death and begins to relinquish a timeless omnipotence. In fact, the feelings of adolescence have led Hurn (1971) to conceptualize this developmental period as a paradigm for the terminal phase of analysis, with a pleasurable need for relinquishing dependency ties and a rehearsal for the future. Similar feelings are utilized in time-limited psychotherapy, which we will discuss later in this chapter.

> These ideas about termination were dramatically brought home to me in a recent session with Mr. E, a depressed young man of 35 whom I saw in weekly psychotherapy for about 16 months. He had worked with a female therapist in group treatment for 8 years, and was ending this treatment by seeking my help. At age 15, he had fractured a cervical vertebrae while wrestling and was immobilized for 5 months, dependent on his understandably anxious mother. In addition, his wife was successfully treated for a cancer of the breast that occurred soon after the birth of a son 2 years previously. His depression responded well to support and fluoxetine, and he eventually decided to remain in individual treatment and terminate his long relationship with Joan, the group therapist, with her full support. Mr. E brought in the following dream:
>
>> I was outdoors. A huge hand appeared from within the overhanging clouds. It seemed to cover the entire land. The hand was reaching down, and I ran, and began to enter the earth. I seemed to go down a flight of stairs, then through a series of labyrinthine tunnels, then down more stairs and tunnels, deepening my penetration into the earth. I eventually came to a cavelike room and suddenly encountered Joan.

> I asked Mr. E what he thought about the dream, and he spontaneously said, "I guess the hand is like death." I asked what it seemed to be reaching for, and he smilingly replied, nodding, "my neck." He was more puzzled about the earth sequence, and I inquired if he recalled a poetic name for earth, and he said "Mother Earth." It was soon clear to Mr. E that Joan was an "Earth Mother" figure to her groups, and this was one reason he felt it was time to leave and "grow up." A dream he had the next night confirmed this insight by being filled with passionate, erotic longings for his wife. (It often occurs that as a patient accepts the ending of treatment, he or she overtly turns with greater need to his or her real objects, to their intense relief.)

Besides its confirmation of the primordial transference as maternal, and its consistency with the previously cited ideas, this material immediately brought to mind a fascinating paper by Max Stern that I had frequently assigned to resident groups in my course on termination. Entitled "Fear of Death and Neurosis" (Stern 1968), this paper describes a group of analytic patients who reexperienced states of "mortal terror as a repetition of early biotraumatic states of object loss" (p. 4). These terrors, stemming from infantile conflicts of the past, were "amalgamated with the fear of future death" (p. 4) as anticipatory anxiety and depression. These patients' transference cravings for "symbiotic fusion with the analyst, the protective mother, as a defense against fear of death" (p. 6) were interpreted and worked through in the end phases of treatment. Even though this paper seemed most relevant to termination, the resident groups, who were enthusiastic participants in most discussions, consistently avoided reading it. Their own anxieties about separation from the "mother institution," with all the built-in, regressive elements of a training situation, had elicited a resonance in each of them.

In my early work teaching a seminar on termination, a particularly cohesive resident group, in the laid-back style of the early 1970s, had a rich social involvement and specifically asked for a continuation of the group as a support in leaving the formal training program. We met monthly in an informal evening session at my home for the next 4 or 5 years until the members had established their own individual careers or entered analytic training. This group was called "the termination seminar that couldn't" by my children, and has continued in our gratifying friendships ever since. The need for a group experience after leaving a training program is ubiquitous and should be gratified. In analytic training, the similar period of 5 years after graduation was always one of some identity diffusion, which has been mitigated by formal seminars or informal peer supervisory groups, many of which have lasted for entire careers.

The reaction of the resident group to the theme of death is equally relevant to other aspects of training. Just as medical students must face their own limitations in their first clinical encounter with the death of a patient, so therapists are confronted by threats to their own omnipotent, narcissistic fantasies. These grandiose creations, which are never totally renounced, occur as defenses against the realities of childhood helplessness. They are prominent components of the rescue fantasies that pervade the world of therapists, many of whom felt overwhelmed in dealing with depressed or disturbed parents and families of their own (Lewin and Ross 1960).

Residents are confronted with a number of interruptions in the treatment of patients. As demonstrated in the vignette cited above, many relevant ideas appear most vividly in the termination of long-term dynamically oriented psychotherapy, and therefore I focus on this type of treatment in greater detail in this first section. In the following sections I comment on the problems in an inpatient service, and conclude with a discussion of time-limited psychotherapy, which intensifies some of the same issues.

Long-Term Psychotherapy

Schafer (1973) has elegantly described long-term treatment and has differentiated it from analysis—an important distinction. Long-term treatment is seen as a situation in which

> [the] therapist tries to establish an exploratory or investigative atmosphere . . . and is particularly alert to signs that the patient is having emotional difficulty in the therapeutic relationship . . . of the sort that entails anxiety, guilt, or shame, and the evident withholding, circumventing or dissimulating of certain experiences. . . . In other words, the therapist pays special attention to manifestations of conflict, resistance and transference. . . . The patient develops a more comprehensive idea of the complexity and scope of the problems, discovers symptoms and inhibitions he was unaware of and feelings of all sorts. . . . In one sense he comes to realize more fully the extent of his illness, but in another, he realizes the extent of his human existence. (Schafer 1973, pp. 137–138)

As termination approaches, the changes "appear as if all were built on sand. With the patient apparently as depressed, morose, provocative or helplessly symptom-ridden as when the work started, the therapist may wonder whether the patient's enlarged and active view of his life was worth anything" (Schafer 1973, p. 139). Resentment flourishes in both the patient and the therapist. Therapists may feel that their despondency is an appropriate countertransference to the patient's aggression or negative therapeutic reaction. They may feel that their work was incomplete, superficial, or totally inadequate, as befitting their lack of full experience. Therapists naturally wonder if more work would rectify the situation, and they may even share some personal feelings in an attempt to enrich the relationship and repair the damage.

Although this type of regression sometimes occurs in the end phases of analysis, it seems more common in psychotherapeutic settings, where endings are more unilateral. The loss of a person with whom one has experienced so much and has grown more human is a profound loss for both parties. Often, residents are stunned by the impact of their loss on the patient, which becomes dramatically apparent at this time. In addition to the ending of training, there is a further blurring of roles with the resident's loss of his or her well-defined professional image. Because the resident's "best patients" are often medical students, psychologists, or other personnel close to the therapist in age, there is both loss and confusion. Fledgling healers must begin to face the limitations of what therapy can do, and start to accept the difference between "life goals and therapeutic goals" (Ticho 1972). They must also accept the idea that the potentiality for working through issues has been more readily available to them through the greater intensity and length of their personal therapy, which is often classical psychoanalysis. Freud went through the same painful acceptance of the limitations of analysis in his essay "Analysis, Terminable and Interminable" (1937/1964), which, although beyond the scope of the current discussion, is worth a careful study for the picture it provides of the modesty and honesty of a great figure.

Schafer's ideas on the goals of psychotherapy are very helpful in this regard, although they have not received the full attention they deserve. In fact, most seminars dealing with termination take on the aspect of a therapeutic group, as the members gain support in their mutual acceptance of their feelings of failure, sadness, and anger, and share their guilt over leaving dependent patients. He argued that one of the best protections against this type of self-criticism and doubt is a "reasonable and stable sense of one's own goodness . . . as having offered something good, having made a sincere effort, and having achieved some results" (Schafer 1973, p. 141) within the limitations of brief psychotherapy. The other sense of goodness is "the archaic or infantile sense that whatever one's faults, one is a worthwhile person" (Schafer 1973, p. 141), akin to the "good enough mother" of Winnicott (1965), "the necessary object representation the child must achieve for satisfactory development" (Schafer 1973, p. 141). Most importantly, in ending treatment with a patient who is only partially improved, therapists must again face the limits of their own concurrent individual therapy or psychoanalysis, as well as recognize its advantages. Ironically, a personal therapeutic experience has been associated with a significantly lower rate of premature termination of patients (Greenspan and Kulish 1985).

In the discovery of aspects and feelings about oneself in working with a patient, a process that continues throughout one's career as a therapist, there is a diminution in the fragmentation of one's sense of self, which can lead to a greater tolerance of painful and irrational feelings in the patient.

Effective treatment often allows the awareness and expression of powerful repressed feelings with the loosening of old defenses. This phenomenon is painfully evident in our work with a growing population of patients who have lived through divorces or other losses, and who seek help at times of major transitions or attempts at intimacy—college, marriage, or parenthood. The working through of some of these feelings can be most meaningful and ultimately reassuring, and can assist these patients to more fully accept earlier figures who have been recipients of bitterness and anger.

As noted previously, unlike long-term therapy or psychoanalysis, in which both parties can eventually concur on the ending, most of these endings in training fall into the category of forced terminations, which lead to a higher incidence of the regressive phenomena noted above. Forced terminations are generally attributable to external factors. The most common situation occurs in the rotation of services in training. Many of these patients react with a preemptive withdrawal from treatment, literally or figuratively.

> Many of these issues were illustrated in my supervision of Dr. F, a rather compulsive, somewhat depressed and overweight young male resident who was confronting his patient Ms. G—a bright, highly perceptive young woman—with the news that he had to terminate with her after two terms of treatment in his rotation through a college clinic. Her parents compounded the problem by refusing to allow her to continue working with him privately at a modest fee, which she knew they could handle. Ms. G had narcissistic, sadomasochistic, and hysterical features in her characterological repertoire, with a history of involvement with a series of highly unsuitable partners of lower class, who abused her on occasion. She teased Dr. F, my supervisee, about his tightness and noted his depression, but consoled him by adding, "I'm sure you have a spark of life somewhere deep inside of you." Relating this interchange to me later, Dr. F said, "She was talking about me as a middle-aged man. I finally asked how old she thought I was. She answered, 'Probably in your early 30s, though you act like 40!' " He confessed that "this happens to be a sensitive spot."
>
> I liked this young resident and had worked with him for a long time. I tried to get back to the transferential element by saying that although the patient "might seem sharp, I don't think your eyes lack a spark. I think she's angry because she's clearly not the gleam in your eye." My support was of limited value, for the patient continued to get to Dr. F by saying, "You can be professional without being cold. I'm not asking you to go to bed with me. I think life could be happier if you would let people get closer to you."

As Schafer noted, this is the kind of provocation that could push a neophyte to revelation of personal material, which is what occurred in this case. At one point, Ms. G told Dr. F that she doubted that she was important to him, and I used this statement to emphasize that "the only question which required an answer was the origin of her feelings of insignificance, in her doubt that she had any impact on you after many months of work together. . . . Her need to attack you was a desperate measure to deal with your rejection, like her need to sleep with a series of unsuitable men to deal with her feelings that she was a 'piece of shit,' as she previously described herself in many earlier sessions."

The sadistic component of this patient's need to punish the abandoning figure seems clear in this case, and was abetted by Dr. F's own masochism. Ms. G's characteristic masochistic proclivity to snatch defeat from the jaws of victory was partially related to her guilt at her sadistic impulses. A history of prior masochistic relationships, such as seen in this patient, should alert the therapist to the probability of a similar unhappy scene, which derives from feelings of being forced to accept an ending of help (Glick 1987).

In other patients, there is often a pressing need to remain sick as a plea for continuation of help. A great deal of acting out also occurs, as was witnessed in this patient's renewal of inappropriate sexual encounters with questionable partners—behavior that is particularly problematic in the present social climate. The more severely disturbed clinic patients may dramatize their rage in suicidal threats, disruptive scenes in the clinic, or an increase in middle-of-the-night telephone calls, and may on occasion require hospitalization. Finally, patients who wish to withhold potentially humiliating or guilt-laden material may experience the knowledge of a limitation of treatment with relief:

> Many years ago, I treated a borderline young woman who had been the recipient of repetitive enemas by her compulsive, anally fixated father. She left me, in anticipation of a marriage, swearing that her fiancee must never be aware of her prior therapy. Her parting gift was the sharing of her masturbatory fantasies, which understandably involved scenes of people defecating. A few years later she reentered treatment, to her chagrin.

In summary, one might say that in both transfer and termination, neophyte therapists must be consistently aware of the identification that they feel with their patients and of the profound countertransferential issues that this generates. It should be comforting to younger clinicians to learn of the depth and intensity of sadness and loss, and the feelings of "not having done enough," that even senior therapists experience in these situations, as reported in a remarkably open series of interviews obtained by Viorst (1982). Issues of guilt and separation anxiety must be acknowledged and the limitations of their goals accepted. These problems have impressed educators sufficiently to lead them to institute workshops or seminars on the issues of "closure or transfer" in the 2 months prior to those events. As Pumpian-Mindlin has suggested, therapy is envisioned as equipping a patient "with a method of facing problems rather than an answer. . . . If we have succeeded in helping patients to find some ways of facing and coping . . . rather than continuing their neurotic, self-destructive ways, . . . this is a modest but on the whole realistic goal" (Pumpian-Mindlin 1958, p. 460).

Transitions on an Inpatient Service

The problem of termination has unique ramifications for trainees who are leaving an inpatient service: not only are they abandoning sick individuals with whom they are identified, but they must also deal with the effects of their departure on the permanent staff. The therapeutic milieu involves a group process. Therapists must work with an outpatient for 1 or 2 years to achieve a knowledge of the patient equivalent to that gained in an intensive inpatient experience of 3 to 4 months. This overidentification can lead to a mutual sense in therapists and patients of being forced to terminate, and to a collusive antagonism against the "system." By blaming the system, therapeutic trainees can both negate the legitimacy of the patient's rage at them and depreciate their therapeutic roles by seeming equally impotent.

The permanent staff and the inpatient form a new alliance against both the old and the new figure. With the average rotation lasting 6 months (or less) these days, the midyear rotation is particularly difficult; as one chief resident put it, "It's my job to rescue January." Certain programs have attempted to lessen these effects by staggering rotations, keeping a chief for an entire year, or preventing senior permanent staff from taking vacations at these periods of transition, which they previously were likely to do.

Most importantly, there is a pervasive emphasis on the issues of beginnings and endings, often to the irritation of the resident staff. In team meetings, announcements are made of patient and staff departures. In one such program, therapists are forced to individually announce their departure 5 weeks before the event, with repetitions at weekly meetings. This procedure helps to minimize the denial, which can still be powerful in the more disturbed group.

The pattern on an inpatient unit varies, but there is always a group of patients on "best behavior" in the weeks before transition who explode in the last few days before the event. There can also be collusions of secrecy that are only brought to light with a new therapist. In one particularly dramatic situation described by a colleague, a patient's pregnancy became understandable only when she revealed to the new therapist that she had been aware of the pregnancy of a female resident, who had been secretly married to the patient's therapist. This announcement occurred during her treatment with the new therapist.

Ravenscroft (1975), in a sensitive essay on the effect of turnover on a milieu, subtitled "The Human Cost of Psychiatric Education," noted that in the week before rotation, speculation about the incoming residents intensified, alternating between a "messianic wish for new saviors" and deep apprehension and foreboding. Such feelings are reflected not only in erratic and problematic behavior on the part of the staff, with some displacement onto patients, but in the general intensification of anxiety that occurs with the loss of a stable object.

A further source of these difficulties may be found in the inpatient's externally provided sense of identity. With a change in that status, either by discharge or by the concrete loss of the therapist, there is a fragmentation of the individual's self: "If I'm not your patient, then who am I?" Tarachow has abetted the acceptance of a substitute by interpreting the transference itself as a form of substitution, and adding, "I seem to be standing in for your father, and you must miss him very much" (Tarachow 1963).

Because of the relative brevity of treatment being provided to inpatients these days, in which hospital stays are often truncated by third-party payers, residents feel frustrated in their goals. It has been helpful for them to feel that they have provided patients with an awareness of their problems, a didactic kind of preparation for the work to be continued in their outpatient therapy over a long period. In addition, it can be helpful for residents to emphasize to patients the elements of progress, by comparing their feelings on admission with their present status. Certain psychotic individuals, at a termination of more extended treatment, express a new rage at the therapist for not having been available "back there" as a protector against their early trauma. Such rage can be used as a means of expressing the wish that the therapist be available as an ally against future blows. As in the previous example of pointing out patients' progress, it can be reassuring to point out their accomplishments in mastering certain situations in current treatment. In general, awareness of the changes that have occurred in treatment, even if minimal, diminishes the therapist's guilt at termination and allows hope for their patients' continued progress. Some therapists suggest to patients that they drop them a note after a specific number of months or carry the therapist's address with them as a kind of transitional object.

Because of the growing number of these types of reactions from a more disturbed clinic population, I have emphasized that the time limitation of all clinic treatment be specified in the initial contact, even if the treatment might last through 2 years of training. Although such statements are often repressed or totally denied by the patient, they have been helpful in enabling the resident group to feel free of any deception. As noted previously, discussion of termination should be reiterated throughout the treatment to diminish these defenses. The tendency of the therapist to deny the significance of forced terminations may let the patient off too easily or allow the therapist to blame him- or herself exclusively. These types of patients, who were unable to face the psychic reality of their own early losses, can turn their transferential feelings of vengefulness and rage onto themselves.

If inpatients are to continue treatment after discharge, it is often beneficial to allow them to meet the new therapist during the last weeks of treatment. This practice is also helpful in transferring borderline outpatients to a subsequent therapist. Whereas in healthier patients such a meeting might lead to a premature focus on the new therapist with concomitant avoidance of feelings about the present one, in more chronically disturbed patients an overlap of this kind is vital.

Inpatients very often become dependent on one member of the permanent staff—for example, an activity therapist—who acts as a kind of "nanny" until an attachment to the new therapist can be formed. The more chronic outpatient or recently discharged inpatient might best be served by being assigned to a permanent staff member, often a social worker. Individual treatment might be concurrent or limited to psychopharmacological maintenance. Many years ago, Reider (1958) astutely identified the value of an "institutional transference" with an object-tie attachment to ancillary personnel and even to the setting itself. Although useful, along with the above-indicated practices, such a maneuver may be employed by the therapist to encourage displacement of the patient's anger and helplessness away from him- or herself, which limits the expression of rage. The same weakening of important transferential feelings is also accomplished by the therapist's saying that the termination affecting both parties was due to "clinical policy," supervisory intervention, or even third-party payers. This acknowledgment of an external castrator (figure of Death) must be dealt with in the termination phase, if possible.

Therapist Relocation: A Natural Experiment in Forced Termination

Besides the arbitrary and forced terminations of clinical programs, a natural experiment occurs when a therapist relocates. DeWald (1965) described the reactions of 12 psychotherapy patients at the news of a major move early in his career. DeWald was also one of the first to describe frankly the intense countertransferential feelings at this acknowledged abandonment, consistent with all that Schafer later noted. In those patients being seen supportively, the verbalized reactions were generally positive, with feelings of sadness, regret, or grief. In four of the patients in longer-term, insight-oriented treatment, rage and anger over sudden rejection were intense and helped these patients work through earlier traumatic object losses.

In patients who had only brief contact with the therapist and who were told of his impending move within the next 6 months, a type of time-limited therapy took place. In one case, the patient resisted any emotional involvement, which only occurred with the subsequent therapist. One woman, who knew she would move concurrently with her therapist due to her husband's reassignment, developed a workable and useful therapeutic partnership and was able to deal with specific issues.

Characterological defenses were most apparent in a 48-year-old man whose wife had been treated for 5 years by DeWald for severe phobic and anxiety symptoms. With his wife's improvement, the man became impotent. He accepted the announced limitation of time as a challenge to economically outdo his crippled partner and was able to express his anger strongly during three hypnotic trances. By attributing the subsequent relief of his impotency—almost magically—to the procedure, this man was able to avoid any acknowledgment of his dependency on the hypnotizing therapist.

A number of patients were able to be reassured by knowledge of DeWald's new location and of where they could reach him in the future. This solution is equally applicable for a resident who is leaving a program for a new location and who wishes to provide appropriate information to a suitable type of patient. A unique variation of this approach is described by Rosenbaum (1977), who continued contact with a few relatively healthy patients by phone or letter for a long period after his move.

Time-Limited Psychotherapy: The Ultimate Test

As noted above, in a number of DeWald's cases, a type of time-limited psychotherapy took place. This type of approach is receiving increased scrutiny in this era of growing concern about cost effectiveness by third-party participants (insurance, private, or governmental) and limitations in time sequences in training programs. Research-oriented psychoanalysts such as Schlesinger (in press) have also been interested in ways of "keeping psychotherapy efficient." He cites instances in which the reassurance in a single consultation is all that is needed. Schlesinger strongly emphasizes the value of dealing with focal issues and avoiding the countertransferential need for perfection as a factor in prolonging treatment.

The earliest attempt at time limitation actually was instituted by Rank (1929), who proposed a 9-month limitation in analytic treatment, since the "trauma of birth" was the basis of all psychopathology. Ironically, elements of this idea are universally seen in the frequent ideas of rebirth that accompany termination of intensive treatment, with classic dreams of water. Even Freud, in "Analysis Terminable and Interminable" (1937/1964), proposed brief spells of analysis for professionals with a return for a refresher at 5-year intervals. With the current obsession for a thorough training analysis, that idea seems outdated.

The idea of interruptions of developmental lines, with a resolution in briefer treatment, has been a major contribution of child and adolescent therapists, who seem satisfied to let youngsters proceed by themselves when they have climbed back onto the "normal" developmental track, with the possibility of a return for help if needed subsequently (Novick 1990). This concept has influenced adult treatment to a major degree and is evident in focal or time-limited psychotherapy as well as in the work of Malan (1976), Sifneos (1972), and Mann (1973), whose ideas I have cited as representative of the field. Mann's work is based on a clear understanding of unconscious determinants, the relation of those determinants to maturational phases, and the acceptance of structural elements in the elaboration of conflict. The central issue to be dealt with in therapy is recurrent, maladaptive, and causes pain.

Mann (1973) noted that he consults a calendar in the initial visit to dramatically establish the "ultimate materialization of separation anxiety" in setting up the 12 sessions and defining the date of the final interview. He accepts the validity of both developmental and narcissistic components in the etiology of psychopathology, and feels that the transferential development in time-limited psychotherapy will reflect "pre-Oedipal and Oedipal parental failure." In a time-limited focus, the patient receives a "second chance to reunite" with a more available object and to separate in an adaptive way. This type of treatment was developed in a college student health setting and focused on the struggle between the wish to be dependent and the wish to remain autonomous that characterizes this stage of development perfectly.

The first four sessions capitalize on an upsurge of unconscious magical expectations that past disappointments will now be undone under the "sustaining golden sunshine of eternal union" (Mann 1973, p. 33). A rapid, positive transference develops, with great symptomatic relief. During this phase, important aspects of the current problem, maladaptive maneuvers, and genetic roots of the conflict will emerge.

In the next four sessions, the therapist consistently limits his or her attention to the central conflict. "The characteristic feature of any middle point is that one more step signifies the point of no return . . . the confrontation that he needs to avoid what he suffered in early life" (Mann 1973, p. 34)—separation from the ambivalently experienced early object. The last four meetings deal with the patient's reaction to termination. Sadness, anger, and guilt, with their "accompanying manifestations in fantasy and in behavior, must be dealt with. The genetic source of these affects is relived in the disappointing termination and separation from the therapist. But this time the appropriate management of the ending will allow the patient to internalize the therapist as a good object or replacement for the earlier ambivalent object" (Mann 1973, p. 35), a type of corrective emotional experience. The ending of any kind of treatment involves a process of internalization, as is evident in Mann's and Schafer's remarks.

Conclusion

In an important paper on termination, Loewald (1962) defined *internalization* as a "general term for certain processes of transformation by which relationships and interactions between the individual psychic apparatus and its environment are changed into inner relationships. . . . The word therefore covers such mechanisms as incorporation, introjection and identification" (p. 489). Relinquishment and internalization of external objects involve a process of loss and restitution in many ways similar to mourning, and are thus relevant to all endings, most profoundly those in an analysis. The internal relationships of the past have been externalized, or projected, onto the figure of the therapist, and "have been replaced by relationships with a new external object" (Loewald 1962, p. 486). With the prospect of an impending separation, there is an accelerated need for a new internalization that will continue and come to relative completion only after termination.

In the termination of a long-term treatment, a sense of emancipation, akin to that experienced in adolescence, "goes hand in hand with the work of internalization which reduces or abolishes the sense of loss" (Hurn 1971, p. 345). More importantly, only at termination can the patient explore and relinquish the residual infantile wishes demanded of the new object (the therapist) based on the patient's early relationships. Such exploration is necessarily compressed in time-limited treatment, played to the fullest in analysis, and dealt with in modified measure in psychotherapy, depending on the intensity of the relationship established and the capacities of both patient and therapist to deal with this material.

If therapy of all kinds can be seen as a developmental experience, then its ending is a process of separation and a "necessary loss," in the felicitous phrase of Judith Viorst (1986). Most importantly, and in an overall sense, therapeutic terminations represent a loss and reinternalization that must be acknowledged and dealt with by both participants, which is why the process of termination has suddenly received greater attention and recognition. But with this loss can also be a gain, if the patient is able to hold on to valuable insights from time past, internalize the valued experience with the therapist in time present, and apply the gained understanding to time future.

For Further Study

Bornstein M (ed): Termination, in Psychoanalytic Inquiry, Vol 2. Hillsdale, NJ, Analytic Press, 1982

Firestein SK: Termination in Psychoanalysis. New York, International Universities Press, 1978

Freud S: Analysis terminable and interminable (1937), in The Standard Edition of the Complete Psychological Works of Sigmund Freud, Vol 23. Translated and edited by Strachey J. London, Hogarth Press, 1964, pp 209–254

References

Bonaparte M: Time and the unconscious. Int J Psychoanal 21:427–468, 1940

DeWald PA: Reactions to the forced termination of therapy. Psychiatr Q 39:102–126, 1965

Freud S: Analysis terminable and interminable (1937), in The Standard Edition of the Complete Psychological Works of Sigmund Freud, Vol 23. Translated and edited by Strachey J. London, Hogarth Press, 1964, pp 209–254

Glick R: Forced terminations. J Am Acad Psychoanal 15:449–463, 1987

Greenspan M, Kulish NM: Factors in premature termination in long-term psychotherapy. Psychotherapy 22:75–82, 1985

Hurn HT: Toward a paradigm of the terminal phase. J Am Psychoanal Assoc 19:332–348, 1971

Lewin B, Ross H: Psychoanalysis in the United States. New York, WW Norton, 1960

Loewald H: Internalization, separation, mourning, and the superego. Psychoanal Q 31:485–504, 1962

Malan DH: Frontier of Brief Psychotherapy. New York, Plenum, 1976

Mann J: Time-Limited Psychotherapy. Cambridge, MA, Harvard University Press, 1973

Novick J: Comments on termination in child, adolescent, and adult analysis. Psychoanal Study Child 45:419–435, 1990

Pumpian-Mindlin E: Comments on technique of termination and transfer in a clinic setting. Am J Psychother 12:455–464, 1958

Rank O: The Trauma of Birth. New York, Harcourt, Brace, 1929

Ravenscroft K Jr: Milieu process during residency turnover: the human cost of psychiatric education. Am J Psychiatry 132:506–511, 1975

Reider N: A type of transference to institutions. Bull Menninger Clin 17:58–65, 1958

Rosenbaum M: Premature interruption of psychotherapy: continuation of contract by telephone and correspondence. Am J Psychiatry 134:20–202, 1977

Schafer R: The termination of brief psychoanalytic psychotherapy. International Journal of Psychoanalytic Psychotherapy 2:135–147, 1973

Schecter DE, Symonds M, Bernstein I: The development of the concept of time in children. J Nerv Ment Dis 121:301–310, 1955

Schlesinger HJ: Keeping Psychotherapy Efficient: How Much Is Enough? (in press)

Sifneos PE: Short-Term Psychotherapy and Emotional Crisis. Cambridge, MA, Harvard University Press, 1972

Stern MM: Fear of Death and Neurosis. J Am Psychoanal Assoc 16:3–31, 1968

Tarachow S: An Introduction to Psychotherapy. New York, International Universities Press, 1963

Ticho E: Termination of psychoanalysis: treatment goals, life goals. Psychoanal Q 41:315–333, 1972

Viorst J: Experiences of loss at the end of analysis: the analyst's response to termination. Psychoanalytic Inquiry 2:399–419, 1982

Viorst J: Necessary Losses. New York, Simon & Schuster, 1986

Winnicott DW: The Maturational Processes and the Facilitating Environment. New York, International Universities Press, 1965

Chapter 27

Research In Psychodynamic Therapy

Robert S. Wallerstein, M.D.

Introduction: Outcome and Process Studies

The central research questions in psychoanalysis and in the expressive and supportive psychoanalytic psychotherapies qua therapies are 1) *what* changes take place during and as a consequence of the therapy (i.e., the *outcome* question), and 2) *how* do those changes come about or how are they brought about—that is, through the interaction of what factors in the patient, in the therapist and treatment, and in the evolving life situation (i.e., the *process* question). In theory, process and outcome are necessarily interlocked. Any study of outcome, even if it counts only the percentage of cases "improved," must establish some criteria for "improvement," and these criteria, in turn, must derive from some conceptualization of the nature of the illness and the process of change, whether or not such a conceptualization is explicitly formulated. Similarly, any study of process, in delineating patterns of change among variables, makes cross-sectional assessments at varying points in time, which, if compared with one another, provide measures of short- or longer-term outcomes.

On practical grounds, however, outcome studies and process studies are usually separated. Although process is conceptually not separable from outcome, methods that yield the best judgments in the one area are often operationally opposed to those that yield the best judgments in the other. For example, judgments of outcome will be scientifically most convincing if bias is minimized and freedom from contamination maintained by keeping those who make the "after" judgments unaware of the "before" judgments and predictions. From the point of view of process judgments about the *same therapy,* such care to minimize contamination would be unnecessary. Indeed, it would be counter to the whole spirit of inquiry into process, in which maximum knowledge of all the known determinants, as these have varied over time, is essential in order to understand the changes that occur.

Given this situation, I divide this chapter into two sections: 1) a recounting of the *outcome research* on psychoanalytic therapies, both because such research is conceptually less complex and because it started prior in time, and 2) an accounting of the *process research.* The primary focus will be on formal and systematic empirical research rather than on the far larger and much antecedent clinical case study and theoretical literature out of which, of course, have grown the questions to which the more formal research studies have been addressed. In both the outcome and the process arenas, only the major empirical studies will be described; as a result, a bias will be created toward American contributions, as well as toward empirical work in Germany and in Great Britain. Finally, I provide a brief overview of the "offset" studies that describes the effect of psychological therapy in reducing utilization of the physical or general health care system—that is, in economic terms, the effect of mental health care in offsetting expenditures for general health care.

But first I should mention some of the considerations related to the topic of process and outcome research in psychoanalytic therapies—issues that, although beyond the scope of this chapter, are nonetheless germane to its central argument. These include:

1. The *goals* of these treatment modalities, both ideal and practical (realizable)
2. The issues of suitability or *treatability* as against *analyzability,* which is not the same thing, although the two are often confounded
3. The *indications* and *contraindications* for this array of treatments as these have evolved over time with increasing experience and expanding theoretical and technical knowledge
4. The role of the initial *diagnostic* and *evaluation* procedures in differential treatment planning (as against the view that only a trial of treatment can lead to proper case formulation and prognostication)
5. The place of *prediction* (and predictability) in relation to issues of change, expectable reach, and limitation
6. The *theory of technique* (how treatment works and achieves its goals—that is, the relationship of means to ends)
7. The *similarities* and *differences* between psychoanalysis and the dynamic psychotherapies, as compared from the viewpoint of different goals projected for different kinds of patients, determining through these differences the specifically appropriate technical approaches from within the available spectrum
8. The *criteria* for satisfactory treatment termination
9. The evaluation of *results* (process and outcome changes, therapeutic benefit, and analytic completeness)
10. The conception of the *ideal state of mental health* and the unavoidable impingements upon its empirical assessment by value judgments as well as by the vantage point and the partisan interests of the judge

11. The place of the *follow-up* study as a desirable, feasible, and appropriate activity (or not) in relation to psychoanalytic therapies, for research and/or for clinical purposes
12. The place of the continuing accretion of knowledge in relation to all these areas by the traditional *case study method* innovated by Freud as against the desirability or necessity for more *formal systematic clinical research* into these issues, by methods of course that are responsive to the subtlety and the complexity of the subjectivistic clinical phenomena, while simultaneously remaining loyal to the canons of empirical science

Early Statistical Studies: First-Generation Outcome Research

As early as 1917, within the first decades of the introduction of psychoanalysis in America, Coriat reported on the therapeutic results achieved in 93 cases, of whom 73% were declared either recovered or much improved; these rates were nearly equal across all his diagnostic categories. As with all the early statistical studies to be noted here, the judgments of improvement were made by the treating clinician, according to (usually) unspecified criteria, and without individual clinical detail or supporting evidence.

In the decade of the 1930s, several comparable but larger-scale reports emerged from the collective experiences of the psychoanalytic treatment centers of some of the pioneering psychoanalytic training institutes. In 1930 Fenichel reported results from the initial decade of the Berlin Institute, the first formally organized psychoanalytic institute in the world. Of 1,955 consultations conducted, 721 patients were accepted for analysis; 60% of the neurotic patients were judged to have received substantial benefit, but only 23% of those who were adjudged "psychotic."[1] Jones in 1936 reported on 73 applicants to the London Psychoanalytic Clinic, of whom 74 were taken into analysis; 28 of the 59 neurotic patients were judged to have benefited substantially, but only one of the 15 so-called psychotic patients. And in 1937, Alexander reported on 157 cases from the Chicago Psychoanalytic Clinic, with 63% of the neurotic patients, 40% of the psychotic patients, and 77% of those designated psychosomatic judged to have received substantial benefit from their treatment. During the same period, Kessel and Hyman (1933), two internists who followed up 29 patients referred for psychoanalysis, reported almost all the neurotic patients to have benefited from the treatment, and all the psychotic ones to be either unchanged or worse.

In a 1941 review article evaluating the overall results of psychoanalysis, Knight combined the findings of all of these studies (except the first one by

[1] *Psychotic* here is to be taken as ambulatory and in some sense functioning in the community, although considered "psychotic" from the standpoint of the quality of mental life.

Coriat) and added 100 patients treated at the Menninger Clinic, where the results were judged to be completely comparable to those of the other studies in the observed outcomes with neurotic and psychotic patients. The overall composite tabulation comprised 952 patients, with the therapeutic benefit rate approximately 60% for the neurotic, close to 80% for the psychosomatic, and only 25% for the psychotic patients. Knight made particular reference to the pitfalls of these simple statistical summaries: the absence of consensually agreed-upon definitions and criteria, the crudity of nomenclature and diagnostic classification, and the failure to address issues of therapeutic skill in relation to cases of varying severity.

The most ambitious study of this first-generation genre was the report of the Central Fact-Gathering Committee of the American Psychoanalytic Association (Hamburg et al. 1967).[2] Data were collected over a 5-year period beginning in 1952; altogether, there were 10,000 initial responses to questionnaires submitted by 800 analysts and candidates, with some 3,000 termination questionnaires submitted upon treatment completion. As with the other studies cited thus far, criteria for diagnosis and improvement were unspecified, and these and other flaws and ambiguities resulted ultimately in a report that was simply an "experience survey" consisting of 1) facts about the demographics of analysts' practices, 2) analysts' *opinions* on their patients' diagnoses, and 3) analysts' *opinions* on the therapeutic results achieved. Not unexpectedly, the great majority of patients were declared substantially improved.

Finally, in the very next year, Feldman (1968) reported on the results of psychoanalysis in 120 patients (selected from 960 evaluations) treated at the clinic of the Southern California Psychoanalytic Institute over its 11-year history. Again, the reported improvement rates were completely comparable to those of all the preceding studies, with two-thirds of the outcomes being in the "good" or "very good" categories; and once more, difficulties were experienced due to the lack of clear and agreed-upon criteria, concepts, and language for diagnostic assessment, analyzability, and analytic results.

Altogether, this sequence of so-called first-generation outcome studies of psychoanalysis, spanning a half-century from 1917 to 1968, was scientifically simplistic and failed to command the interest of the psychoanalytic clinical world. Most practitioners agreed with Glover (1954) in his dour assessment: "Like most psycho-therapists, the psycho-analyst is a reluctant and inexpert statistician" (p. 393)—and, we could add, researcher. It was such conclusions that spurred what I call the second-generation studies—the efforts at more formal and systematic outcome research geared toward overcoming the glaring methodological simplicity that marked each of the studies described to this point.

---

[2] Although the span from Coriat (1917) to this study (1967) is a half-century, I call all of these studies "first generation" in terms of their degree of conceptual and methodological sophistication rather than in temporal terms—although, of course, each "generation" started at a later point in time than its predecessor or spanned a later period of time.

Formal and Systematic Outcome Studies: Second-Generation Research

The methodological flaws in the first-generation statistical enumerations of psychoanalytic outcomes have already been indicated. In addition to the lack of consensually agreed-upon criteria at almost every step—from initial assessments to outcome judgments of therapeutic benefit and analytic result—and the use of these judgments (derived from unspecified, and even unformulated, criteria) by the (necessarily biased) therapist, as the (usually) sole evidential primary database, there was also the methodological difficulty that these studies were all retrospective, with all the potential therein for bias, confounding and contamination of judgments, *post hoc ergo propter hoc* reasoning, and the like. Efforts to address these issues, including the introduction of prospective inquiry and even the fashioning of predictions to be validated or refuted by subsequent assessment, began in earnest in the 1950s and 1960s. Three major projects based on studies of clinic cases from the Boston, Columbia, and New York Psychoanalytic Institutes are described from this second-generation research approach.

Group-Aggregated Studies

Boston Institute. In 1960, Knapp et al. reported on 100 supervised psychoanalytic patients from the Boston Institute clinic, rated initially for suitability for analysis, of whom 27 were followed up a year later with questionnaires addressed to the treating analysts in order to ascertain just how suitable the patients had indeed turned out to be. The evaluation procedures (i.e., the initial judgments and the subsequent questionnaire responses) were "blind." There turned out to be fair but limited success in this assessment of suitability for analysis from the initial evaluation. However, two significant limitations of this study should be mentioned. First, the testing of the predictions took place only at the 1-year mark rather than more suitably upon treatment termination; clearly, much can change in this regard—in both directions—at later points in analysis. Second, and this is a problem with all research on this model, the patients selected by psychoanalytic clinic committees are already carefully screened, with obviously unsuitable cases already rejected. The range of variability in the accepted cases is thus considerably narrowed, making differential prediction within that group inherently less reliable.

Sashin et al. (1975), inspired by this work, subsequently studied 183 patients treated at the same clinic from 1959 to 1966. Final data were collected on 130 (72%) of these patients after an average of 675 treatment hours and at a point averaging 6 years after treatment termination. Predictor variables were assessed with a 103-item evaluation questionnaire and via six major outcome criteria: 1) restriction of functioning by symptoms, 2) subjective discomfort, 3) work productivity, 4) sexual adjustment, 5) interpersonal relations, and 6) availability of insight. Only 10 of the predictor items demonstrated some predictive value in relation to assessed outcomes and that only with modest (albeit statistically significant) correlations. As a group, however, these predictor variables "made little clinical sense." Overall, the Boston Institute studies yielded only fair prediction to judgments of analyzability as assessed at the 1-year mark in treatment, and no effective prediction at all to treatment outcomes from the patient's characteristics as judged at initial evaluation.

Columbia Psychoanalytic Center. The Columbia Psychoanalytic Center project, contemporaneous with the Boston studies, was written up in final accounting in a series of published reports in 1985 (Bachrach et al. 1985; Weber et al. 1985a, 1985b, 1985c). This project consisted of prospective studies of a large number of patients (1,348 in sample 1 and 237 in the later sample 2), all treated by the same body of therapists. Data were collected from multiple perspectives over time (initially and at termination), with opportunities to compare findings in psychoanalysis (about 40% of the total) with those in psychoanalytic psychotherapy (the other 60%). The authors stated that all previous studies had been limited in at least one of the following ways: small sample size, inadequate range of information about outcomes, not based on terminated cases, or restricted to retrospective data. Further, no other studies had permitted comparison between large numbers of terminated analyses and psychotherapies conducted by the same analysts, in which all pertinent information had not been retrospectively assessed. In addition, criteria for therapeutic benefit were established distinct from separate criteria for the evolution of a psychoanalytic process.

The most striking finding from this project was that across every category of patient, the therapeutic benefit measures always substantially exceeded the measures of an evolved analytic process. For example, only 40% of those who completed analyses with good therapeutic benefit were characterized as having been "analyzed" by the project criteria. An equally striking finding was that the outcomes of these treatments, in terms of both therapeutic benefit and analyzability, were only marginally predictable from the perspective of the initial evaluation. This finding was, of course, in keeping with those of the Boston studies just cited—and for the same reasons. As noted by the authors (Weber et al. 1985a), "The prudent conclusion . . . is *not* that therapeutic benefit or analyzability are *per se* unpredictable, but that once a case has been carefully selected as suitable for analysis by a candidate, its eventual fate remains relatively indeterminate" (p. 135).

Another significant finding was that "retrospective assessments of patient qualities by the treating analyst show a more substantial relationship to outcome than assessments made at the beginning of treatment" (Weber et al. 1985a, p. 136). Expectedly, those selected for psychoanalysis were assessed initially as functioning at higher levels than those selected for psychotherapy, and those in psychoanalysis achieved greater therapeutic benefits than those in psychotherapy. In conclusion, the authors stated that sample 1 was three times larger than that in any previously published study, and that the project was the first to have a psychotherapy comparison group and one of the first to make the conceptual distinction between analyzability and therapeutic benefit. Sample 2 was a smaller sample gathered a decade later with some refinements in methods of data collection and some differences in observational vantage points, but in almost every particular, all the findings of sample 1 were replicated. From both studies, the authors concluded "that a substantially greater proportion of analysands derive therapeutic benefit than develop an analytic process, and that the development of an analytic process is associated with the highest levels of therapeutic benefit. Yet, what we do not yet know precisely is the nature and quality of benefit associated with the development of an analytic process and without its development" (Weber et al. 1985b, p. 261).

The final article in this series (Bachrach et al. 1985) was devoted to a review of clinical and methodological considerations. The authors stressed the advantages of their project over other comparable studies: 1) the *N* was very large; 2) it was a prospective study with predictive evaluations performed before outcomes were known; 3) they used many (clinically meaningful) scales; 4) aside from evaluations by patients and therapists, they used independent judges; and 5) psychoanalysis and psychotherapy were comparatively assessed.

New York Psychoanalytic Institute (Erle and Goldberg). The New York Psychoanalytic Institute studies (Erle 1979; Erle and Goldberg 1979, 1984) were similarly constituted, although with more of a focus on the study of treatments carried out by more experienced analysts. There were two studies. The first (Erle 1979) consisted of 40 supervised analytic patients selected from 870 applicants to the Treatment Center of the New York Psychoanalytic Institute. The results were completely comparable with those of the Boston and Columbia centers. Twenty-five of the patients terminated satisfactorily but only 11 of these were considered to have completed treatment; 24 of the patients were judged to have benefited substantially, but only 17 were judged to have been involved in a proper psychoanalytic process. A sample of 42 *private* patients from 7 analyst colleagues of the author who began treatment in the same period and were assessed in the same manner as the Treatment Center patients showed substantially comparable results. The second study (Erle and Goldberg 1984) extended the work to a sample of 160 private patients gathered over a subsequent 5-year span from 16 cooperating experienced analysts. The outcomes from these experienced analysts were completely comparable to the results of their own (and of all other) earlier studies of clinic patients treated by candidates.

Individually Focused Studies

New York Psychoanalytic Institute (Pfeffer). Over a time span parallel to that of these relatively large-sample outcome studies of psychoanalytic clinic patient populations (as well as some comparison private patients) assessed by pre- and/or posttreatment rating scales and grouped statistically, Pfeffer at the same New York Psychoanalytic Institute Treatment Center initiated a wholly other kind of outcome and follow-up study of terminated psychoanalyses by intensive individual case studies of a research-procured population (Pfeffer 1959, 1961, 1963). He first reported on nine patients who had completed analyses under Treatment Center auspices and had agreed to a series of follow-up interviews by a "follow-up analyst" who had not conducted the treatment. The interviews were open-ended, once a week, "analytic" in character, and ranged from two to seven in number before the participants agreed upon a natural close. The chief finding, and that in *all* instances, consisted of the rapid reactivation of characteristic analytic transferences, including even transitory symptom flare-ups, as if in relation to the original treating analyst, with subsequent rapid subsidence, at times aided by pertinent interpretations, and in a manner that indicated the new ways of neurotic conflict management that had been achieved in the analysis.

In the last of this sequence of three reports (1963), Pfeffer attempted a metapsychological explanation of these "follow-up study transference phenomena" (p. 23). His overall conclusion was that "The recurrence in the follow-up study of the major preanalytic symptomatology in the context of a revived transference neurosis as well as the quick subsidence of symptoms appear to support the idea that conflicts underlying symptoms are not actually shattered or obliterated by analysis but rather are only better mastered with new and more adequate solutions" (p. 234). The neurotic conflicts thus "lose their poignancy" (p. 237).

San Francisco and Chicago research groups. Two other research groups, one in San Francisco (Norman et al. 1976; Oremland et al. 1975) and one in Chicago (Schlessinger and Robbins 1974, 1975, 1983), replicated the Pfeffer studies, with some slight alterations in method, and in both instances confirmed what has come to be called "the Pfeffer phenomenon." The San Francisco group concluded that "the infantile neurosis had not disappeared. What had changed was the degree to which it affected [the patient's] everyday life" (Norman et al. 1976, p. 492). The Chicago group concluded that "psychic conflicts were not eliminated in the analytic process . . . the more significant outcome of the analysis appeared to be the development of a preconsciously active self-analytic function, in identification with the analyzing function of the analyst, as a learned mode of coping with conflicts" (Schlessinger and Robbins 1983, p. 9). This overall finding from all three groups—that even in analyses considered highly successful, neurotic conflicts are not obliterated or shattered, as was once felt, but rather are tamed, muted, or lose their poignancy—is echoed in the well-known analytic quip that we all still recognize our good friends after their analyses.

I note one final consideration: A shared characteristic of these second-generation studies—whether the group-aggregated broad statistical accountings (the Boston, the Columbia, Erle and Goldberg in New York) or the individually focused, in-depth research studies (Pfeffer in New York, the San Francisco, the Chicago)—was the failure to segregate outcome results discerned at treatment termination from the issue of the stability (or not) of these results as revealed at some established follow-up point subsequent to termination, with all the different possibilities—for consolidation and further enhancement of treatment gains, for the simple maintenance of treatment achievements, or for actual regression back toward the pretreatment state.

Conceptually, this was a failure to accord specific theoretical status to what Rangell (1966/1990) has called the "postanalytic phase." Rangell described a variety of possible courses that can characterize this phase and concluded that "the desired goal should be a transition to a normal interchange in which the analyst can be seen and reacted to as a normal figure and no longer as an object for continued transference displacement" (p. 722). In the third-generation studies next to be described, the distinction between results at the termination study point and those at a subsequent prearranged follow-up study point (anywhere from 2 to 5 years later) becomes a clearly demarcated research focus—among the advances over the second-generation studies. A considerable variety of posttermination therapist-patient contact or interaction patterns are delineated in these studies.

Combined Process and Outcome Studies: Third-Generation Research

What I am calling the third-generation studies of the outcomes of psychoanalysis have actually been contemporaneous in time with the (conceptually) second-generation studies just described. These are systematic and formal psychoanalytic therapy research projects that have attempted both to assess analytic outcomes across a significant array of cases *and* to examine the processes through which these outcomes have been reached via the intensive longitudinal study of each of the individual cases. In this, these studies have combined the methodological approaches of the group-aggregated studies (the Boston, the Columbia, and the New York—Erle and Goldberg) with those of the individually focused studies (the New York—Pfeffer, the San Francisco, and the Chicago). Like the best of the second-generation studies, they have carefully defined their terms, constructed rating scales, and tried to operationalize their criteria at each assessment point. These third-generation studies have been constructed prospectively, starting with pretreatment assessment of patients. Unlike the second-generation studies, they have carefully separated outcomes at termination from functioning at a specified subsequent follow-up point and have attempted to account for the further changes, in either direction, that took place during this "postanalytic phase." Bachrach and colleagues (1991), in a comprehensive survey of research on the efficacy of psychoanalysis, singled out the newer Boston Psychoanalytic Society and Institute studies (Kantrowitz 1986; Kantrowitz et al. 1986, 1987a, 1987b, 1989, 1990a, 1990b, 1990c) and the Psychotherapy Research Project of The Menninger Foundation (Wallerstein 1986, 1988) as the only ones to fully meet their array of state-of-the-art specifications.

Boston Psychoanalytic Society and Institute Studies

The Boston studies were undertaken in the 1970s and came to publication in the following decade. Twenty-two supervised analytic cases at the Boston Institute clinic were selected for prospective study, with the initial assessment based on a projective test battery used to yield measures of 1) affect availability and modulation, 2) quality of object relations, 3) adequacy of reality testing, and 4) motivation for change. Approximately a year after treatment termination, the initial test battery was repeated; both the patient and the treating analyst were interviewed.

A series of three papers (Kantrowitz et al. 1986, 1987a, 1987b) described the results. Nine of the 22 patients were felt to have had a successful analytic outcome, 5 to have had a limited analytic outcome, and 8 to be unanalyzed. Nonetheless, the greater number achieved therapeutic benefits along each of the change and outcome dimensions, and along each dimension the therapeutic benefit *exceeded* the analytic result in terms of the degree of successfully completed analytic work. That is, a consistent and important finding was that therapeutic benefit was achieved by the majority of the patients and was regularly in excess of what could be accounted for by the evocation and the interpretive resolution of the transference neurosis. However, although most patients derived significant therapeutic benefit from their analytic experience, successful outcome could not be predicted from any of the predictor variables. This finding led these investigators to speculate that "a particularly important omission (from the predictor variables) might have been consideration of the effect of the [therapist-patient] match in shaping the two-person psychoanalytic interaction" (Kantrowitz et al. 1989, p. 899). By "match," they meant "an interactional concept; it refers to a spectrum of compatibility and incompatibility of the patient and analyst which is relevant to the analytic work" (p. 894). They further noted that although "this mesh of the analyst's personal qualities with those of the patient has rarely been a special focus of attention, . . . most analysts when making referrals do consider it; few assume that equally well-trained analysts are completely interchangeable" (Kantrowitz 1986, p. 273).

This same team then returned for follow-up interviews with the same patient cohort in 1987, now 5 to 10 years after the treatment terminations, this time including the retrospective assessment of the goodness of the analyst-patient match as one of the variables contributing to the patient outcomes (Kantrowitz et al. 1990a, 1990b, 1990c). Nineteen of the original 22 patients could be located and of these, 18 agreed to be interviewed. Again, a variety of change measures were used: global improvement ratings, affect management, quality of object relations, adequacy of reality testing, work accomplishment, and overall self-esteem. Overall results at the follow-up point comprised 3 patients further improved, 4 stable, 6 deteriorated but restored with additional treatment, 4 deteriorated despite additional treatment, and one returned to the original analyst and still in treatment and therefore not counted.

The most striking finding, however, was that again, the stability of achieved gains in the follow-up period could not be predicted from the assessments at termination—that is, according to Kantrowitz and colleagues (1990a), "psychological changes were no more stable over time for the group of patients assessed as having achieved a successful analytic outcome concomitant with considerable therapeutic benefit than for the other group of patients assessed as having achieved therapeutic benefit alone" (p. 493). In focusing on the assessment of analyst-patient match (Kantrowitz et al. 1990c), the authors concluded that with 12 of the 17 patients, the kind of match (impeding or facilitating) did play a role in the outcome achieved. They gave examples of facilitating matches with good outcomes, impeding matches with poor outcomes, and more complex situations in which the kind of match was at first facilitating to the unfolding of the analytic process but later seemed to have an influence in preventing the completion of the analytic work.

Psychotherapy Research Project (The Menninger Foundation)

The other so-called third-generation psychoanalytic therapy research study to be described here is the Psychotherapy Research Project (PRP) of The Menninger Foundation, the most comprehensive and ambitious such research program ever carried out (Wallerstein 1986, 1988; Wallerstein et al. 1956). The intent of the PRP was to follow the treatment careers and subsequent life careers of a cohort of patients (ultimately 42 in number), half in psychoanalysis, and half in other psychoanalytic psychotherapies—and each in the treatment deemed *clinically* indicated—from the initial pretreatment comprehensive psychiatric evaluation, through the entire natural span of their treatments (for however many years that entailed), and then into formal follow-up inquiries at several years after the treatment terminations, and with as much of an open-ended follow-up thereafter as circumstances might make possible and as the span of interested observation might last. The patients entered into their treatment over the span of the mid-1950s (contemporaneous with the bulk of the second-generation studies); their periods of treatment ranged from 6 months to a full 12 years; all were reached—100%—for formal follow-up study at the 2- to 3-year mark; and more than one-third could be followed for periods ranging from 12 to 24 years beyond their treatment terminations (with four still in ongoing treatment).

The aim of the PRP was to learn as much as possible about 1) *what* changes actually take place in psychoanalysis and other psychoanalytic psychotherapies (the outcome question), and 2) *how* those changes come about—through the interactions over time of what variables in the patient, in the therapy and the therapist, and in the patient's evolving life situation that together co-determine those changes (the process question). Three overall treatment groups were set up—psychoanalysis, expressive psychoanalytic psychotherapy, and supportive psychoanalytic psychotherapy—in accordance with the then-consensus in the psychoanalytic literature regarding the defining characteristics of these therapeutic modes, together with differential indications derived from the dynamic formulations of the nature of the patients' lives, history, character, and illness structure.

The project goals within this framework were to specify in detail the particular reach and limitation of the therapeutic outcome for each kind of patient appropriately treated within each of the proffered therapeutic approaches. There was a special interest in the more empirical elaboration of the psychological change mechanisms operative within both the uncovering (expressive) and the "ego-strengthening" (supportive) therapeutic modes. The 784-page book *Forty-Two Lives in Treatment,* written over the period 1981–1982, represents the full statement of the project's findings and conclusions (Wallerstein 1986). For an overall capsule summarization of the main highlights here, I can best report by paraphrasing (and sharply condensing) a lengthy segment from the concluding part of a summarizing paper about the project (Wallerstein 1988, pp. 144–149).

PRP conclusions. The overall conclusions can be brought together as a series of sequential propositions regarding the appropriateness, efficacy, reach, and limitations of psychoanalysis and of psychoanalytic psychotherapies (variously expressive and supportive)—always, of course, with the caveat that this segment of the overall patient population (i.e., those [usually sicker] individuals who were brought to or who sought their intensive analytic treatment within a psychoanalytic sanatorium setting) was not representative of the usual outpatient psychoanalytic therapy population.

1. The first proposition concerns the distinction so regularly made between true "structural change," presumably based on the interpretive resolution of unconscious intrapsychic conflicts, and "behavioral change," based on "just altered techniques of adjustment" and presumably all that can come out of the other, noninterpretive, non-insight-aiming change mechanisms. Intrinsic to this way of dichotomizing change has always been the easy assumption that only structural change, as brought about through conflict resolution marked by appropriately achieved insight, can have some guarantee of inherent stability, durability, and capacity to weather at least ordinary future environmental vicissitude. The PRP experience clearly and strongly questioned the continued usefulness of this effort to so tightly link the *kind* of changes achieved with the intervention mode—expressive or supportive—by which they are brought about. The changes reached in the more supportive therapies seemed often enough to represent just as much structural change, in the terms indicated, as the changes reached in the most expressive-analytic cases.
2. The second proposition concerns the conventional proportionality argument—that therapeutic change will be *at least* proportional to the degree of achieved conflict resolution. This proposition is, of course, almost unexceptionable, since it is clear that there can be significantly more change than there is true conflict resolution, on all the varying (supportive) bases through which change can be brought about, as well as properly proportionate change in which the change is on the basis of conflict resolution with accompanying insight—if such an ideal type ever actually exists in practice. Conversely, it would be hard to imagine real conflict resolution (and accompanying insight) without at least proportional concomitant change in behaviors, dispositions, and symptoms.

3. The third proposition, often linked to the proportionality argument but much more debatable and clearly separated from it, concerns the necessity argument—that effective conflict resolution is a necessary condition for at least certain kinds of change. It is clear that an overall PRP finding—and almost an overriding one—has been the repeated demonstration that a substantial range of changes—in symptoms, in personality functioning, and in lifestyle—have been brought about via the more supportive psychotherapeutic modes, cutting across the gamut of declared supportive *and* expressive (even analytic) therapies, and that in terms of the usual criteria, these changes can be (in many instances) quite indistinguishable from the changes brought about by typically expressive-analytic means.
4. A counterpart to the proposition based on the tendency to overestimate the necessity of the expressive (analytic) treatment mode's operating via conflict resolution in order to effect therapeutically desired change has been the other proposition, based on the happy finding that the supportive therapeutic approaches so often achieved far more than was expected of them—and, indeed, often enough reached the kinds of changes expected to depend on more expressive and insightful conflict resolutions—and did so in ways that represented indistinguishably "structural" changes. In fact, proportionately, each within its own category, the designated psychotherapy cases did as well as the designated psychoanalytic ones. More to the point, the good results in the one modality were not overall less stable or less enduring or less proof against subsequent environmental vicissitude than in the other. And, more important still, within both the psychotherapy and the psychoanalysis groups, the changes predicted, although more often predicated on the more expressive techniques, in fact were achieved to a greater-than-expected degree (often the same changes) on the basis of the more supportive techniques.
5. Considering these PRP treatments from the point of view of psychoanalysis as a treatment modality, just as more was accomplished than expected with psychotherapy, especially in its more supportive modes, so psychoanalysis, as the quintessentially expressive therapeutic mode, achieved less—at least with these patients—than had been anticipated or predicted. This more limited success in part reflected the ethos of the psychoanalytic sanatorium and the psychoanalytic treatment opportunities this setting is intended to make possible—that is, the protection and life management of those temporarily disorganized and incompetent individuals who cannot be helped sufficiently with any other or lesser treatment approach than psychoanalysis, but who cannot tolerate the rigors of psychoanalytic treatment within the usual outpatient setting.

   This is the concept of so-called heroic indications for psychoanalysis, and in the PRP experience, these particular patients characteristically did very poorly with the psychoanalytic treatment method, however modified by parameters or buttressed by concomitant hospitalization. And there were certainly enough instances of very good outcomes with these "sicker" patients in an appropriately modulated supportive-expressive psychotherapy, especially when we could ensure truly adequate concomitant life management. The shift is in the departure from the effort at psychoanalysis per se (even modified analysis) as the treatment of choice for these "sicker" patients in that setting. On this basis, we can speak of the failing of the so-called heroic indications for *psychoanalysis* and can invite a repositioning of the pendulum, in its swings over time around this issue, more in the direction of "narrowing indications" for (proper) psychoanalysis.

6. The predictions made for prospective courses and outcomes tended to be for more substantial and more enduring change (more "structural change") where the treatment was to be more expressive-analytic; *pari passu,* the more supportive the treatment was intended to be (had to be), the more limited and inherently unstable the anticipated changes were expected to be. All of this speculation was consistently tempered and altered in the actual implementation in the treatment courses. Psychoanalysis and the expressive psychotherapies as a whole were systematically modified to introduce more supportive components—they by and large accomplished less than anticipated, with a varying but often substantial amount of their successful outcomes achieved by supportive means. The supportive psychotherapies, on the other hand, often accomplished a fair amount more—and sometimes a great deal more—than initially expected, again, with much of the change on the basis of more supportive techniques than originally specified.

In conclusion, these overall results can be generalized as follows: 1) the treatment results in psychoanalysis and in varying mixes of expressive-supportive psychotherapies tend to converge, rather than diverge, in outcome; 2) across the whole spectrum of treatment courses, from the most analytic-expressive to the most single-mindedly supportive, the treatment carried more supportive elements than originally projected, and these elements accounted for substantially more of the changes achieved than had been originally anticipated; 3) the supportive aspects of psychotherapy, as conceptualized within a psychoanalytic theoretical framework, deserve far more respectful specification than they have usually been accorded in the psychodynamic literature; and 4) from the study of the kinds of changes achieved by this patient cohort, partly on an uncovering insight-aiming basis and partly on the basis of the opposed covering-up varieties of supportive techniques, the changes themselves—divorced from how they were brought about—often seemed quite indistinguishable from each other in terms of being so-called real or structural changes in personality functioning.

Psychoanalytic Therapy Process Research

Because of inherently greater conceptual and methodological complexity, counterpart research into the nature of the *processes* by which change comes about or is brought about in psychoanalytic therapies—the answer to the *how* question, through the interaction of what factors in the patient, in the therapy and the therapist, and in the concomitantly evolving life situation—has been more recent in origin and has not yet undergone generational transformations. Also, since it necessarily (at least usually) entails more detailed focus on moment-to-moment therapeutic interactions, such research has only been rendered feasible on a significant scale by the recent development and deployment of suitable technology—namely, the possibilities for audio (and video) recording and of computerization and high-speed computer word or situation searches.

Audio recording was actually introduced into clinical psychoanalytic research as early as 1933, when Earl Zinn was known to have made dictaphone recordings of psychoanalytic sessions with a patient at Worcester State Hospital (Carmichael 1956). Since then, recordings have been advocated and used by a widening array of analytic investigators. In a major overview of "Issues in Research in the Psychoanalytic Process," Wallerstein and Sampson (1971) reviewed the literature to that date on the use of audio recording in therapy sessions and discussed the various arguments for and against such use. The major arguments pro are the greater completeness, verbatim accuracy, permanence, and public character of the database, as well as the facilitation of the separation of the therapeutic from the research responsibility with the possibility of thus bypassing the inevitable biases of the analyst as a contaminant of the data filter. The major arguments con are the indeterminate impact of this (research) intrusion upon the "naturalness" of the therapeutic process (including the compromise of full confidentiality and the insertion of goals other than therapeutic) and the sheer enormity, complexity, and cost of the database thus made available (cost being not just for audio recording but for faithful transcription that includes prosodic elements as much as possible in addition to lexical accuracy).

It is only within the past two decades that an adequate consensus has emerged that analytic theory *can* go on under these observed circumstances—that is, that a properly therapeutic analytic process can nonetheless evolve—and that computer technology has advanced to where the enormous database generated can be feasibly managed. This has led to the recent (almost explosive) proliferation of psychoanalytic therapy process research, mainly in the United States and Germany (centered there especially at the University of Ulm), but also in Great Britain and elsewhere. The proceedings of a major Workshop [of American and German researchers] on Empirical Research in Psychoanalysis held just prior to the 1985 International Psycho-Analytical Association Congress in Hamburg were brought together in a 1988 book, *Psychoanalytic Process Research Strategies,* edited by Dahl, Kächele, and Thomä. The proposed conceptual framework of this workshop was in the principle enunciated in the initial chapter by Strupp, Schacht, and Henry: "that the description and representation, theoretically *and* operationally, of a *patient's conflicts*, of the *patient's treatment*, and of the *assessment of the outcome*, must be congruent, which is to say, must be represented in comparable, if not identical terms" (Dahl et al. 1988, p. ix). This fundamental integrative principle—proposed to subsume conceptually the entire array of process researches, however seemingly disparate their concepts and their instruments—is termed the Principle of Problem-Treatment-Outcome Congruence ("P-T-O congruence" for short; Strupp et al. 1988, p. 7).

Here I will only very briefly (alphabetically) indicate those (American) psychoanalytic therapy process research studies (13 in number) that are linked under the auspices of the American Psychoanalytic Association as components of a Collaborative Multi-Site Program of Psychoanalytic Therapy Research.[3] The Dahl et al. volume provides comparable access to the major German studies within this same arena. All of these process research studies are based on the use of (research-accurate) transcribed audiotaped psychoanalytic therapy session hours.

1. Wilma Bucci of Adelphi University (Long Island, New York) reformulates psychoanalytic theory in the context of a dual-code model of mental representation. The major research instruments are measures of *Referential Activity (RA),* defined as activity of the system of referential connections between verbal and nonverbal (emotional) representations. RA measures provide objective indicators reflecting variation in degree of access to emotional experience and its expression in linguistic forms. The measures may be applied to both patient and therapist speech. There are RA peaks and troughs; the peaks usually coincide with stories of past events activated and experienced emotionally by the patient in the here and now, and characteristically embody references to the transference.
2. Hartvig Dahl of the SUNY Health Science Center (Brooklyn, New York) focuses on *three* major propositions: 1) the Principle of P-T-O Congruence; 2) the Therapeutic Change Hypothesis—that therapeutic change is a causal result of specific changes in "ME" emotions (affects) that function as beliefs about the status of fulfillment of "IT" emotions and other significant appetitive wishes; and 3) the Principle of Task-Goal-Technique Congruence—that treatment success is a function of the congruence of the patient's *task* in the treatment (i.e., to free-associate), the patient's *goal* for the treatment (i.e., to "become free"), and the therapist's technique (i.e., to analyze transference and resistance with a neutral stance). These propositions are studied via the interaction of three sets of measures: 1) *Frames,* which are recurrent, structured sequences of events that represent significant wishes and beliefs manifested in perceptions, thoughts, and actions and explicitly represented in the discrete narratives told by patients in therapy; 2) *Emotions*; and 3) *Defenses* (the latter two described by separate E/D measures).

---

[3] Organized by Wallerstein; see Wallerstein RS: "Proposal to the Ludwig Foundation for a Collaborative Multi-Site Program of Psychoanalytic Therapy Research," 1991 (unpublished report; available from author) for the overall program design integrating these studies plus other, outcome studies into a unifying framework, and also for bibliographic access to major presentations of the research strategies and the research findings to date of each component project within the collaborative program.

3. Stuart Hauser of Harvard Medical School and Boston University (Cambridge and Boston, Massachusetts) codes *Constraining and Enabling Interactions* between analysts and patients—ways of measuring speech qualities that facilitate and inhibit communication in therapeutic dialogues—and correlates these with findings from specifically designed psychological tests and interviews administered before and after termination of psychoanalytic treatments. These assessments include 1) the patient's overall ego development using the Loevinger Sentence Completion Test, 2) the attachment representations of patient and analyst using Mary Main's new approach, and 3) the ego defenses and other ego strengths of the patient using scales stimulated by the work of Vaillant, Valenstein, and Prelinger.
4. Mardi Horowitz of the University of California at San Francisco applies his *Role Relationship Model Configuration (RRMC)* to the formulation of transferences and recurrent maladaptive interpersonal patterns. The RRMC is based on the conception that persons have multiple self-concepts and relationship scenarios in dynamic layering. The RRMC formats the desired, the dreaded, the defensive compromise, and the coping compromise sectors of these person schemata. As a process measure, it is likely to show shifts in transferences and resistance and in recurrent maladaptive interpersonal patterns throughout the treatment phases. Predictions at the beginning of treatment concerning RRMCs inferred to be warded off as unconscious fantasies can be checked for validity or refuted in later phases, and may also be used as outcome-during-process measures relative to strategies of interpretive intervention.
5. Leonard Horwitz of The Menninger Foundation (Topeka, Kansas) studies shifts in the *Therapeutic Alliance (TA)* by assessing changes in the patient's collaboration with the therapist (a basic component of the TA) using a scale with two components, one rating the extent to which the patient is bringing in significant material and the other rating the extent to which the patient is using the analyst's help. Shifts on the collaboration scale are related to the analyst's preceding interventions to ascertain whether these enhanced or diminished the patient's collaboration, and different intervention methods (more supportive or more expressive) are related to differential suitability for different kinds of patients.
6. Enrico Jones of the University of California at Berkeley studies the relation between analytic process and outcome by means of his *Psychotherapy Process Q-Sort,* which is designed to provide a basic language for describing the analytic process in a form suitable for quantitative analysis, thus beginning to construct an empirical/descriptive base for how psychoanalytic treatments are actually conducted. These data will allow intensive analysis of cases in a manner that provides detailed descriptions of the analytic process and can therefore begin to address the problem of individual differences in response to treatment. In addition, a new method for assessing changes other than changes in symptoms—an *Inventory for Psychological Functioning (IPF)*—is being developed as a measure of structural change and treatment outcome.

7. Otto Kernberg and Harold Koenigsberg of the Cornell Medical Center (Westchester Division, White Plains, New York) apply a rating system for assessing the therapist's adherence to proper psychoanalytic technique as well as a system for rating therapeutic skill variables in the conduct of treatment sessions. These scales (a *Treatment Contract Rating Scale*, a *Therapist's Attitudes and Qualities Rating Scale*, and a *Therapist Verbal Intervention Inventory*) have been piloted in a study of the psychotherapy of borderline patients and are now being applied across the larger psychopathological spectrum in individual psychoanalytic treatments.
8. Lester Luborsky, Paul Crits-Christoph, and Jacques Barber of the University of Pennsylvania (Philadelphia) apply their *Core Conflictual Relationship Theme (CCRT)* measure to study 1) the nature of the therapeutic relationship, especially the therapeutic alliance, 2) the main transference patterns in the analysis (assessed by the CCRT), 3) the degree of focus on the transference in the analyst's interpretations, 4) the accuracy of the analyst's interpretations, and 5) the type and degree of patient-achieved insight. The CCRT is a guided clinical judgment system for evaluating the transference concept by identifying three components in relationship episodes described in therapy: 1) the patient's main wishes, needs, or intentions toward the other person, 2) the expected or actual responses of the other person, and 3) the responses of the self. Changes in these measures are correlated with therapeutic change.
9. Christopher Perry and Steven Cooper of Cambridge Hospital and Harvard Medical School (Cambridge, Massachusetts) focus on two cornerstones of psychoanalytic theory: 1) that conscious and unconscious motives underlie behavior and 2) that defenses operate to protect the individual from awareness of certain motives in conflict. They apply measures of motives and defenses, *Wishes and Fears: A Standard List* and *Guidelines for Assessing Dynamic Motives,* and their *Defense Mechanism Rating Scales* to empirically test hierarchical arrangements for motive and defense development and to allow the calculation of overall "maturity scores" for both over the course of psychoanalytic therapies.
10. Herbert J. Schlesinger of the New School for Social Research (New York, New York) focuses on the relationship between the lexical content and the prosodic elements (the "music") of speech in treatment sessions. The words and "music" can be concordant—enhancing the patients' intended meanings—or discordant—conveying conflict and signaling unstated and contradictory meanings. Audio-recorded sessions are dubbed onto the same computer disk as the transcribed text so that the text can be read on the screen while one listens to the spoken words. Prosodic elements that are rated include pitch, word frequency, and loudness as well as other nonlexical elements (length of pauses, rate of speech, coughing, sighing, and crying) and various dysfluencies (false starts to sentences and characteristic nonword vocalizations). Algorithms will be developed that use both the lexical and the prosodic elements to describe speech segments that clinicians have identified as conveying a particular affect or intent.

11. George Silberschatz and John Curtis of Mt. Zion Hospital (San Francisco, California) base their studies on the concept of the *Plan Formulation,* a reliably derived case formulation that includes the patient's goals in the therapy, the obstructions (belief systems) that have kept the patient from achieving these goals, the insights that it will be helpful for the patient to achieve, and how the patient can work in therapy to overcome the obstructions and achieve the goals. The investigators study 1) the effects of interpretations on the immediate therapeutic process, with accuracy of interpretation defined as adherence to the Plan Formulation as measured by the *Plan Compatibility Scale*; 2) the impact of plan-compatible interpretations on the treatment outcome; and 3) the application of a case-specific measure of outcome that correlates the Plan Formulation for each case with the individually tailored measure of outcome, the *Plan Attainment Scale,* derived from the Plan Formulation.
12. Donald Spence of the Robert Wood Johnson Medical School of Rutgers University (New Brunswick, New Jersey) studies *Lexical Co-occurrence Density (LCD)*—a measure of the closeness of appearance of highly associated nouns and adjectives (e.g., man-woman, large-small) within an arbitrary textual search space; the greater the associative freedom, the more co-occurrences. LCD should therefore be lower in phases of resistance than in phases of freer association. It can be used to track association fluency and referential specificity throughout various phases of psychoanalytic treatments.
13. Sherwood Waldron, Jr., of the New York Psychoanalytic Society and Institute studies *Rating Scales of Analyst Segments* (8 subscales) and *Rating Scales of Patient Segments* (7 subscales). The scales of Analyst Segments assess how well and/or how much the analyst addresses resistances, addresses transferences, is optimally supportive, avails him- or herself of opportunities to convey understanding, encourages the development of an analytic process, follows the patient's material, expresses interfering difficulties, and uses an approach that is or is not similar to the one the rater would use. The scales of patient segments assess how clearly the patient conveys experiences, conveys feelings, maintains self-observation, expresses transference themes, shows awareness of transference experiences, is overall analytically productive, and is identifiably responding to the analyst's interventions in a potentially productive way.

It is these 13 process-focused studies, which, together with the two successor projects to the two described third-generation outcome studies[4] and one child-

[4] The group headed by Judy Kantrowitz of the Boston Psychoanalytic Society and Institute studying the quality of patient-analyst "match" in relation to analytic treatment outcomes, and the group headed by Robert Wallerstein of the University of California at San Francisco studying structural change in the array of psychoanalytic psychotherapies and psychoanalysis through the use of 17 *Scales of Psychological Capacities (SPC)* devised to measure personality attributes that as a set correlate with mature achievements and satisfactions in life.

therapy–focused study in England (George Moran and Peter Fonagy of the Anna Freud Centre in London), are all gathered into the proposed Collaborative Multi-Site Program of Psychoanalytic Therapy Research (Wallerstein 1991).

The collaborative multisite PRP program incorporates a design in which all 16 member groups will each use their own concepts and instruments upon a common agreed-upon database of available audiotaped and transcribed psychoanalytic session hours from already-completed psychoanalytic treatments, as well as upon session hours from new psychoanalytic cases, so that appropriate before-and-after studies (as well as planned follow-ups) can be prospectively built in. The comparing and contrasting of findings in relation to the same database by all of these process and outcome study groups will finally make it possible to determine the degrees of convergence of the concepts and instruments elaborated to this point by the different groups, and also to determine the degree and the nature of the imbrication of process and outcome studies—that is, the degree to which the Principle of P-T-O Congruence in fact holds. This is the direction that what I call the fourth-generation studies are taking—a direction which, if successful, promises not only to integrate the various psychoanalytic process studies carried out more or less independently over the past two decades, but also to integrate process studies with outcome studies to achieve a more complete fulfillment of the aim articulated in the introduction to this chapter.

"Offset" Research Relating Mental Health and General Health Care

In the 1950s and 1960s, Duehrssen and her co-workers in West Germany published a series of papers based on the health care records of the Berlin General Health Insurance Office that demonstrated, in a large patient cohort, that the cost of intensive outpatient psychoanalytic therapy was significantly offset by savings in medical expenditures for general health care by these patients and by their reduced use of hospitalization over a 5-year period (see especially Duehrssen and Jorswiek 1965).[5] These studies were picked up and extended by a considerable variety of American investigators, most notably in the 1970s and 1980s, by Mumford, Schlesinger, Glass, and their co-workers, whose work both reviewed and summarized the rapidly burgeoning literature in this field and added their own studies concerning the impact of psychological interventions on recovery from surgery and from severe medical illness, as well as the impact of mental health treatment on medical care utilization in patients with various chronic somatic diseases.

---

[5] These studies were not published in English, but English translations were made available by the National Institute of Mental Health, and they thus became widely known and cited in the United States.

The comprehensive literature reviewed (Mumford et al. 1984) included two data sources: 1) 58 controlled studies (between 1978 and 1953) subjected to meta-analysis[6] and 2) the massive fee-for-service research database derived from the health insurance claims file of the Blue Cross/Blue Shield Federal Employees Program (FEP) for the years 1974–1978. In addition to offering complementary perspectives, these sources provided mutually supporting evidence of the cost-offset effects of outpatient mental health treatment. The reductions in use of medical services were found to be associated with inpatient rather than outpatient utilization and tended to be larger for older persons. The authors felt that these findings argued both for the inseparability of mind and body in health care and for the likelihood that mental health treatment improved patients' ability to stay healthy enough to avoid hospital admission for physical illness.

A comparable quantitative review of 34 controlled studies (Mumford et al. 1982) demonstrated that surgical or coronary patients who are provided information or emotional support to help them master their medical crises do better than patients who receive only ordinary care. On the average, psychological intervention reduced hospitalization to approximately 2 days below the control group's average, although most of the interventions were modest and most were not matched in any way to the needs of particular patients or to their coping styles. In another article on the same subject (Schlesinger et al. 1980), the authors concluded that studies "testing the effects of psychologically informed intervention on the quality and speed of recovery of surgical patients show that a wide range of such interventions is effective in helping patients master the stresses of surgery, results in an improved sense of well-being and satisfaction, and also speeds the recovery of patients and shortens hospital stays . . . however brief or circumscribed these measures may be, a beneficial effect upon surgical outcome as defined by various parameters . . . almost invariably occurs" (p. 15).

In still another study, Schlesinger and colleagues (1983) reviewed the records for medical services covered by the Blue Cross/Blue Shield FEP from 1974–1978 for patients who were first diagnosed as having one of four chronic diseases in which psychological factors have been implicated in causation, aggravation, or maintenance, and for which the course may be responsive to lifestyle and health behavior: airflow limitation disease, diabetes, ischemic heart disease, and hypertension. They compared the group who had started some form of mental health treatment (MHT) within a year of this diagnosis with a comparison group who had no MHT, and found that those who had MHT incurred significantly lower medical treatment costs over the span of the study. The authors concluded that the inclusion of outpatient psychotherapy in medical care systems can improve the quality and appropriateness of care and can also lower the cost of providing such care. They did add the caveat that for some individuals, emotional illness leads to self-neglect, including neglect of health and avoidance

---

[6] For the theory and techniques of meta-analysis as a method of combining data from multiple reported studies, see the seminal book by Smith et al. (1980).

of medical services except for emergencies. As such individuals benefit from MHT, their use of medical services would be expected to rise somewhat, but it would be more appropriate use.

Two major implications or consequences can be drawn from these "offset studies." The first is in the public policy realm in regard to the economics as well as the humanity of providing for adequate mental health (i.e., psychotherapeutic) treatment coverage as our nation moves increasingly in the direction of universal health care insurance. The second is scientific and will emerge more fully as these "offset studies" move beyond aggregated statistical outcome studies to more individual process-oriented studies built around the intensive and in-depth case study method, including psychotherapeutic intervention and treatment. Such a move should result in a deeper knowledge of the interactive psychological and physiological mechanisms in the psychosomatic (or somatopsychic) disease process and, in a more basic sense, a more fundamental knowledge of the nature of the mind-body relationship.

Conclusion

In this chapter I have presented a review of the major formal and systematic research studies into the processes and outcomes of psychoanalysis and related psychoanalytic psychotherapies. Outcome research was the earliest undertaken and was presented first, divided into three "generations" characterized by increasing complexity and sophistication, from first-generation early statistical studies, through second-generation more formal and systematic outcome studies, and into third-generation combined process and outcome studies. This was followed by an overview of 13 major (American) psychoanalytic therapy process research studies now being coordinated within the Collaborative Multi-Site Program of Psychoanalytic Therapy Research. A final section has described "offset"research relating mental health care to utilization patterns of general health care. It should be clear overall that research into the nature of psychoanalytic therapies has finally come into its own as a significant component of the discipline of psychoanalysis as both science and profession.

For Further Study

Appelbaum SA: The Anatomy of Change. New York, Plenum, 1977

Dahl H, Kächele H, Thomä H (eds): Psychoanalytic Process Research Strategies. Berlin, Springer-Verlag, 1988

Horowitz MJ: Stress Response Syndromes. New York, Jason Aronson, 1976

Horwitz L: Clinical Prediction in Psychotherapy. New York, Jason Aronson, 1974

Kernberg OF, Burstein ED, Coyne L, et al: Psychotherapy and psychoanalysis. Bull Menninger Clin 36:1–275, 1972

Luborsky L, Crits-Christoph P: Understanding Transference: The CCRT Method. New York, Basic Books, 1990
Malan DH: A Study of Brief Psychotherapy. London, Tavistock, 1963
Wallerstein RS: Forty-Two Lives in Treatment: A Study of Psychoanalysis and Psychotherapy. New York, Guilford, 1986

References

Alexander F: Five Year Report of the Chicago Institute for Psychoanalysis: 1932–1937. Chicago, IL, Chicago Institute for Psychoanalysis, 1937
Bachrach HM, Weber JJ, Solomon M: Factors associated with the outcome of psychoanalysis (clinical and methodological considerations): report of the Columbia Psychoanalytic Center Research Project (IV). International Review of Psycho-Analysis 12:379–388, 1985
Bachrach HM, Galatzer-Levy R, Skolnikoff AZ, et al: On the efficacy of psychoanalysis. J Am Psychoanal Assoc 39:871–916, 1991
Carmichael HT: Sound film recording of psychoanalytic therapy: a therapist's experiences and reactions (1956), in Methods of Research in Psychotherapy. Edited by Gottschalk LA, Auerbach AH. New York, Appleton-Century-Crofts, 1966, pp 50–59
Coriat I: Some statistical results of the psychoanalytical treatment of the psychoneuroses. Psychoanal Rev 4:209–216, 1917
Dahl H, Kächele H, Thomä H (eds): Psychoanalytic Process Research Strategies. Berlin, Springer-Verlag, 1988
Duehrssen A, Jorswiek E: An empirical and statistical inquiry into the therapeutic potential of psychoanalytic treatment. Der Nervenarzt 36:166–169, 1965
Erle JB: An approach to the study of analyzability and analysis: the course of forty consecutive cases selected for supervised analysis. Psychoanal Q 48:198–228, 1979
Erle JB, Goldberg DA: Problems in the assessment of analyzability. Psychoanal Q 48:48–84, 1979
Erle JB, Goldberg DA: Observations on assessment of analyzability by experienced analysts. J Am Psychoanal Assoc 32:715–737, 1984
Feldman F: Results of psychoanalysis in clinic case assignments. J Am Psychoanal Assoc 16:274–300, 1968
Fenichel O: Statistischer bericht uber die therapeutische tatigkeit 1920–1930, in zehn jahre Berliner Psychoanalytisches Institut. Internazionale Psychoanalytischer Verlag 13–19, 1930
Glover E: The indications for psycho-analysis. Journal of Mental Science 100:393–401, 1954
Hamburg DA, Bibring GL, Fisher C, et al: Report of ad hoc committee on central fact-gathering data of the American Psychoanalytic Association. J Am Psychoanal Assoc 15:841–861, 1967

Jones E: Decannual report of the London Clinic of Psychoanalysis, 1926–1936. London, London Clinic of Psychoanalysis, 1936

Kantrowitz JL: The role of the patient-analyst "match" in the outcome of psychoanalysis. Annual of Psychoanalysis 14:273–297, 1986

Kantrowitz JL, Katz AL, Greenman DA, et al: The patient-analyst match and the outcome of psychoanalysis: a pilot study. J Am Psychoanal Assoc 37:893–919, 1989

Kantrowitz JL, Katz AL, Paolitto F: Follow-up of psychoanalysis five to ten years after termination, I: stability of change. J Am Psychoanal Assoc 38:471–496, 1990a

Kantrowitz JL, Katz AL, Paolitto F: Follow-up of psychoanalysis five to ten years after termination, II: development of the self-analytic function. J Am Psychoanal Assoc 38:637–654, 1990b

Kantrowitz JL, Katz AL, Paolitto F: Follow-up of psychoanalysis five to ten years after termination, III: the relation between resolution of the transference and the patient-analyst match. J Am Psychoanal Assoc 38:655–678, 1990c

Kantrowitz JL, Katz AL, Paolitto F, et al: Changes in the level and quality of object relations in psychoanalysis: follow-up of a longitudinal, prospective study. J Am Psychoanal Assoc 35:23–46, 1987a

Kantrowitz JL, Katz AL, Paolitto F, et al: The role of reality testing in psychoanalysis: follow-up of 22 cases. J Am Psychoanal Assoc 35:367–385, 1987b

Kantrowitz JL, Paolitto F, Sashin J, et al: Affect availability, tolerance, complexity, and modulation in psychoanalysis: follow-up of a longitudinal, prospective study. J Am Psychoanal Assoc 34:529–559, 1986

Kessel L, Hyman H: The value of psychoanalysis as a therapeutic procedure. JAMA 101:1612–1615, 1933

Knapp PH, Levin S, McCarter RH, et al: Suitability for psychoanalysis: a review of one hundred supervised analytic cases. Psychoanal Q 29:459–477, 1960

Knight RP: Evaluation of the results of psychoanalytic therapy. Am J Psychiatry 98:434–446, 1941

Mumford E, Schlesinger HJ, Glass GV: The effects of psychological intervention on recovery from surgery and heart attacks: an analysis of the literature. Am J Public Health 72:141–151, 1982

Mumford E, Schlesinger HJ, Glass GV, et al: A new look at evidence about reduced cost of medical utilization following mental health treatment. Am J Psychiatry 141:1145–1158, 1984

Norman HF, Blacker KH, Oremland JD, et al: The fate of the transference neurosis after termination of a satisfactory analysis. J Am Psychoanal Assoc 24:471–498, 1976

Oremland JD, Blacker KH, Norman HF: Incompleteness in "successful" psychoanalyses: a follow-up study. J Am Psychoanal Assoc 23:819–844, 1975

Pfeffer AZ: A procedure for evaluating the results of psychoanalysis: a preliminary report. J Am Psychoanal Assoc 7:418–444, 1959

Pfeffer AZ: Follow-up study of a satisfactory analysis. J Am Psychoanal Assoc 9:698–718, 1961

Pfeffer AZ: The meaning of the analyst after analysis: a contribution to the theory of therapeutic results. J Am Psychoanal Assoc 11:229–244, 1963

Rangell L: An overview of the ending of an analysis, in Psychoanalysis in the Americas. Edited by Litman RE. New York, International Universities Press, 1966, pp 141–165 (reprinted in Rangell L: The Human Core: The Intrapsychic Base of Behavior, Vol 2. Madison, CT, International Universities Press, 1990, pp 703–725)

Sashin JI, Eldred SH, van Amerongen ST: A search for predictive factors in institute supervised cases: a retrospective study of 183 cases from 1959 to 1966 at the Boston Psychoanalytic Society and Institute. Int J Psychoanal 56:343–359, 1975

Schlesinger HJ, Mumford E, Glass GV: Effects of psychological intervention on recovery from surgery, in Emotional and Psychological Responses to Anesthesia and Surgery. Edited by Guerra F, Aldrete JA. New York, Grune & Stratton, 1980, pp 9–18

Schlesinger HJ, Mumford E, Glass GV, et al: Mental health treatment and medical care utilization in a fee-for-service system: outpatient mental health treatment following the onset of a chronic disease. Am J Public Health 73:422–429, 1983

Schlessinger N, Robbins FP: Assessment and follow-up in psychoanalysis. J Am Psychoanal Assoc 22:542–567, 1974

Schlessinger N, Robbins FP: The psychoanalytic process: recurrent patterns of conflict and changes in ego functions. J Am Psychoanal Assoc 23:761–782, 1975

Schlessinger N, Robbins FP: A Developmental View of the Psychoanalytic Process: Follow-up Studies and their Consequences. New York, International Universities Press, 1983

Smith ML, Glass GV, Miller TI: The Benefits of Psychotherapy. Baltimore, MD, Johns Hopkins University Press, 1980, p 269

Strupp HH, Schacht TE, Henry WP: Problem-Treatment-Outcome congruence: a principle whose time has come, in Psychoanalytic Process Research Strategies. Edited by Dahl H, Kächele H, Thomä H. Berlin, Springer-Verlag, 1988, pp 1–14

Wallerstein RS: Forty-Two Lives in Treatment: A Study of Psychoanalysis and Psychotherapy. New York, Guilford, 1986, p 784

Wallerstein RS: Psychoanalysis and psychotherapy: relative roles reconsidered. Annual of Psychoanalysis 16:129–151, 1988

Wallerstein RS, Robbins LL, Sargent HD, et al: The Psychotherapy Research Project of The Menninger Foundation: rationale, method and sample use. Bull Menninger Clin 20:221–278, 1956

Wallerstein RS, Sampson H: Issues in research in the psychoanalytic process. Int J Psychoanal 52:11–50, 1971

Weber JJ, Bachrach HM, Solomon M: Factors associated with the outcome of psychoanalysis: report of the Columbia Psychoanalytic Center Research Project (II). International Review of Psycho-Analysis 12:127–141, 1985a

Weber JJ, Bachrach HM, Solomon M: Factors associated with the outcome of psychoanalysis: report of the Columbia Psychoanalytic Center Research Project (III). International Review of Psycho-Analysis 12:251–262, 1985b

Weber JJ, Solomon M, Bachrach HM: Characteristics of psychoanalytic clinic patients: report of the Columbia Psychoanalytic Center Research Project (I). International Review of Psycho-Analysis 12:13–26, 1985c

Chapter 28

A Recommended Curriculum for Psychodynamic Psychiatry

Allan Tasman, M.D.

The place of psychodynamic psychotherapy in modern psychiatric treatment is changing; whereas it was the central modality during the 1950s, it now is only one of several treatment modalities that psychiatrists may employ. The exact role of psychodynamic psychotherapy in future practice and training has been a point of discussion, and in recent years there have been public debates at the American Psychiatric Association annual meeting on the subject. Invariably, the neurobiologists seem less radical than the dynamicists fear, and the psychodynamic psychiatrists are far less dualistic and threatened than the biological psychiatrists imagine. Nonetheless, one can still hear that psychiatrists should not be practicing psychotherapy anymore—or, conversely, that psychiatry is "losing the mind" (Reiser 1988).

At stake is our vision of the future psychiatrist. Do we think that the future psychiatrist should/will be an applied neurobiologist who should know only the *indications* for exploratory psychotherapy, so as to make appropriate referrals to psychologists and social workers, as many neurologists and family practitioners

---

This chapter is a modified version of a curriculum proposal by Drs. Paul C. Mohl, James Lomax, Allan Tasman, Carlyle Chan, William Sledge, Paul Summergrad, and Malkah T. Notman: "Psychotherapy Training for the Psychiatrist of the Future," *American Journal of Psychiatry* 147:7–13, 1990. It is printed here with permission of the authors and the American Psychiatric Association.

now do? Do we think that the remarkable new knowledge in neurobiology, including in such areas as personality disorders (Cloninger 1987), will render psychotherapy obsolete? Do we think that a psychiatrist poorly versed in psychotherapeutic perspectives will be at a competitive disadvantage with other mental health professionals? What effects do we think the radical economic restructuring of American medicine and mental health will have on patterns of practice? We are clearly at a historic scientific watershed, but should the psychiatrists who teach psychodynamic psychotherapy be viewed as the medieval alchemists and astrologers, only grudgingly giving way to the Newtons and Galileos of neurobiology, or should they be regarded as the medieval monks carefully preserving the writings of Aristotle lest the wisdom be lost?

Psychiatric educators, who are always attempting to forecast the future so that they can prepare young psychiatrists for it, are particularly concerned with this issue. The choices they make will simultaneously influence the answers to these questions and lay the groundwork for the future success or failure of the field, depending on how prescient the forecasts turn out to be. Psychiatric educators are as uncertain about the future as everyone else—a fact that was highlighted by two recent studies. One (Langsley and Yager 1988), a survey of attitudes and opinions among department chairpersons, residency training directors, and practitioners, found that knowledge of psychodynamic theory and its application to such skills as countertransference management and psychodynamically informed supportive therapy was viewed as central to the training of all psychiatrists by more than 90% of the respondents. However, specific knowledge about and skill in conducting expressive psychotherapy was less valued.

Similarly, a survey (Tasman and Kay 1987) of current residency training programs showed that although many of these are carefully preserving a place for psychodynamic psychotherapy, that place is far smaller than previously. Most programs offer such training during outpatient rotations, which average 9 months and occupy three-fourths of the resident's time during postgraduate year 3 (PGY-3). Usually, a couple of hours are available to continue following patients beyond the rotation, but it is unusual for a resident to be able to treat a patient longer than 18 months. Furthermore, the teaching and supervising of long-term psychodynamic psychotherapy is increasingly relegated to part-time unpaid clinical faculty. Thus, the primary role models for residents do not necessarily convey the sense that a psychodynamically informed perspective is part of every psychiatrist's identity, regardless of his or her primary area of interest.

These trends in psychiatric training led the Association for Academic Psychiatry and the American Association of Directors of Psychiatry Residency Training to form a joint task force in 1987 to consider the case for the continued importance of training in psychodynamic psychotherapy in current general psychiatric education and to devise a realistic, reasonable model curriculum for it. The result of those deliberations was the development of a model curriculum that was presented in an article published in the *American Journal of Psychiatry* entitled "Psychotherapy Training for the Psychiatrist of the Future" (Mohl et al.

1990). This chapter, a slightly modified version of that original article, presents a model curriculum for training in psychodynamic psychiatry and psychotherapy. While what follows emphasizes specific experiences related to psychotherapy training, it is assumed that such training would occur within a broad-based curriculum that emphasizes a biopsychosocial approach. Many educators feel strongly that such an emphasis not only is the best way of understanding patients but also goes a long way toward reducing the dichotomy between psychodynamic and neurobiological understanding and treatments that has permeated academic departments for too long. Adhering to a biopsychosocial approach ensures that dynamic concepts and treatment approaches are integrated throughout psychiatric education and not just confined to outpatient experiences.

The group did not consider psychotherapy broadly, but rather focused on long-term psychodynamic psychotherapy. Other therapies—for example, brief, dynamic treatments, long-term supportive modalities, and group and family dynamic therapy—were seen as deriving from, and thereby educationally building on, individual expressive therapy. Obviously, the treatment setting dictates in large part the particular modality of psychotherapy that will be chosen. The focus of the group was on what has been variously called "expressive," "exploratory," "reconstructive," "psychodynamic," "psychoanalytic," or "insight-oriented" psychotherapy. After much discussion, the task force concluded that psychotherapy in which the goal is to explore, understand, and alter the inner experience of another human being is not only the best way, but perhaps the *only* way to learn and consolidate various core concepts and experiences. It is only after these concepts have been consolidated that answers to the technical questions "What is support?," "What is an appropriate brief focus?," and "Is individual, group, and/or family therapy the preferred intervention?" can be learned and effectively implemented by residents.

The task force also did not consider specific modifications and modernizations of the traditional didactic curriculum in psychodynamic psychotherapy. Reading lists and recommended texts are current only when originally prepared. The thoughtful psychotherapy educator must continually integrate new information into training program curricula. Although there have been exciting research developments in the study of psychodynamic psychotherapy—for example, the evolution of manuals (Luborsky 1984; Strupp and Binder 1984) and the identification of useful tactics in treatment (Foreman and Marmar 1985; Luborsky et al. 1985)—that will affect its practice and should influence training, the task force addressed only two questions: "Should long-term individual psychodynamic psychotherapy continue to be a significant part of a psychiatric residency?" and "What should a modern curriculum contain, given the diverse demands of training?" *In dealing with this latter question, the task force was intent on producing a curriculum that would be realistic and usable in virtually all programs, not an ideal that would be shelved because it was out of touch with day-to-day training realities.* In the end, we developed two curricula: one that should be applicable to the vast majority of residencies and one that represents a minimum for resource-poor programs. The rationale, the model curriculum, and the minimum curriculum were each reviewed by both the Association for Academic Psychiatry and the American Association of Directors of Psychiatry Residency Training.

Rationale

The task force identified 10 major reasons for continuing to teach psychodynamic psychotherapy. The first three involve the acquisition of skills directly related to the delivery of psychodynamic psychotherapy to psychiatric patients. The next seven are related to the acquisition of skills, knowledge, and experience important to other aspects of psychiatric and medical clinical practice.

1. Psychodynamic psychotherapy is an effective treatment for many medical disorders, and all well-trained psychiatrists should be familiar with—and achieve a basic level of competence in—its principles and techniques.
2. Training in psychodynamic psychotherapy provides the resident with a unique opportunity for professional growth by promoting the full development of skills of a complete psychiatrist.
3. Many nonmedical mental health professionals who are supervised by psychiatrists use psychodynamic psychotherapy; therefore, for the psychiatrist to responsibly supervise such work, he or she should possess basic psychotherapeutic competence.
4. The principles of psychodynamic psychotherapy are intimately related to the psychological and social concepts that underlie all doctor-patient relationships. The psychotherapeutically competent psychiatrist will be able both to provide more effective consultation to medical colleagues and to manage his or her own nonpsychotherapy doctor-patient relationships more effectively.
5. Psychodynamic psychotherapy training provides the resident with experiences that enhance learning about and management of other dyadic relationships within psychiatry, such as in supervision, consultation, and mental health administration.
6. Training in psychodynamic psychotherapy enhances basic interviewing expertise by providing the resident with an opportunity to observe longitudinally the course of psychopathological and nonpathological mental phenomena present in an initial interview. This experience makes it possible for the resident to recognize emerging mental phenomena earlier, more accurately, and more confidently.
7. Training in psychodynamic psychotherapy provides the resident with an in-depth and longitudinal study of both conscious and unconscious mental functioning—either nonpathological or pathological—that is related to the effort to change thinking, feeling, and behavior. Such an effort requires an ongoing relationship between therapist and patient and involves the inevitable obstacles, resistances, strengths, and opportunities related to such an ef-

fort. Understanding these phenomena is essential to treatment planning and management of virtually all psychiatric disorders.

8. Psychodynamic psychotherapy allows observation of complex pathological and nonpathological mental functioning over time. In so doing, it complements the observation of similar mechanisms in inpatient, consultation, and emergency room settings. Furthermore, it provides access to the primary materials that form the basis of general psychodynamic theory. In this way, psychotherapy training enhances the learning of psychodynamics as a basic science within psychiatry.
9. Many ethical difficulties result from psychiatrists' problems in managing their feelings and reactions to patients. With its emphasis on the complex dyadic emotional interplay between psychiatrist and patient, psychodynamic psychotherapy training enhances psychiatrists' ability to anticipate, analyze, and avoid ethical dilemmas and transgressions.
10. Practicing psychodynamic psychotherapy compels the psychiatrist in training to observe, analyze, and attempt to understand extremely complex interactive phenomena. This effort imposes an intellectual rigor and discipline in observing behavior, developing hypotheses, and analyzing theories and data.

In these rationales, a clear philosophy was at work. The exciting developments in clinical neuroscience do not displace the importance of the experiential meanings that behavioral and mental phenomena have to patients. After all, some of the most promising developments in neuroscience are at the interface of mental experience and biochemical phenomena (Hofer 1984; Kandel 1983; McGuire et al. 1984; Reiser 1984; Winson 1985). Not only clinical experience but also empirical data support the notion that psychotherapy alone or in combination with pharmacological treatment is effective for many patients (Weissman et al. 1987). Although many psychiatrists may choose to delegate the psychological treatment to others, just as in the past many psychiatrists delegated the pharmacological treatment to others, a solid grounding in those treatments is essential. In short, a deep, usable understanding of and ability to apply clinically the concepts of the dynamic unconscious, transference/countertransference, and mental defense mechanisms is central to being an effective pharmacotherapist, behavior therapist, inpatient psychiatrist, consultation psychiatrist, psychotherapist, community psychiatrist, neuropsychiatrist, emergency psychiatrist, geriatric psychiatrist, and, perhaps, even a laboratory research psychiatrist.

How can these principles be taught effectively yet reasonably concisely in residencies as they now exist?

Model Curriculum

Residency curriculum structure provides a coordinated set of experiences to develop the core knowledge and skills of psychiatrists. The task force developed the following core curriculum in individual psychotherapy; for each postgraduate year (PGY), the curriculum specifies terminal and enabling objectives for the resident, a set of learning experiences to be used by the resident to meet the objectives, and evaluation instruments for determining whether the resident has acquired the pertinent knowledge, skills, and attitudes. The learning experiences are divided into seminars, case conferences, supervision, and clinical care. Although space constraints limit the detail presented, clearly each clinical rotation allows for specific modifications and/or elaborations of the principles discussed here. For example, acute inpatient units or consultation-liaison rotations emphasize brief, focal therapeutic interventions with both individuals and families; substance abuse programs emphasize group modalities. Furthermore, although beyond the scope of this chapter, there is the necessity of learning to integrate dynamic principles and interventions with other forms of treatment such as pharmacological or cognitive/behavioral therapies. Teaching of dynamic principles can and should take place through appropriate supervision and didactic work in all clinical sites in a way that emphasizes a biopsychosocial approach. The ideas of Jerry Lewis (1978) were influential in the development of the curriculum presented below.

PGY-1

Goals. The resident should be able to conduct open-ended diagnostic psychiatric interviews that both generate adequate information for initial psychiatric assessment and enlist the patient in a collaborative manner to participate in treatment. The resident should be able to facilitate increasingly more personal revelations by the patient about interpersonal and intrapsychic experiences and the patient's subjective responses to the experiences. The resident should appreciate the importance of a detailed personal history as it relates to symptom development. The resident should make salient observations about the patient's relationships, including the doctor-patient relationship.

Learning experiences. The resident should perform a large number of (at least 20–25) initial interviews with a variety of patients and should likewise conduct a large number of follow-up interviews. Because of the usual clinical rotation sequence, most of these interviews will take place with hospitalized patients. Each resident should videotape one of his or her psychiatric interviews to be viewed by a faculty member and members of the residency group. Each resident should interview a substantial number of psychiatric inpatients in front of faculty and other residents. Each resident should also see and critique videotape interviews conducted by faculty and should observe such interviews in person. In a seminar on psychiatric interviewing, the resident should be assigned a list of readings on both diagnostic and process aspects of the psychiatric interview.

Case conferences in the first postgraduate year should emphasize diagnosis and broad areas of treatment planning. The case conferences should include discussions, at least in general terms, of the roles of supportive and expressive psychotherapy. Whenever possible, some conferences might be chaired or attended by faculty with a predominant psychodynamic orientation. To avoid educational splitting, such individuals should emphasize the importance of dynamic approaches within the biopsychosocial model.

The emphasis in PGY-1 supervision is on consolidation of the resident's identity as a physician and psychiatrist rather than on psychotherapy. Supervision is used to deepen understanding of the patient's psychopathology and to begin introducing the resident to psychodynamic principles and the impact of physician behavior and communication on the patient.

Clinical care given by first-year residents emphasizes diagnosis, crisis intervention, pharmacotherapy, and extensive history taking and treatment planning in both medical and psychiatric settings, most often in hospital settings. Residents follow hospitalized psychiatric patients with a primary focus on understanding the natural course and resolution with treatment of major psychiatric illness rather than on providing psychotherapeutic treatment. On a medical service, the focus is obviously on medical illness. There can be, however, important lessons to be learned regarding dynamic issues in patients and families related to the psychological impact of serious medical illness and its sequelae.

Evaluation. The relevant evaluation of PGY-1 residents covers psychiatric assessment and interviewing and focuses on the residents' ability to provide appropriate clinical intervention. The PGY-1 evaluation instrument should specify the skills and abilities under consideration.

PGY-2

Goals. During the second year, the resident should develop an understanding of core psychodynamic concepts, become familiar with transference and countertransference phenomena, gain sophistication in observing the process of psychotherapy, and develop an understanding of the definitions and roles of key concepts and interventions in psychotherapy (e.g., therapeutic alliance, empathy, clarification, interpretation). The resident should learn to recognize the patient's emotional states and his or her own reactions that interfere with or facilitate deeper patient revelation. The resident should be able to vicariously experience the patient's feelings while maintaining separateness and to subsequently communicate empathic understanding. The resident should recognize that empathy enables the patient to feel understood. The resident should become aware of multiple meanings of symptoms, thoughts, and feelings through his or her understanding of the patient's relevant past experiences, current situations, and relationship to the therapist. The resident should be able to detect conflict in patient behavior or thought. By the end of the second postgraduate year, the resident should be able to establish a therapeutic contract, recognize defense and resistance, and coordinate psychotherapy with other interventions, including medications, with patients with a wide variety of diagnostic conditions. The resident should be able both to identify and deal effectively with emergent issues in therapy and to use supervisory or consultative feedback in ongoing psychotherapeutic work.

Learning experiences. Seminars and case conferences during the second postgraduate year should provide ample opportunity both to learn and to practice the basic principles of psychodynamics and psychotherapy. Didactic seminars should review in detail the basic knowledge entailed in core clinical concepts. It is extremely helpful to have the opportunity to review psychotherapy conducted by a senior attending psychotherapist, particularly with a patient who might otherwise not be seen by a resident in the program. Watching edited videotapes of psychotherapy sessions and observing live sessions are both useful. Such observation is often easily done on inpatient units, which are the predominant PG-2 clinical sites. In conferences that use videotaped materials or live interviews by a senior psychiatrist, the presence of another faculty member with a somewhat different orientation or style enriches the opportunities for learning.

A structured introduction to psychotherapy skills is also useful. In such conferences, residents and faculty members are asked to respond to videotaped and audiotaped patient material. Early in the seminar participant responses may be written, and subsequently they may be verbal. Eventually, seminar participants conduct videotaped interviews with patients or actors. Throughout the course of the seminar, the residents have opportunities to experiment with different responses and to receive feedback from their peers and the faculty members about those responses.

Clinical care in the second postgraduate year largely involves hospitalized patients, but assignments should also include at least two patients for whom outpatient psychotherapy is the predominant or exclusive form of treatment. Optimally, these first patients will have sought treatment because of psychological conflict. There should be at least 2 hours of weekly individual supervision during the second postgraduate year.

Evaluation. In the second postgraduate year, the evaluation takes place at the patient's bedside as well as in seminars, case conferences, and supervision. Seminar evaluations focus on the resident's ability to present concepts in a coherent manner that reflects understanding of the theoretical materials involved. In experiential learning situations, such as the psychotherapy case conference, it is often more important for supervisors to give extensive verbal feedback while downplaying formal written evaluation. Supervisors, however, should complete a narrative evaluation form that addresses the goals and objectives enumerated in the curriculum.

PGY-3

Goals. By the end of the third postgraduate year, the resident should have been able to involve at least two patients in the middle phase of insight-oriented dynamic psychotherapy. The resident should be able to manage silence, anxiety, aggression, and seductive behavior by psychotherapy patients. The resident should appreciate the basic theoretical and technical differences among the major approaches to psychotherapy and should have a more sophisticated appreciation of multiple levels of psychological development and meaning. The resident should have the knowledge and skill to understand and establish a therapeutic alliance with a variety of patients. The resident should demonstrate competence with empathic functions in psychotherapy and should be able to handle fee setting and collection in the outpatient clinic. The resident should recognize and deal with resistance—particularly positive or negative transference reactions—and acting out. The resident should be aware of countertransference responses and should be able to put these to use in understanding patients. The resident should understand major dynamic themes in individual sessions as well as organizing themes over the course of therapy and should be able to identify progress and stalemates. The resident should be able to avoid competition, overidentification, and moralizing with patients and should understand mental mechanisms and defensive structure. The resident should be able to recognize and learn from mistakes without counterproductive defensive responses. The resident should also begin to apprehend the importance of various forms of therapy termination and to anticipate difficulties that can emerge in the termination phase. The resident should be able to understand the role of character in the patient's participation in treatment.

Learning experiences. Seminars in the third postgraduate year should deepen and broaden the resident's sophistication about psychotherapy. A core textbook with a variety of assigned readings is one way to both provide a unifying structure for seminars and help the resident become familiar with a range of topics and perspectives as well as essential principles.

Case conferences during the early part of PGY-3 should emphasize the problems inherent in engaging a wide variety of patients in psychotherapeutic treatment. It is also useful to have a continuous case conference in which the progress in ongoing psychotherapy with one or two patients receives special attention.

Clinical care during PGY-3 consists of 4–7 psychotherapy hours per week and at least one patient who is seen more than once per week. These patients should represent diverse experiences in terms of gender, diagnosis, age, phase of life, developmental level, and cognitive style. Each resident should have 2 hours of individual supervision and at least 1 other hour for a case conference. In addition to work with specific psychotherapy patients, residents should have learning experiences structured to teach applications of dynamic principles with other patients, such as those seen for medication follow-up, or in other settings, such as a consultation-liaison rotation. Consultation-liaison experiences can provide an excellent opportunity to illustrate the value of psychodynamic understanding in an acutely ill, hospital-based population.

Evaluation. Again, evaluation takes place in direct observation of residents' clinical interventions as well as in seminars, case conferences, and individual supervision. Evaluation in the case conferences and seminars is based on the same principles as for PGY-2. In individual supervision, greater sophistication is expected of the resident during this year, and this expectation should be reflected in the evaluation guidelines.

PGY-4

Goals. Goals for the fourth postgraduate year include development of the ability to function autonomously as a psychotherapist and of the capacity to achieve continuing educational growth and development. By the end of this year, the resident should also be proficient in at least one subspecialized psychotherapeutic technique, such as time-limited, group, family, behavioral, cognitive, or hypnotherapy.

Learning experiences. In PGY-4, there should be one seminar on advanced individual psychotherapy and at least one seminar that introduces the resident to a psychotherapeutic subspecialty (e.g., brief psychotherapy, hypnosis, cognitive therapy, sexual therapy). The individual psychotherapy seminar should help the resident relate psychotherapy to other forms of treatment and should emphasize management of the middle and termination phases of psychotherapy.

The case conferences during PGY-4 should include a second continuous case conference in which the residents describe ongoing individual psychotherapy. A case conference emphasizing a particular psychotherapy subspecialty should also be offered that focuses on the practice and evaluation of that form of therapy.

In PGY-4, most residents will not add new long-term cases but will add some that provide the opportunity to use a subspecialty form of psychotherapy. There should also be some unsupervised cases during this year. Each resident should have at least two individual supervisors in addition to participating in the case conferences.

In addition to clinical experiences, many PGY-4 residents will have administrative and supervisory experiences. With appropriate supervision, such experiences can provide an excellent opportunity to appreciate the value of a psychodynamic understanding of group process from another perspective.

Evaluation. The evaluation of PGY-4 residents should include an assessment of their ability to terminate therapy and to ask for consultation in psychotherapy.

General Issues of Implementation

In PGY-1, no more than 2 hours per week are required for activities exclusively related to this curriculum. In PGY-2, this requirement increases to 6 hours per week: 1 hour of didactic seminar, 1 hour for the case conference, 2 hours of psychotherapy, and 2 hours of supervision. In PGY-3, the time needed for this curriculum peaks at approximately 8–11 hours per week: 1 hour of didactic seminar, 1 hour for the case conference, 2 hours of supervision, and 4–7 hours of cases. There would probably be a slight drop in hours in PGY-4 as the cases terminate and the didactic seminars become more episodic.

The task force emphasized the cumulative nature of training in expressive psychotherapy, which makes the consolidating experiences of PGY-4 especially important. Besides the incremental addition of specific knowledge and clinical skills, the cumulative and transforming nature of the experience produces a depth of understanding such that by the time of graduation, the way a psychodynamically informed psychiatrist hears patients is radically different from the way he or she heard them in PGY-1.

Specific Considerations

It is worth noting what is not included in the curriculum presented above. The task force did not recommend personal psychotherapy for residents, individual work with a latency-aged child, more cases, a specific structure (e.g., many thought there should be an outpatient rotation in PGY-2), more activities during PGY-1, or specific activities for rotations in settings involving other specific teaching tasks (e.g., consultation-liaison, inpatient units, emergency room).

In general, the task force members were convinced that what should be expected of all residents and what is optimal could not be identical and, further, that the proposals had to be broad enough and flexible enough to be implemented in very different programs with very different structures, priorities, and resources. Personal psychotherapy remains one of the very best routes to psychodynamic sophistication but can no longer be a general requirement of residents, who now enter psychiatry for widely varied motives. A long-term child case is one of the best ways to consolidate the developmental perspective on adult behavior and could be one of the added PGY-3 cases, but this simply cannot be done in many programs. A greater caseload is optimal for achieving a certain competence and greater sophistication in all residents, but the goal is no longer to teach all residents how to practice psychoanalytic psychotherapy. Rather, the goal is to turn out psychodynamically informed and sophisticated psychiatrists.

Given the issues of 3-year versus 4-year programs, we felt that the bulk of the training had to be accomplished after the internship year. Likewise, given the widely varied resources and skills available on different services at different programs, we could not insist on a specific structure or specific content. For instance, consultation-liaison services have a strong psychodynamic bent in some programs and almost none at all in others. It was assumed that learning activities at various sites would encourage the application of principles mastered while conducting individual dynamic therapy to other situations, but that the curriculum needed to stand on its own as the primary means of formally teaching these principles. To repeat a point made earlier, the best way to ensure integration of a psychodynamic perspective throughout training is to ensure that the biopsychosocial model forms the basis for teaching and supervision.

The task force also considered how a psychotherapy training curriculum could be applied in a program with either limited resources or such a strong commitment to other areas of psychiatry that few resources are directed to psychotherapy training. Although the model curriculum already represented a distinct compromise of some members' standards, the task force saw the need to establish standards for a minimal training experience as well. In this endeavor, the structural variability of programs again became a concern, so the focus became hours of exposure.

Model Curriculum for Minimum Training

This curriculum was designed for training programs that have limited resources to devote to training in psychodynamic psychotherapy. In the opinion of the task force, this curriculum represents the minimum that would meet the requirements of the Residency Review Committee for Psychiatry extant at the time of publication. The goal of such a curriculum would be to provide an awareness, knowledge, and appreciation of psychodynamic issues that meet a minimum standard and that could be built upon through ongoing educational activities. The task force members believe that some knowledge of the unconscious, transference, and therapeutic process is more desirable than ignorance or misunderstanding. The objectives of this curriculum are as follows:

1. Provide an adequate basic background for the general psychiatrist so that he or she can later achieve competence as a psychodynamic psychotherapist with additional supervision and training.
2. Provide the general psychiatrist with a beginning language and basic concepts for understanding dyadic interactions and unconscious forces.
3. Provide the general psychiatrist with an awareness of the ongoing and omnipresent role of unconscious forces in all clinical situations.
4. Sensitize the general psychiatrist to the complicated process and evolution of the clinical relationship in all therapeutic settings.

To meet these objectives, each resident must spend a minimum of 200 hours treating patients with psychodynamic psychotherapy. These sessions must be at least weekly and should last at least 45 minutes, and the purpose of each session must be to engage in psychodynamic, expressive, exploratory psychotherapy. Preferably, these 200 or more hours of experience will extend over the entire training period of the general psychiatrist. Each resident should treat at least four different patients, at least one for more than 50 sessions and at least one (and preferably more than one) until termination; the termination should be planned and dealt with as part of the treatment. A minimum of 100 hours of supervision by well-trained psychodynamic psychiatrists is expected. There must be at least 1 year of weekly didactic seminars on theory and technique and 1 year of weekly case conferences. The readings for the didactic seminars should include at least one widely respected basic text on psychotherapy and one widely respected basic text (or collection of classic papers) on the core concepts of psychodynamic theory.

In addition, there must be an application experience in which the principles learned while practicing psychodynamic psychotherapy are explicitly applied to other settings. This application experience will usually be in the form of a case conference. In the emergency room, emphasis would be on the psychodynamic forces leading to a patient's decompensation at a particular time, the family and interpersonal dynamics interfering with a patient's support system, the psychodynamics of suicidal behavior, and the dynamic basis for specific crisis intervention interpretations. In an inpatient setting, the following issues should be covered: the dynamic meaning of psychotic content, family dynamics, psychodynamics of acting-out behavior, psychodynamic underpinnings of milieu therapy, psychodynamics of control and authority issues in the doctor-patient relationship, and the definition and psychodynamic basis of "psychosocial support." In a medication clinic, the application conference should deal with the dynamics of compliance and noncompliance, institutional transference, covert positive transference, the unconscious meaning of medication and medication adjustments, and the role of family dynamics in maintenance of stability. On a consultation-liaison rotation, the conference should address the dynamics of the doctor-patient relationship, the unconscious meanings of hospitalization and illness, the adaptive and maladaptive uses of regression, the psychodynamics of grieving and dying, and psychotherapeutic interventions to deal with such issues.

Conclusions

The curricula presented in this chapter reflect the task force's shared vision of the psychiatrist of the future. There was a consensus that psychiatrists must continue to be applied psychologists as well as become applied neuroscientists, as is implicit in the biopsychosocial model. Furthermore, psychiatrists must be synthesizers and integrators of these fields. This vision is justified from clinical, intellectual, and economic perspectives. Despite the changes in third-party coverage, patients will continue to need and find psychotherapy as best they can, regardless of what system is in place. The task force encountered a large body of anecdotal evidence that young psychiatrists going into practice who integrate psychotherapy into their treatments have more success than those who must refer patients once the hospitalization is over or medication maintenance is achieved.

In addition to the specific training recommendations elucidated in this chapter, the reader will note that repeated reference is made to the biopsychosocial model. This emphasis is deliberate, since that model provides the best way of integrating several different approaches to understanding human behavior. The implications for training are legion, but in reference to the aim of this chapter, several points are worthy of emphasis. The didactic curriculum should include phase-specific and site-appropriate materials regarding psychodynamic theory and practice at all levels of training. In addition, clinical supervision in all service sites, flowing from a biopsychosocial approach, should include an appropriate focus on dynamic issues and interventions.

One major controversy in the task force meetings was over whether the model curriculum for psychotherapy training should be designed so that every psychiatric resident would achieve a full level of competence as a psychodynamic psychotherapist. It was agreed that the curriculum should be thorough enough so that gifted, committed residents could become competent by its completion and so that all residents should achieve a level of skill allowing generalization, wide application, and ongoing learning of principles—that is, they should become psychodynamically informed psychiatrists.

The task force gave much attention to the details of the minimum curriculum, because we wished to avoid fostering biologically oriented clinicians who are able to offer only an intuitive, unsophisticated form of supportive therapy. The task force members recognized the possibility that the minimum standard might be interpreted as the average expectable standard.

Some might claim that the expressive psychotherapy experience itself is not necessary to produce a psychodynamically informed psychiatrist. These critics might suggest that site-based experiences are sufficient to enable residents to apply psychodynamic principles to supportive therapy, brief therapy, milieu management, and the like. What the long-term individual psychotherapy experience uniquely offers, however, is the opportunity to explore, struggle with, and actually use unconscious forces and transference-countertransference interactions in open, explicit ways. It is this process that solidifies both the experiential and the intellectual learning, making the applications more effective, sophisticated, alive, and human.

The task force concluded that the psychiatrist of the future must be deeply and effectively psychodynamically informed and must have the opportunity to become psychotherapeutically competent. Such competence can only be achieved with formal training in expressive, insight-oriented psychoanalytic psychotherapy. This training can be accomplished with a carefully planned curriculum—spanning 3, or all 4, residency years—that requires approximately 13% of training time (based on a 50-hour week). More than this may be desirable but may not be realistic. Less than this may be inevitable in a few settings but is acceptable only if very specific criteria are met.

References

Cloninger CR: A systematic method for clinical description and classification of personality variants. Arch Gen Psychiatry 44:573–587, 1987

Foreman SA, Marmar CF: Therapist actions that address initially poor therapeutic alliances in psychotherapy. Am J Psychiatry 142:922–926, 1985

Hofer MA: Relationships as regulators: a psychobiologic perspective on bereavement. Psychosom Med 46:183–197, 1984

Kandel ER: From metapsychology to molecular biology: explorations into the nature of anxiety. Am J Psychiatry 140:1277–1293, 1983

Langsley DG, Yager J: The definition of a psychiatrist: eight years later. Am J Psychiatry 145:469–475, 1988

Lewis J: To Be a Therapist: The Teaching and Learning. New York, Brunner/Mazel, 1978

Luborsky L: Principles of Psychoanalytic Psychotherapy: A Manual for Supportive-Expressive Treatment. New York, Basic Books, 1984

Luborsky L, McLellan AT, Woody DE, et al: Therapist success and its determinants. Arch Gen Psychiatry 42:602–611, 1985

McGuire MT, Raleigh MJ, Brammer GL: Adaptation, selection, and benefit-cost balances: implications of behavioral-physiological studies of social dominance in male vervet monkeys. Ethology and Sociobiology 5:269–277, 1984

Mohl PC, Lomax J, Tasman A, et al: Psychotherapy training for the psychiatrist of the future. Am J Psychiatry 147:7–13, 1990

Reiser MF: Mind, Brain, Body. New York, Basic Books, 1984

Reiser MF: Are psychiatric educators "losing the mind"? Am J Psychiatry 145:148–153, 1988

Strupp HH, Binder JL: Psychotherapy in a New Key: A Guide to Time-Limited Dynamic Psychotherapy. New York, Basic Books, 1984

Tasman A, Kay J: Setting the stage: residency training in 1986, in Training Psychiatrists for the 90s: Issues and Recommendations. Edited by Nadelson CC, Robinowitz CB. Washington, DC, American Psychiatric Press, 1987, pp 49–59

Weissman MM, Jarrett RB, Rush JA: Psychotherapy and its relevance to the pharmacotherapy of major depression: a decade later (1976–1985), in Psychopharmacology: The Third Generation of Progress. Edited by Meltzer HY. New York, Raven, 1987, pp 1059–1069

Winson J: Brain and Psyche. New York, Anchor Press/Doubleday, 1985

Index

*Page numbers printed in **boldface** type refer to tables or figures.*